Manual of

CARE OF CRITICAL NEWBORN

Second Edition

Editor

J.N. Sharma
Ex. Professor and Head
Dept. of Pediatrics
Gauhati Medical College
Guwahati, Assam

PEEPEE PUBLISHERS AND DISTRIBUTORS (P) LTD.®

Manual of Care of Critical Newborn

Published by
Pawaninder P. Vij

Peepee Publishers and Distributors (P) Ltd.
Head Office: 160, Shakti Vihar, Pitam Pura, Delhi-110 034 (India)

Correspondence Address:

7/31, First Floor, Ansari Road, Daryaganj,
New Delhi-110 002 (India)

Ph: 41512412, 23246245, 9811156083

e-mail: peepee160@yahoo.co.in

e-mail: peepee160@gmail.com

www.peepeepub.com

First Edition: **2007**

Second Edition Reprint: **2021**

ISBN: 978-81-8445-099-6

PREFACE TO SECOND EDITION

It is important that textbooks have to be revised in view of the rapid changes as well as advances in the management issues of medical problems. Neonatology is a rapidly developing area of pediatrics and hence needs revision and additions.

It is really a matter of satisfaction that the second edition of this book will be delivered to the students. Two chapters have been added and changes have been made in few chapters in this edition. Hope the readers will like it.

I would take this opportunity to thank the students all over India for accepting this book as a reference book in postgraduate level. I would like to extend my heartfelt thanks and gratitude once again to all the authors of this book. I am greatly indebted to Dr. Saumendu Bhattacharjee and Dr. Vivek Choudhury for their suggestions and active support during preparation of the second edition. Last but not the least, I am grateful to Mr. Pawaninder Pal Vij, Director, Peepee Publishers (P) Ltd, New Delhi, for taking the task of successfully distributing the book in most parts of the country and for publishing the second edition.

PREFACE TO FIRST EDITION

The infant mortality rate of a country is the most sensitive indicator of health and level of living in that country. The infant mortality has two components– neonatal and post neonatal deaths. Neonatal deaths account for 60% of total infant death. Fifty percent of total neonatal deaths occur during the first week and 25% death occur within the first 24 hours of birth. With the introduction of national programmes, viz. Universal Immunization programme, Diarrhoeal disease control programme, Acute respiratory infection control programme etc., there has been a significant decrease in the post neonatal deaths .This has largely contributed to the lowering of the infant mortality rate in our country in comparison to the preindependent and early post independent era. On the other hand, the neonatal mortality rate has virtually remained static. The high and static neonatal mortality has been the most important deterrent factor in further lowering the infant mortality rate. Hence, the national priority should be to look into measures to bring down the neonatal mortality in order to bring down the high infant mortality.

More than 80% of newborn babies require level I or primary care i.e. minimal care. Newborn babies weighing 2000 gms or more or have a gestational age of 37 weeks or more belong to this category. Care can be provided to these babies at home, at subcentres or at primary health centres by mothers under supervision of basic health professionals. Thus it is needless to say that primary care by the grass roots health workers is the cornerstone to improve salvage of the newborn.

In developed countries where primary care has been successful, priority has been given to develop the secondary and tertiary care because primary, secondary or tertiary care cannot be developed in isolation.

There must be simultaneous development at all levels. This will necessitate the need to create neonatal services at all hospitals where maternity services are available irrespective of the hospital whether it is a private or government concern.

Eighty percent of deliveries, in our country, still take place in rural areas and the babies born are taken care of by the mothers, family members, untrained or trained dais and in a small percentage by nurses and doctors mostly in an unscientific manner. One of the major constraints in imparting appropriate neonatal care is paucity of trained personnel in the field. The basic doctor who is responsible for training the grass roots workers is himself ill-equipped with the knowledge of newborn care. This paucity of knowledge can be directly attributed to the poorly developed medical curriculum. However, recently the curriculum for undergraduate teaching has been revised with proper representation of pediatrics including newborn care. It is time for the concerned authorities to give a serious thought for the basic doctors who are already working in the peripheral areas. Reorientation training programmes, organised at intervals, throughout the year, in batches, will enable the basic doctors to get equipped with the knowledge. They in turn will have to take the responsibility to train the grass roots workers, who actually form the pivot of primary care.

A comprehensive compilation of some important chapters of newborn care has been a need for the practising pediatricians and the basic doctors who look after the newborn in the grass roots level. Such a compilation was published by the NNF, Assam state branch in 1998. This book was highly appreciated by the doctors of this region. This was the impetus for coming up with the present compilation. Most of the common and important aspects of care of the critically ill newborn have been included in this book, with a hope to help the practising doctors to look after the neonates rationally.

I would like to extend my heartfelt thanks and gratitude to all the contributors of this book. I am greatly indebted to Dr. Pradipta Sanker Guha for typing out the manuscript and Dr. Shaumendu Bhattacharjee for his suggestions, assistance and active support during the preparation of the book. I must thank Dr. Himesh Barman for helping out with the photographs included in the book and Dr. Sanjib Gogoi for composing the cover design. Last but not the least I am grateful to Mr. Pawaninder Pal Vij, Director, Peepee Publishers (P) Ltd., New Delhi for taking the task of publishing the book.

LIST OF CONTRIBUTORS

A.K. Dutta
Professor and Head
Department of Pediatrics
Kalawati Saran Children Hospital and
Lady Hardinge's Medical College, New Delhi

A.L. Saha
Senior Pediatrician
International Hospital, Guwahati, Assam

A. Saili
Professor of Pediatrics
Kalawati Saran Children Hospital and
Lady Hardinge's Medical College, New Delhi

Abhinandan Das
Professor and Head, Pediatrics
Jorhat Medical College, Assam

Ajoy Kumar Sarma
Pediatrician
Oil India Hospital, Duliajan, Assam

Anupama Deka Ray
Assoc. Professor of Pediatrics
Silchar Medical College, Silchar, Assam

Arati Deka
Professor and Head, Pediatrics
Silchar Medical College, Silchar, Assam

Bijan Saha
Pediatrician
Central Railway Hospital, Maligaon, Assam

D.K. Patgiri
Professor of Pediatrics and Vice Principal
Assam Medical College, Dibrugarh, Assam

Gautam Medhi
Assistant Professor, Pediatrics
Gauhati Medical College, Guwahati, Assam

H.K. Borah
Retd. Professor and Head
Dept. of Pediatric Surgery, Gauhati Medical College
Guwahati, Assam

J.N. Sharma
Professor and Head
Dept. of Pediatrics, Gauhati Medical College
Guwahati, Assam

P. Bishwanath
Associate Professor
Department of Pediatrics, Assam Medical College
Dibrugarh

Palash Ranjan Gogoi
Pediatrician
Nazareth Hospital
Shillong, Meghalaya

Pradipta S. Guha
Registrar of Pediatrics,
Gauhati Medical College, Assam

R.K. Kayal
Visiting Pediatrician
Central Railway Hospital, Maligaon, Guwahati, Assam

Rukeya Begum
Associate Professor of Pediatrics
Gauhati Medical College, Gauhati, Assam

Shaumendu Bhattacharjee
Pediatrician
Arya Hospital, Guwahati, Assam

CONTENTS

1 *Perinatal Asphyxia*

J.N. Sharma

The term asphyxia in the newborn has long been used to indicate failure on the part of a newborn to establish spontaneous respiration immediately following complete delivery. The first consequence of failure to breathe is lack of oxygen (hypoxia) rapidly followed by excess accumulation of carbon dioxide, and a fall in blood pH. Perinatal asphyxia is an insult to the fetus or newborn due to hypoxia and /or ischemia to various organs.

Definition of Birth Asphyxia/Perinatal Asphyxia

The WHO has defined perinatal asphyxia as "a failure to initiate and sustain breathing at birth". The National Neonatology forum of India has suggested that birth asphyxia should be diagnosed when a 'baby has gasping and inadequate breathing or no breathing at 1 minute after birth. It corresponds to 1 minute Apgar score of 3 or less. It is a simple definition, which can be used in the community as well as for purposes of estimating the incidence of birth asphyxia. The National Neonatal Perinatal database also defined moderate asphyxia as slow gasping breathing or an Apgar score of 4-6 at 1 minute and severe asphyxia as no breathing or an Apgar score of 0-3 at 1 minute.

The American Academy of Pediatrics has proposed that the term perinatal asphyxia should be reserved to describe a neonate who manifests with all the following features:

1. Cord umbilical artery pH of < 7.0 with a base deficit of >10 mEq/L.
2. Neonatal neurological manifestations suggestive of Hypoxic ischemic encephalopathy (HIE).
3. Evidences of multisystem organ dysfunction (e.g. cardiovascular, renal, gastro intestinal, hematologic, pulmonary).

Etiology

Ninety percent of asphyxial insult occurs in the antepartum and intrapartum periods, due to various causes, resulting in an inability to provide oxygen to and remove carbondioxide and hydrogen ion from the fetus. The remainder is postpartum, usually secondary to pulmonary, cardiovascular or neurologic insufficiency. Hypoxia in the intra uterine period may result from anoxic anoxia, anemic anoxia, stagnant anoxia or histotoxic anoxia.

Anoxic *anoxia* is a result of inadequate supply of oxygen which may arise from diminution of oxygen tension in the mother's circulation. Such a situation result in mothers who suffer from congestive heart failure, pneumonia, emphysema, during an eclamptic convulsion, use of inhalational anesthesia or abrupt fall of blood pressure during spinal anesthesia. It may also result from placental insufficiency as a result of pre eclampsia, pregnancy induced hypertension. Premature separation of placenta due to placenta praevia or accidental hemorrhage may lead to sudden, severe anoxia leading to death of the fetus. The fetus is in danger of anoxia if labour is prolonged because oxygen supply is reduced during every uterine contraction.

***Anemic** anoxia* is said to exist when the fetal blood is so anemic that it is unable to carry sufficient oxygen to meet the needs of the body tissues. This may result from hemolysis in Rh incompatibility or from fetal hemorrhage associated with vasa praevia or from twin to twin and materno fetal transfusion.

Stagnant anoxia can arise from compression, prolapse or knotting of the umbilical cord. Such a situation leads to stagnation of blood resulting in anoxia.

Histotoxic anoxia results when fetal tissues are so poisoned by drugs (e.g. morphine, pethidine) or so damaged by hemorrhage that the cells can no longer utilize the oxygen delivered to them. This type of anoxia is more common in preterm labours.

In majority of cases of natal and postnatal anoxia, the causes of fetal anoxia often produce the circumstances in which further anoxia becomes inevitable during or immediately after birth. Infrequently, asphyxia may appear for the first time after birth due to some congenital abnormality like congenital laryngeal web or a congenital diaphragmatic hernia. These conditions do not affect the fetus in the intra uterine life.

Physiology of Perinatal Asphyxia

A sequence of changes takes place in asphyxiated babies at birth. An initial period of rapid breathing is followed by a period of cessation of respiration called *Primary Apnea*. During this period, the heart rate begins to fall. Exposure to oxygen and stimulation during this period of primary apnea, in most instances, induce respiration. If the asphyxia continues, the newborn develops deep gasping respiration and the heart rate continues to decrease and blood pressure begins to fall. The respiration become weaker until the infant takes a last gasp and enters a period of apnea called *Secondary apnea*. In this phase, the newborn becomes unresponsive to stimulation and positive pressure ventilation is necessary for revival.

An important point to note is that in the case of intrauterine asphyxia, the fetus may go through the phases of primary and secondary apnea in utero. So all cases of apnea at birth should be considered as secondary apnea and resuscitation must begin immediately.

Effects of Asphyxia on Various Organs

When a fetus or neonate is subjected to asphyxia, there is redistribution of blood flow. This is achieved by neurogenic vasoconstriction occurring in the non-vital organs like skin, muscles, gut, liver and kidney in an effort to increase the blood flow to the vital organs – the brain, heart and the adrenals. But under progressive hypoxia, myocardial pump failure occurs leading to fall in cardiac output and blood pressure ultimately leading to decreased cerebral blood flow. So, a number of organs are involved in asphyxia. The changes in different systems are as follows:

Central nervous system—Hypoxic ischaemic encephalopathy, infarction, intracranial hemorrhage, seizures.

Cardiovascular system—Myocardial ischaemia, poor contractility, cardiac failure, tricuspid insufficiency, Hypotension.

Pulmonary—Persistent fetal circulation, pulmonary hemorrhage, respiratory distress syndrome.

Renal—Acute tubular necrosis or cortical necrosis.

Adrenal—Adrenal hemorrhage.

Metabolic—SIADH, Hyponatremia, hypoglycaemia, hypocalcemia, cryoglobinuria.

Skin—Subcutaneous fat necrosis.

Hematological—Disseminated intravascular coagulation.

Pathophysiology of Hypoxic Ischaemic Encephalopathy (HIE)

The pathophysiology of HIE has been chiefly studied by creating two experimental states:

1. Prolonged partial asphyxia.
2. Acute total asphyxia.

In prolonged partial asphyxia, at first there is redistribution of fetal blood flow from nonvital to vital organs. As the duration and degree of fetal hypoxemia progresses the fetal blood pressure drops and a second redistribution of blood flow—this time within the brain occurs. Here the blood flow to the cerebral hemispheres (anterior circulation) is found to decrease relative to blood flow to the thalamus, brain stem and cerebellum (posterior circulation). The cerebral hemispheres then become most vulnerable. In full term neonate, the first areas to be compromised are the parasaggital cortex and the underlying white matter. In preterm infant periventricular white matter necrosis occurs. Patterns of changes seen in term infants include selective neuronal necrosis, status marmoratus, parasaggital cerebral injury, focal and multifocal ischaemic brain injury. In preterm infants there is periventricular leukomalacia.

In near total asphyxia (as in cord prolapse), hypoxia is so abrupt that any compensatory inter organ and intra brain shunting is ineffective and the areas of highest metabolic demand and least reserves—the thalamus and certain brain stem nuclei are most vulnerable. Cerebral hemispheres are usually spared.

It has been shown that the presence of preceeding partial asphyxia followed by total asphyxia results in more rapid physiologic deterioration and neuro-pathological damage predominating in the basal ganglia with variable damage to parasaggital cerebrum, thalamus and brain stem.

Mechanism of Hypoxic Ischaemic Brain Damage at Cellular Level

An asphyxial insult precipitates an intricate array of reactions in distinct sequences and they are interrelated on many levels. Under physiologic conditions, levels of cellular ATP, the primary energy source of the cell, are maintained stable as energy consumption is balanced by ATP production. When oxygen availability is limited, oxidative phosphorylation ceases and cells shift to anaerobic glycolysis, which is much less efficient than aerobic metabolism. When this also cannot maintain adequate ATP production, existing ATP breaks down. This leads to depletion of high-energy compounds, in turn making it increasingly difficult to maintain intracellular ion concentration and cellular integrity. Failure of the ATP dependant Na^+K^+ pump leads to depolarization of cells, allowing the influx of Na^+ and Ca^{++} and there by producing cytotoxic oedema. Increased cytosolic calcium, arising from influx across plasma membranes as well as from release of intracellular stores, in turn elicits numerous other intracellular metabolic pathways, which includes activation of phospholipases, release of prostaglandins, lipases, proteases and endonucleases all of which injure various structural components of the cells, culminating in further cytotoxity. High intracellular calcium also contributes to the formation of oxygen free radicals.

During reperfusion, a burst of ROS (reactive oxygen species) is generated, mainly by the activity of xanthine oxidase and primarily in endothelial cells. ROS are in high-energy state with the potential to directly damage almost all types of molecules in living cells (phospholipids, sugars, amino acids and nucleic acids). Of the various neurotransmitters, excessive release of endogenous excitatory neurotransmitter glutamate and failure of its reuptake from the synaptic cleft leads to neuronal injury. Glutamate acts through NMDA receptors resulting in influx of sodium and calcium ions into the cells inducing neuronal death from the osmolar load. In summary, asphyxia triggers a cascade of biologic processes culminating in cell death.

Management of Perinatal Asphyxia

Perinatal asphyxia has been associated with hypoxic ischemic injury to multi organ systems leading to a high mortality and serious long term sequelae among survivors. The newborn has to be assessed for the degree of asphyxia immediately after birth to determine which of the babies require specialized neonatal care and long term followup. This may be done by the Apgar scoring system.

Apgar Scoring System as a Tool for Assessment of Perinatal Asphyxia

The Apgar score consists of the total points assigned to five objective signs in the newborn as shown in the table below:

Apgar scoring system

	score		
Sign	*0*	*1*	*2*
Heart rate	Absent	< 100/min	> 100/min
Respiratory effort	Absent	Slow (irregular)	good crying
Muscle tone	Limp	Some flexion of Extremities	Active movements
Reflex irritability	No response	Grimace	Cough/sneeze
Color	Blue, pale	Pink body Blue extremities	All pink

The five objective signs are evaluated and given a score of 0, 1 and 2. The scores at 1 and 5 minutes after birth are usually noted. If the five minute Apgar score is equal to or less than 6, the score should continue to be noted at 5 minute intervals until it is greater than 6. A score of 10 indicates an infant in perfect condition, but this is quite unusual, because most babies have some degree of acro cyanosis. If the scoring is done properly it yields the following informations:

1. **One minute apgar score:** This score generally correlates with the umbilical pH and a score of 3 or less is an index of intrapartum asphyxia. However, it should be noted that such a low Apgar score may not indicate asphyxia in the very low birth weight babies who are more likely to be hypotonic, have cyanotic extremities, and have diminished response. A very low birth weight baby with an apgar score of 3 or less cannot be assumed to be severely asphyxiated. None the less, such neonates should be resuscitated actively at birth and will usually respond more promptly and to less invasive measures than the baby who is asphyxiated.
2. **Apgar score beyond 1 minute:** Beyond 1 minute, the Apgar score is reflective of:
   a. Infant's changing condition and the adequacy of resuscitative efforts. Persistence of a low Apgar score indicates that further therapeutic efforts are needed.
   b. The more prolonged the period of severe depression (i.e., Apgar score 3 or less), the more likely is an abnormal long term neurologic outcome. Never the less, many babies with prolonged depression (> 15 minutes) are normal

in follow up. Moreover, most babies with long term neuromotor abnormalities do not give a history of neonatal asphyxia.

How Important is Apgar Scoring in Management of Asphyxia?

The Apgar scoring system has limitations in assessing the newborn at birth:

1. It does not help to take decision regarding resuscitation.
2. Assessment of the VLBW baby by Apgar score is fallacious.
3. Recent evidence suggests that there is poor correlation between Apgar score at birth, cord blood pH and long term outcome.

On the other hand, the Apgar score at 1 minute and beyond:

1. Helps in diagnosis of degree of asphyxia.
2. Helps in decisions regarding post resuscitation management of asphyxiated newborns.
3. Helps in assessment of long term neonatal outcome.

Which Asphyxiated Neonate Requires Specialized Care and LONG-TERM Followup?

Specialised neonatal care and long term followup for developmental assessment are indicated in neonates who fail to establish effective breathing at 5 minutes or the 5 minute Apgar score is 3 or less.

Differential Diagnosis

The differential diagnosis of acute asphyxia in a newborn includes maternal drugs or anesthesia; acute blood loss; acute intra cranial bleeding, CNS malformation, neuromuscular disease, cardio pulmonary disease, malformation or hypoplasia, airway obstruction, pneumothorax, hydrops, pleural effusion, ascites, diaphragmatic hernia and septic shock. These problems may be the cause of asphyxia or merely a coincident with it.

Markers of Perinatal Asphyxia

1. *Irregularities of fetal heart rate:* Intermittent auscultation or continuous electronic fetal monitoring are a gold standard of fetal monitoring.
2. Meconium staining of amniotic fluid.
3. *Apgar score*: the Apgar scores assigned at 1 & 5 minutes have for long been used to define asphyxia. But persistent low Apgar scores at 10, 15, and 20 minutes have been associated with adverse long-term outcome.
4. *Biochemical markers:*
   a. Umbilical artery pH < 7.0 is associated with adverse outcome.
   b. Serum lactate pyruvate and creatinine kinase brain isoenzyme (CPK—BB > 5 I U), neuron specific enolase.
   c. Cord erythropoietin elevated levels have been found in asphyxiated infants.
   d. *Hypoxanthine:* which is a breakdown product of ATP, is nowadays being used as the new gold standard for perinatal asphyxia. The recommended cord blood hypoxanthine levels for defining asphyxia is > 16 mmol/L.
5. *Electroencephalogram:* A burst suppression interictal pattern in light sleep and awake stage is ominous.
6. *USG of brain:* Is best done during 4-7 days of life for the diagnosis of periventricular and intraventricular hemorrhage and leukomalacia.

7. *CT scan*: It continues to be the gold standard among imaging studies in term neonates with HIE. CT is useful in assessing the degree of oedema when performed early (2 to 4 days after insult) and the extent of cerebral injury (i.e. encephalomalacia) when performed late (at least 2-4 weeks after insult).
8. *Evoked responses*: Abnormal visual evoked responses (VER) and brainstem auditory evoked responses (BAER) during the first 2 weeks of life have been correlated with poor outcome.
9. Newer imaging techniques like Magnetic Resonance Imaging (MRI), Nuclear Magnetic Resonance Spectroscopy, Near Infrared Spectroscopy (NIRS), Single Proton Emission Computed Tomography (SPECT), and Positron Emission Tomography (PET) have been used mainly to prognosticate the disease.

Target Organs of Perinatal Asphyxia

The target organs of perinatal asphyxia are the brain, heart, lung, kidney, liver, bone marrow and bowel. The most frequent abnormalities involve the kidneys followed by the brain, cardiovascular and pulmonary. Often asphyxiated neonates will succumb to dysfunctions of organs other than the CNS showing minimal evidence of hypoxic ischemic brain injury. In such instances the brain was spared in expense of cardiac output to the affected organ (diving reflex). The degree of asphyxia required to cause permanent neurologic impairment is just below that which is lethal for multisystem failure.

1. **Hypoxic-ischemic encephalopathy** is the most important consequence of perinatal asphyxia. It has a spectrum of clinical manifestations from mild to severe.
   a. Within 12 hours after the insult the infants show signs of cerebral dysfunction and are stuporous or comatose, have periodic breathing or irregular respiratory effort, are hypotonic, and have lost all complex reflexes viz. Moro's reflex, sucking reflex. They have roving eye movements but the pupillary

responses are intact. Subtle, tonic, or multifocal clonic seizures may occur within 6-24 hours in around 50% of cases of moderate or severely asphyxiated infants.

b. Between 12-24 hours there may be apnoea requiring respiratory support.

c. Over 24 to 72 hours following the insult, the severely affected infant may have prolonged apnoea, abnormalities of pupillary reactivity, loss of oculomotor and caloric responses. Brain death may ensue between 24-72 hours later. In most severe cases, in which the incidence of death or significant neurologic sequelae is greatest, other organ systems inevitably show evidence of asphyxial damage. Persistant oliguria (< 1 ml/kg/hr for the first 36 hours) has been found to be significantly associated with severe HIE and poor outcome. To estimate the severity of asphyxial insult, the Saranat clinical stages can be used in infants more than 36 weeks of gestation. For practical purpose, the Levene clinical classification of HIE is useful.

Table 1.1: Clinical severity of HIE (Levene)

Clinical features	*Mild*	*Moderate*	*Severe*
Consciousness	Irritability	Lethargy	Comatose
Tone	Mild Hypotonia	Marked abnormality of tone	Severe hypotonia
Sucking/ Respiration	Poor sucking	Require tube feed	Not possible as spontaneous respiration is absent
Seizures	No seizure	Seizures present	Prolonged seizures

Prevention of hypoxic ischemic brain injury: Perinatal assessment of risk factors and perinatal monitoring should be done vigorously in high-risk pregnancies.

Delivery room management—Vigorous resuscitation of asphyxiated newborns should be done and the protocol currently recommended by the American Heart association should be followed.

2. **Cardiovascular manifestations:** Infants with perinatal asphyxia may have transient myocardial ischemia manifested by respiratory distress and cyanosis shortly after birth. They have signs of congestive cardiac failure viz. tachycardia, tachypnoea, an enlarged soft, tender liver and a gallop rhythm. Many infants will have a systolic murmur at the lower left sternal border (tricuspid regurgitation) and some will have a murmur at the apex (mitral regurgitation). The chest X-ray will show cardiomegaly with or without pulmonary venous congestion.

   The ECG may show ST depression in mid precordium and T wave inversion in left precordial leads.

   The echocardiogram/Doppler will show normal cardiac structures but decreased left ventricular contractions, especially of the posterior wall and signs of persistant pulmonary hypertension. The ventricular end diastolic pressures are usually elevated. Some infants may show tricuspid regurgitation with right to left shunting at the atrial level. Some may show mitral regurgitation.
3. **Renal effects and manifestations:** The asphyxiated infant is at risk of acute tubular necrosis and SIADH.
4. **Gastrointestinal effects and manifestations:** The asphyxiated infant is at risk of bowel ischemia and necrotizing enterocolitis, early signs of which are

intestinal stasis, presence of reducing substances and occult blood in stool.

5. **Hematologic effects and manifestations:** Disseminated intravascular coagulation (DIC) may occur as a result of damage to blood vessels, failure of the liver to produce clotting factors and bone marrow to produce platelets. Spontaneous bleeding from venepuncture site may be earliest sign of DIC, followed by bleeding manifestations.
6. **Liver:** The infant may present with a 'shock liver', (i.e. a severely damaged liver unable to provide even the basic functions) or signs of liver failure.
7. **Pulmonary effects:** The pulmonary effects of asphyxia include increased pulmonary vascular resistance, pulmonary hemorrhage, pulmonary edema secondary to cardiac failure, and possibly due to failure of surfactant production with secondary hyaline membrane disease (Acute respiratory distress syndrome).

Management

Management of perinatal asphyxia should start in the labour room with resuscitation of all newborns that are unable to initiate spontaneous respiration after complete delivery. The following babies are to be transferred to the special care newborn unit:

1. Babies with severe birth asphyxia.
2. Babies who required prolonged bag and mask ventilation.
3. Babies who suffered from moderate asphyxia when monitoring is not possible in the post natal ward.

It should be noted that no specific interventions have yet been shown to improve the out come following perinatal asphyxia although potential therapies are being evaluated. Therefore, careful anticipatory supportive management is recommended.

Maintenance of Temperature

The baby should be placed under a radiant warmer and nursed in a thermoneutral environment and temperature monitored.

Check Vital Signs and Record Base Line Data

The vital signs to be checked include respiration, heart rate, blood pressure/Capillary refill time (CRT), temperature, oxygen saturation and urine output. The base line data should be recorded.

Fluids

Start intravenous fluids in babies with severe birth asphyxia with two third of maintenance fluid. Consider infusion of volume expander (Normal saline/Ringers lactate 10 ml/kg over 5-10 minutes, repeated if necessary up to 3 such) if the CRT is > 3 seconds or there is presence of metabolic acidosis or Apgar score less than 3 at 5 minutes.

Poor perfusion may be due to hypovolemia or secondary to myocardial ischemia. If poor perfusion persists after the initial bolus, ionotropes should be started. Dopamine should be started 3-5 microgram/kg/min. The dose should be increased stepwise upto the rate of 10 microgram/kg/min. If perfusion is still poor dobutamine should be added at the rate of 5 micrograms /kg/min. The maximum dose of each drug is 20 microgram /kg/min.

Fluid overload should be avoided. It may exacerbate cardiac dysfunction and cerebral edema or lead to hyponatremia, which increases cerebral irritability and the risk of convulsion.

Fluids should be restricted in the first 24 hours, as oliguria is likely as a result of ADH secretion and renal ischemia. Fluid balance should be assessed by monitoring:

a. Urine output (Normal urine output 1 ml/kg/hr) and specific gravity.
b. Urine sodium, potassium, chloride and urea.
c. Plasma urea, sodium, potassium, chloride and creatinine.
d. Weight daily.
e. Blood pressure/Capillary refill time (normal < 3 seconds).

Electrolytes

Hyponatremia without excessive urinary sodium loss is likely to be due to excess ADH secretion. It can be managed with fluid restriction. *Hyperkalemia* may occur during the acidotic phase. Potassium should not be added to the IV fluids until good urine flow is established. *Hypokalemia* may occur as result of secondary hyperaldosteronism. Potassium has to be added to intravenous fluid in time. *Hypocalcemia:* Calcium level should be maintained in the normal range. 10% calcium gluconate should be given 4 ml/kg/day for 1- 2 days as continuous infusion or as bolus diluted 1:1 under ECG monitoring.

Acidosis

Acidosis should be treated by improving perfusion and maintaining oxygen saturation. There is no evidence that correction of acidosis with buffer improves the condition. However, if problems with perfusion persist despite treatment with fluids and oxygen, then sodium bicarbonate should be given in the dose of 2-3 meq/ kg diluted in equal volumes of distilled water.

Blood Gases, Blood Glucose and Hematocrit

Blood gases, blood glucose and the hematocrit should be monitored so that all parameters are maintained in the normal range for the first 48-72 hours.

Oxygen

Oxygen levels should be kept in the normal range by monitoring of trans cutaneous or arterial pO_2 or percent oxygen saturation by pulse oximeter. Blood gases should be monitored with an aim to keep $PaO_2 > 60$ mm Hg and $PaCO_2 < 40$ mmHg. In babies with adequate spontaneous respiration, oxygenation is maintained by oxygen delivery by a oxygen hood.

Assisted ventilation is indicated in presence of apnoea, inadequate spontaneous respiration and continuing hypoxia or hypercarbia. Target PaO_2 is 80-100 torr in term and 60–80 torr in preterm babies. Target $PaCO_2$ is 40-45 torr. Oxygen saturation should be maintained in the range of 90-95% in term and 90- 93% in preterm babies.

Blood Glucose

Hypoglycemia is often seen in asphyxiated neonates. It is due to glycogen depletion secondary to catecholamine release and to an unexplained hyperinsulinemic state. An initial phase of hyperglycemia and hypoinsulinemia may be followed by profound hypoglycemia within 2-3 hours. Blood glucose level should be kept at 60-100 mg/dl as hypoglycemia may worsen CNS damage and hyperglycemia may exacerbate acidosis. Blood glucose levels should be monitored and treatment of hypoglycemia should be instituted as and when necessary. Rapid glucose bolus should be avoided. Hence serum glucose levels should be monitored frequently (Dextrosticks) for adjustments of glucose concentration of the fluid for infusion.

Hematocrit

Hematocrit should be maintained at > 40% in ventilated babies. If hematocrit is > 65% it should be brought down to 55% by partial exchange transfusion using normal saline.

Subsequent monitoring of the asphyxiated baby includes:

1. Record of urine output.
2. Blood sugar estimation at 2, 6, 12, 24, 48 and 72 hours of age.
3. Hematocrit once a day for first few days.
4. Serum sodium, potassium, calcium once a day.
5. ABG as often as required.
6. Neurological status viz. sensorium, tone, reflexes, seizure, autonomic disturbances every 4-6 hours.

Treatment of Seizures

Seizures are typically focal or multifocal. They occur in about 50% of cases, characteristically on the first or second day, usually in stage II, rarely in stage III, and almost never in stage I HIE. Seizures may be associated with increase in cerebral metabolic rate, which in absence of adequate oxygen and perfusion, may lead to fall in blood glucose level, an increase in brain lactate level and fall in high energy phosphate levels. In infants not mechanically ventilated, seizures may be associated with hypoxemia and/or hypercapnia. Seizures should be distinguished from jitteriness (rhythmic segmental myoclonus), seen frequently in stage I and even stage II HIE. Slight flexion and extension of the joint in the affected limb will arrest the clonus but does not alter true seizure activity.

When seizures are diagnosed, phenobarbitone should be loaded 20 mg/kg/dose IV slowly over 20 minutes. If there is no response, two additional doses of 10 mg/kg can be given every 15 minutes followed by maintenance dose of 5 mg/kg/day. The maximum loading dose is 40 mg/kg. The rate of infusion of phenobarbitone should not exceed 1mg/kg/min and preferably an infusion pump should be used to deliver the drug. One should always be vigilant for respiratory depression, and/or cardiovascular compromise with hypotension during phenobarbitone injection. There is no role of intramuscular phenobarbitone because of its slow and erratic absorption. If seizures persist, phenytoin should be administered slowly as a second drug, 20 mg/kg IV loading dose slowly over 20 minutes, followed by 5 mg/kg per day maintenance dose. The maintenance doses for both phenobarbitone and phenytoin should be started 12 hours after the loading dose in a single daily dose. If seizure still persists then lorezepam 0.05 mg/kg/dose IV may be given as the third drug. If an IV access cannot be obtained, per rectal diazepam or valproate or paraldehyde can be given as a stopgap measure.

When the infant is stable for 3-4 days, all anti-convulsant are weaned except phenobarbitone. All anti-convulsant are stopped by 14 days. Seizures following severe asphyxia are difficult to control and are often resistant to aggressive anticonvulsant therapy in the first 72 hours .It should be noted that once the conventional anticonvulsant are given in the maximum dosage, there is little utility in eliminating every twitch or EEG seizure. For unexplained reasons, even refractory seizures cease after approximately 48 hours.

In the event of a seizure, one should also exclude metabolic disorders that may complicate asphyxia and cause seizure viz. hypoglycemia, hypocalcemia and hyponatremia, hypomagnesemia. Pyridoxine dependency and local anesthetic toxicity may mimic post asphyxia seizures and should be considered in the differential diagnosis.

Cerebral Edema

Cerebral edema and raised intracranial pressure are uncommon concomitants of perinatal asphyxia. They peak at 36 to 72 hours after the insult. They are more properly regarded as an effect rather than a cause of brain damage. They reflect prior cerebral necrosis rather than swelling of intact cells. Their presence indicates a bad prognosis. Present literature has shown that efforts to reduce cerebral edema or ICP do not affect outcome. Hence interventions previously used as anti edema agents do not have much use. It is believed that the infant's patent sutures and open fontanel are protective of any acute rise of ICP that might occur.

Cardiac Effects

The treatment consists of adequate ventilation with correction of hypoxemia, acidosis and hypoglycemia. Volume overload should be avoided. These babies require continuous monitoring of mean arterial pressure, central venous pressure and mixed venous saturation and urine out put. Infants with cardiac collapse will require treatment with dopamine and dobutamine. Some infants in great distress may require after load reduction with peripheral beta agonist (isoproterenol), a peripheral alpha blocker (e.g. tolazoline), or nitroprusside.

Hepatic, GIT, Hematologic and Pulmonary System Effects

Liver function tests should be monitored. Serum ammonia level should be measured. Serum glucose should be kept at 60-100 mg/dl. Drugs that are detoxified in the liver should be avoided. If used, blood levels monitored. Treatment of liver failure should be instituted if present. It is preferable not to start oral feeds in an asphyxiated infant till 5-7 days. NEC should be treated in the usual lines. Clotting factors, fibrinogen, and platelets should be monitored and replaced if need be in case the baby develops DIC. Besides oxygenation and ventilation, extra corporeal membrane oxygenation (ECMO) provides a recent therapeutic modality in an asphyxiated infant who's CNS appears otherwise intact.

Newer Treatment Modalities for the Treatment of Birth Asphyxia

1. Opioid antagonist—post ischaemic blood brain barrier disruption and enhanced endogenous opioid have been implicated in the pathogenesis of ischaemic neuronal injury. The potential for use of naloxone is under evaluation.
2. Free oxygen radical scavengers and inhibitors- it has been shown that super oxide desmutase, vitamin E, mannitol and allopurinol, xanthine oxidase inhibitor have neuroprotective roles in animal studies.
3. Calcium channel antagonist—the use of calcium channel blockers like flunarizine and nimodepine could prevent neuronal injury and death by preventing calcium influx into cells.
4. Excitatory amino acid antagonist—pretreatment of animals with agents such as MK801, Ketamine and

dextromethhorphan has produced variable results when used prior to asphyxia.

5. Selective head cooling has been shown to decrease cerebral energy demands and is an attractive option.

Selective Head Cooling

In instances of HIE, following the termination of the insult, a cascade of deleterious events result in cell death. Two fundamental modes of cell death occur. They are ***necrosis*** and ***apoptosis***. Hypoxic ischemic insults may lead to necrosis or apoptosis, or both, depending on the severity of the insult, the local environment of the affected region of the brain, and the maturational state of the brain cell.

Necrosis occurs during and for a period following the injury and is characterized by cell swelling, membrane disintegration, cell rupture, release of intracellular contents, and as a consequence inflammation and phagocytosis.

Necrotic cell death then triggers a series of biochemical cascades. During the next 24-48 hours, a secondary energy failure initiates, leading to apoptotic cell death.

Apoptosis is a secondary energy failure starting within ~ 24 hours of birth and may last for more than 48 hours. It is characterized by cell shrinkage, relative preservation of the cellular membrane, and death without inflammation. Apoptotic cell death requires the activation of specific death genes – cell suicide.

See Fig. on the next Page

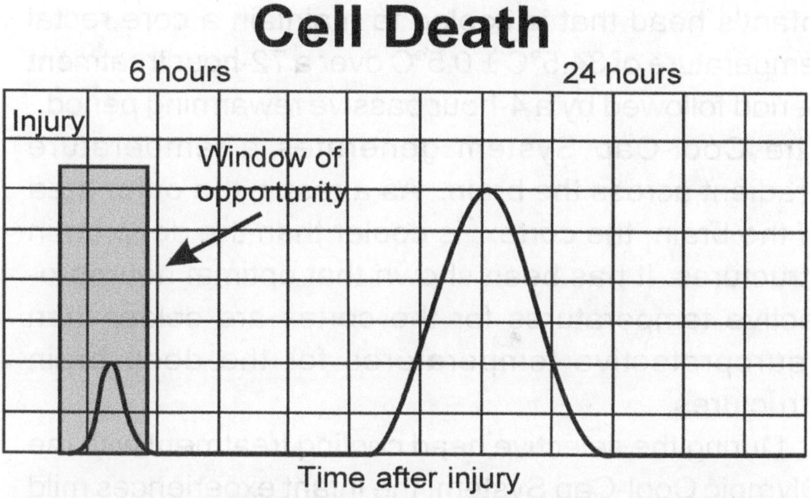

Fig. 1.1: Sequence of brain cell death after the perinatal insult

HIE is a progressive injury developing over hours to days. There are two major areas of the brain that can be affected by the asphyxial event and the resultant hypoxia and/or ischemia. They are the cortical "watershed" area, and the deep structures – the basal ganglia and thalamus.

There is a therapeutic window of opportunity during which hypothermic intervention can decrease the amount of cell death resulting from secondary energy failure. If selective brain cooling can be initiated during the first 6 hours after the injury and the baby's brain is kept cool for the duration of the secondary energy failure state, it has been demonstrated that selective head cooling can interrupt the second phase of the injury and have a significant effect on the severity of the secondary cell death. Further, animal studies have also shown that if selective head cooling is started sooner (< 3 hours) results are even more significant.

Selective head cooling with the Olympic Cool-Cap System utilizes a sealed water cap placed over the infant's head that is cooled to maintain a core rectal temperature of 34.5°C ± 0.5°C over a 72-hour treatment period followed by a 4-hour passive rewarming period. The Cool-Cap System generates a temperature gradient across the brain. As a result, the outer area of the brain, the cortex, is cooler than the deep brain structures. It has been shown that optimal neuroprotective temperatures for the cortex are colder than neuroprotective temperatures for the deep brain structures.

During the selective head cooling treatment with the Olympic Cool-Cap System, the infant experiences mild *systemic* hypothermia and receives warmth through the radiant warmer. The goal is to adjust the cap water appropriately in order to maintain the infant's core rectal temperature at 34.0°C – 35.0°C.

There are two expected benign side effects associated with selective head cooling (although not all babies will experience these side effects). The first is minor cardiac arrhythmias. Sinus bradycardia is known to be associated with hypothermia. The second side effect is head or scalp edema, which generally resolves with no action, or with scalp massage, through adjustments to the cooling cap, or by positioning.

Selection Criteria for Selective Head Cooling with the Olympic Cool-Cap System

Once an infant has suffered a hypoxic and/or ischemic event, selective head cooling with the Olympic Cool-Cap System may be considered for treatment to prevent or reduce the severity of neurological injury associated with HIE for an infant that is:

Full-term infant with clinical evidence of moderate to severe hypoxic-ischemic encephalopathy (HIE) as defined by criteria A, B and C.

Criteria A

Infant at $\geq$ 36 weeks gestational age and at least one of the following:

- Apgar score $\leq$ 5 at 10 minutes.
- Continued need for resuscitation, including endotracheal or mask ventilation, at 10 minutes after birth.
- Acidosis defined as either umbilical cord pH or any arterial pH < 7.00 within 60 minutes of birth.
- Base deficit $\geq$ 16 mmol/L (or Base excess $\leq$ 16 mmol/L) in umbilical cord blood sample or any blood sample within 60 minutes of birth (arterial or venous blood).

Criteria B

Infant with moderate to severe encephalopathy consisting of altered state of consciousness (as shown by lethargy, stupor or coma) and at least one of the following:

- Hypotonia.
- Abnormal reflexes, including oculomotor or papillary abnormalities.
- Absent or weak suck.
- Clinical seizures.

Criteria C

Infant has an amplitude-integrated encephalogram/ cerebral function monitor (aEEG/CFM) recording of at least 20 minutes duration that shows either moderately/

severely abnormal aEEG background activity (score of 2 or 3 in a HIE Scoring Technique) or seizures.

If all three criteria are met, selective head cooling with the Olympic Cool-Cap System should be started within six hours of birth. Whenever possible, treatment should be started as early as possible.

Contraindications

Selective head cooling is contraindicated in the presence of the following conditions:

- Imperforate anus.
- Evidence of head trauma or skull fracture causing major intracranial hemorrhage.
- Birth weight < 1,800 grams.

Precautions

- Monitor and correct all blood gases and pH values for core temperature.
- Do not initiate oral feeding during treatment.
- Care should be taken to monitor these conditions especially when administering medications that would further prolong the QT interval or increase the effects of hyperglycemia. The potential adverse effects of hypothermia include increased oxygen consumption, transient hyperglycemia, prolongation of the QT interval.
- Maintain skin integrity using selective head cooling only on unbroken skin or covered lesions, using only the scalp sensor under the water cap and maintaining at least 12-hour scalp checks.
- Do not set the radiant warmer above 37.5°C.
- Larger infants may require less heat to re-warm or may re-warm faster than 0.5°C per hour. These infants should be closely monitored. One should

not attempt re-cooling to slow down the rate of re-warming.

Warnings

When following the criteria and treatment parameters, selective head cooling with the Cool-Cap System is FDA approved and safe for the treatment of HIE. Safety is not known for off-label use.

Hypothermia has been known to prolong the half-lives of medications, inhibit antimicrobial activity and create anticoagulant effects. Care should be taken to monitor these conditions.

Significant overcooling (– 32°C) may result in a shut down of the infant's peripheral circulation and the infant will no longer be taking in body warmth from the radiant warmer. Infants should be carefully rewarmed to the target range by removal of the cooling cap before cooling is resumed. Rewarming rate should not exceed 0.5°C per hour to prevent vasodilatation, hypotension, and possible seizures (as seen in some animal studies).

Prognosis

Overall, full term asphyxiated infants have a mortality of 10-20%. The incidence of neurologic sequelae in survivors is 20-45% (approximately 40% of these are minimal; 60% severe) i.e. the majority will be normal. The risk of CP is 5-10 % among asphyxiated newborns.

Indicators of poor outcome are low (0-3) extended Apgar score, Sarnat Stage III encephalopathy, seizure of early onset and difficult to control, elevated ICP. (>10 mm of Hg), persistence of abnormal neurologic signs specially absence of Moro's reflex after 1-2 weeks, persistence of extensive hypodensity on CT., elevated CK-Bb level (>5 IU), persistent oliguria (<1ml/kg/hr) for first 36 hours of life, interictal EEG with extreme burst suppression activity.

CONCLUSION

It is note worthy that birth asphyxia severe enough to damage the fetal brain usually kills before or soon after birth. Approximately 25% of asphyxiated term newborn will die. The remainder, even those with seizures will be normal. The only group with significant neurological impairment will be those who were severely asphyxiated yet narrowly escaped death, which is a relatively small group. Therefore, death on one hand and intact survival on the other are more likely outcomes than survival with brain damage.

Given this, no infant will have undergone an asphyxial insult severe enough to cause permanent brain damage without other organs being equally severely affected. Thus a diagnosis and management of asphyxia must hinge on assessment of other systems in addition to CNS. Prevention of asphyxia, which is possible upto 100% with proper antenatal care of the mother and efficient care of the newborn immediately after birth need top priority to prevent neonatal mortality as a result of birth asphyxia.

SUGGESTED READINGS

1. James H. Hutchison and Forrester Cockburn. Asphyxia Neonatorum in Practical Pediatric Problems Sixth edition, 1986. P 1–10. Published by Singapore National Printers.
2. Armida Fernandez, Jayshree Mondkar, RuchNanavati, Perinatal Asphyxia in Recent Advances in Pediatrics Vol-6, edited by Suraj Gupte; P-241-257.
3. Evan Y, Synder and John P. Cloherty. Perinatal asphyxia; Manual of Neonatal Care: Edited by John P.

Cloherty, Eric C Eichenwald and Ann R. Stark. 5 th., 2004, P-515-532.
4. Sanglcae Chamnanavanakij, Jaffrey M. Periman; Management of Perinatal hypoxic ischemic encephalopathy in Recent Advances in pediatrics; edited by T.J.David; P-33-44.
5. John Kattwinkel; Textbook of neonatal resuscitation, 4th edition 2000.
6. Costello A, Francis V, Byrne A, Puddephatt C. State of the world's newborns. Kinetik Communications 2001.
7. World Health Organization. Perinatal mortality: A listing of available information. FRH/MSM.96.7. Geneva: WHO 1996.
8. Report of National Neonatal Perinatal Database (National Neonatology Forum, India) 2000.
9. American Academy of Pediatrics, American College of Obstetricians and Gynecologists: Relationship between perinatal factors and neurological outcome in Poland RL, Truman RK,(Eds): Guidelines for perinatal care 3rd edition, Elk Grove Village, Illinois: American Academy of Pediatrics,1992; 221-24.
10. Meherban Singh Care of the baby in the labour room in Care of the Newborn 5th edition 1999, Sagar Publication, New Delhi.
11. Michael F. Epstein Resuscitation in delivery room in Manual of Neonatal care edited by John P. Cloherty and Ann R. Stark 3rd edition 1993. Little, Brown and company. Boston/Toronto/London.
12. Evan Y. Snyder and John P Cloherty. Perinatal Asphyxia. In Manual Of neonatal care edited by John P Cloherty and Ann R Stark 3 rd edition 1993. Little Brown and Company. Boston/Toronto/London.
13. Textbook of Neonatal resuscitation edited by John Kattwinkel 4th edition 2000 American Academy of Pediatrics and American Heart Association.
14. Rajiv Agarwal, Ashok K Deorari and Vinod Paul. Post resuscitation management of asphyxiated newborn, Indian J Pediatrics; 68: 12, 2001 1149-1153.

15. A Neonatal Vade–Mecum edited by Brian Speidel, Peter Fleming, John Henderson *et al.* 3rd edition 1998 published by Oxford University Press Inc., New York.
16. Selective Head Cooling With Mild Systemic Hypothermia after Neonatal Encephalopathy: Multicentre Randomized Trial. Gluckman PD, Wyatt JS, Azzopardi D. Lancet vol. 365, 663 - 670, 2005.

2 Neonatal Shock

P. Biswanath

Circulatory shock or acute circulatory failure is a serious neonatal emergency. By definition, it is a complex clinical syndrome caused by an acute failure of blood circulation, which is characterized by inadequate tissue perfusion, and inefficient removal of toxins and metabolic waste products at the cellular level. It remains a major cause of neonatal morbidity and mortality without any racial or sex predilection.

The high mortality of neonatal shock can be attributable to difficult early diagnosis of the condition and associated primary organic immaturity of the newborn baby. Another important practical problem is that—lowest acceptable blood pressure value for the newborn is not well established. So the blood pressure that triggers a decision to treat a newborn that do not have acidosis is somewhat arbitrary.

The aetiology is multifactorial and the syndrome is frequently complicated by secondary involvement of many organ systems.

Etiological Classification

Neonatal shock is classified according to the underlying etiology as:

Hypovolemic Shock

Decreased circulating blood volume is the most common cause of shock in the neonate. The decrease in blood volume can result from whole blood, plasma or extra vascular fluid loss due to the following:

1. Placental hemorrhage: Abruptio, previa, velamentous insertion.
2. Fetal to maternal transfusion.
3. Donor fetus in a twin-to-twin transfusion.
4. Birth injuries that result in neonatal blood loss.
5. Intracranial hemorrhage.
6. Intra-abdominal bleeding.
7. Disseminated intravascular coagulation (DIC) or other coagulation disorders.
8. Plasma loss into the extra vascular compartment seen in conditions such as sepsis and hypoproteinaemia.
9. Excessive fluid and electrolyte losses seen in dehydration (from insensible loss or inappropriate diuresis) causes: Diarrhea, vomiting, heat stress, skin disorders, gastrointestinal (G.I.) abnormalities.
10. Asphyxia.

Cardiogenic Shock

Inadequate tissue perfusion may result from defects of the pump function as occurs in asphyxia, arrhythmias, cardiomyopathy, myocarditis, PDA, congenital heart disease, myocardial ischemia, hypoglycemia, acidosis and sepsis.

Distributive Shock

Abnormalities within the vascular beds may also result in shock as in septicemia, use of vasodilators and muscle relaxants, endothelial injury and adrenal insufficiency.

The precise mechanisms operative in septic shock are unclear. Probably a combination of factors are operating (endotoxins from bacteria, vasoactive agents secreted such as serotonin, prostaglandins, histamine and endorphins) all resulting in peripheral vasodilatation and relative hypovolemia.

Obstructive Shock

Flow restriction due to interference with venous return and subsequently cardiac output results in obstructive shock. This may occur due to tension pneumothorax, pulmonary interstitial emphysema, cardiac tamponade, congenital diaphragmatic hernia.

Dissociative Shock

Inadequate oxygen releasing capacity results in dissociative shock and is seen in profound anemia and methemoglobinemia.

Stages of Shock and Clinical Features

Shock is a progressive disorder, but it can generally be divided into 3 phases: Compensated, Uncompensated and Irreversible.

Compensated Stage

In compensated shock, perfusion to vital organs, such as the brain, heart, and adrenal glands is preserved by sympathetic reflexes, which increase systemic arterial resistance. Derangement of vital signs, such as heart rate, respiratory rate, blood pressure, and temperature, is absent or minimal. Increased secretion of angiotensin and vasopressin allows the kidneys to conserve water and salt, the release of catecholamines enhances myocardial contractility, and decreased spontaneous activity reduces oxygen consumption.

Clinical Features: Clinical signs of compensated phase include pallor, tachycardia, cool peripheral skin, poorly felt pulses, prolonged capillary refilled time (>3secs), core—skin temperature gradient > 2°C, and poor activity. Warm extremities and a widened pulse pressure are features of early-compensated phase of shock. As these homeostatic mechanisms are exhausted or become inadequate to meet the metabolic demands of the tissues, the uncompensated stage ensues.

Uncompensated Stage

In uncompensated stage, delivery of oxygen and nutrients to tissues becomes marginal or insufficient to meet demands. Anaerobic metabolism becomes the major source of energy production, and production of lactic acid is excessive, which leads to systemic metabolic acidosis. Numerous chemical mediators, enzymes, and other substances are released, including histamine, cytokines (especially tumor necrosis factor and interleukin-1), xanthine oxidase (which generates oxygen free radicals), platelet-aggregating factor, and bacterial toxins in the case of septic shock. This cascade of metabolic changes further reduces tissue perfusion and oxidative phosphorylation.

Anaerobic metabolism results in failure of the energy-dependent sodium-potassium pump, which maintains the normal homeostatic environment in which cells function. The integrity of the capillary endothelium is disrupted, and plasma proteins leak, with the resultant loss of oncotic pressure and intravascular fluids in the extra vascular space. Sluggish flow of blood and chemical changes in small blood vessels lead to platelet adhesion and activation of the coagulation cascade, which may eventually produce a bleeding tendency and further blood volume depletion.

Clinical Features: Clinically, patients with uncompensated shock present with falling blood pressure, prolonged capillary refill time, tachycardia, mottling of skin, cold skin, rapid breathing (to compensate for the metabolic acidosis), and reduced or absent urine output. If effective intervention is not promptly instituted, progression to irreversible shock follows.

Irreversible Stage

A diagnosis of irreversible shock is actually retrospective. Major vital organs, such as the heart and brain, are so extensively damaged that death occurs despite adequate restoration of the circulation. Early recognition and effective treatment of shock are crucial.

Pathophysiology of Shock

Maintenance of adequate tissue perfusion depends on a pump (the heart), delivering the correct type of fluid (blood), through controlled vessels (arteries, veins, capillaries) without obstruction to flow. So inadequate tissue perfusion resulting in impaired cellular respiration may result from any of the factors mentioned below:

- Defect in the pump —— Cardiogenic shock.
- Loss of fluid ——— hypovolemic shock.
- Abnormal vasculature —— distributive shock.
- Flow resistance —— obstruction at the level of great vessels.
- Inadequate oxygen release—Dissociative shock.

Points to be Noted

1. Septic shock should be suspected in any newborn with respiratory distress and reduced perfusion, particularly in the presence of maternal history of chorioamnionitis or premature rupture of membrane.

Flow diagram of pathophysiology of shock

Poor tissue perfusion
↓

Compensated Shock

Improved adaptive homeostatic mechanism
↑ sympathetic reflexes
↑ Catecholamine secretion
↑ secretion of Angiotensin and AVP
↓ spontaneous activity
↓
Splanchnic vasoconstriction

Preserved vital organ perfusion
Improved systemic arterial pressure
Enhanced myocardial contractility
↓ O_2 consumption
Not intervened
↓
Exhaustion of adaptive mechanism
↓

Uncompensated Shock

Further reduction of perfusion
↑ anaerobic metabolism (lactic acidosis)
Release of chemical pro-inflammatory mediators
↓
Impaired oxidative phosphorylation
Na^+/K^+ pump failure
Disruption of capillary endothelial cells
Stimulation of coagulation cascade
↓

Irreversible shock

Organ dysfunction

2. Cardiogenic shock can result from closure of the PDA in newborn with ductal dependent cardiac anomaly. Suspicion of such a situation needs intravenous or oral PGE_1 therapy which will be a life saving alternative till appropriate surgery is undertaken.
3. Distributive shock presents with a hyper dynamic state of tachycardia, bounding pulse in the initial period.

4. Shock can occur in presence of normal blood pressure. Hypotension is a late and often sudden sign of decompensation. In very premature infants there may be bradycardia with acute hypotension.

Laboratory Studies

1. Blood for hematocrit, electrolytes, sepsis screen, blood culture, and glucose as soon as vascular access is obtained.
2. Among laboratory investigations, supportive data include metabolic acidosis in the face of reasonable oxygenation on an arterial blood specimen. Mixed venous blood gases may be more helpful because this reflects oxygen extraction and waste products at the tissue level, compared to arterial blood, which reflects lung function and the composition of blood before it is delivered to the tissues. Comparison of simultaneous arterial and mixed venous blood gas determinations may be more useful in assessing cardiac output, tissue oxygenation, and acid-base balance. The value of capillary blood gas determinations is severely limited because they may only reflect diminished perfusion to the periphery and not reflect central perfusion.
3. Elevated plasma lactate with a normal pyruvate also suggests anaerobic metabolism triggered by tissue hypoxia-ischemia.
4. Specific studies must be performed to rule out both the causes (e.g. sepsis, cardiac lesions, and anemia) as well as the sequelae (e.g., renal, hepatic, endocrine) of shock.
5. Other tests include APT test, coagulation profile.

Imaging Studies

1. Echocardiography and Doppler flow velocimetry may provide semi quantitative and semi qualitative

noninvasive analysis of myocardial function. Automated Doppler provides blood pressure readings through a noninvasive method.

Management of Shock

Prevention, early diagnosis and aggressive management are the cornerstones of care. Once the secondary complications of shock (SIRS etc.) are established it is very difficult to reverse shock. The key goal is the establishment of adequate tissue perfusion and oxygenation.

Therapeutic End Points

- Capillary refill < 2 secs.
- Normal pulse with no difference between peripheral and central pulse.
- Warm extremities.
- Urine output > 1ml/kg/min.
- Normal mental status and normal blood pressure for age.
- > 95% SaO_2.
- < 5% difference in preductal and post ductal saturation and central venous O_2 saturation > 70%.

Monitoring

1. Vitals viz. heart rate, respiratory rate, temperature (peripheral to gradient), capillary refill time and blood pressure on an hourly basis.
2. Fluid status viz. daily weight or preferably 12 hourly, intake output charting, estimation of serum sodium, blood urea and serum creatinine.
3. Oxygenation and ventilation viz. arterial blood gas, transcutaneous oxygenation and carbon dioxide estimation as and when required.

4. Central venous pressure to differentiate between hypovolemic and cardiogenic shock.
5. Urine output should be monitored on an hourly basis and maintained over 1 ml/kg/hour.

Establishing Airway, Breathing, Circulation

Position the baby supine with neck in slight extension to ensure a patent airway. Provide supplemental oxygen. Sick, clinically shocked neonates should be intubated and ventilated before they meet conventional ventilation criteria if this can be achieved safely. Intubation may precipitate decompensation in the critically ill child. It should be performed once circulation is stabilised, especially if using induction agents. Any bleeding should be stopped.

Establishing Reliable Intravenous Access

If peripheral access is difficult to achieve, umbilical venous catheterization (5F for preterm, 5-8 F for term or 5-8F sterile feeding tube) or an interosseous line can be considered. The intra osseous line is as good as an IV line for the purpose of any fluid or medication administration necessary for the acute resuscitation of a compromised infant in shock.

Administration of Oxygen as Needed

The oxygen saturation has to be monitored as well as arterial blood gas. ABG helps to determine the patient's acid-base status, which reflects the degree of systemic shock and the patient's response to therapy.

Measurement of Central Venous Pressure

CVP is measured using a catheter introduced through the umbilical vein or percutaneous through external or internal jugular or subclavian vein with its tip in the right atrium or in the intrathoracic superior vena cava. The CVP is maintained at 5-8 cm of water.

Ensuring Adequate Volume Replacement

Normal saline, 10-20 ml/kg is administered. May be repeated according to response except when there is cardiogenic shock. If clinical evidence of major blood or fluid loss exist, use of appropriate higher volumes. Severe sepsis may require 40-60 ml/kg to establish adequate blood volume. There is **no** evidence of advantage of colloid over normal saline in **initial** resuscitation. If there is blood loss, early replacement with blood, initially packed cells, urgently cross matched if available in time or O-negative uncrossmatched. Once initially stabilised need for other blood products (fresh frozen plasma, platelets) on the basis of active bleeding or abnormality on investigation may be considered.

Treatment of Hypoglycaemia

Neonates have limited glycogen stores that may become rapidly depleted during shock, resulting in hypoglycemia. Because glucose is the major metabolic substrate, a rapid bedside glucose test is performed on all patients presenting in shock. If the glucose level is low, they are provided replacement therapy with IV 10% dextrose. The dose of dextrose is 200 mg/kg IV over 1 min. Dextrose is best provided as a continuous IV infusion at a rate of 6-8 mg/kg/hour.

Treatment of Cause (Including Iatrogenic Problems)

In cases with suspected sepsis, broad spectrum antibiotics, on the basis of the nursery protocol should be started after sending blood specimen for sepsis screen, blood and CSF culture. Should consider herpes and need for acyclovir as well as use of immunoglobulin, exchange transfusion in established sepsis. One should also exclude pneumothorax, pericardial tamponade and occult bleeding and treat accordingly.

Treatment of Hypocalcaemia

Shock may cause alterations in available serum ionized calcium levels, despite normal total serum calcium. Furthermore, administered blood products (which contain citrate) may bind free available calcium, additionally decreasing available ionized calcium levels. Therefore, calcium therapy may be useful when treating shock in a patient with documented hypocalcaemia. Dose: 1-2 ml of 10% Calcium gluconate.

Treatment of Acidosis

The primary goal is establishment of stable circulation, perfusion and ventilation. Once these are addressed and CO_2 is normal, if metabolic acidosis is present with pH below 7.2, acidosis is corrected using Sodium Bicarbonate 1-2mEq/kg IV.

Inotropic Agents

Inotropic agents should be used in shock early in the course of the illness as institution of this therapy after profound hypotension has set in does not seem to benefit. Dopamine can be used alone or in combination with dobutamine in a dose of 5 -20 ug/kg/minute as a continuous infusion. Epinephrine can be used if there is no response to dopamine and dobutamine especially in sepsis when low perfusion is due to peripheral vasodilatation. The starting dose is 0.05 to 0.1 microgram/kg/minute and can be increased rapidly as needed while dopamine infusion rates are decreased. A poor response to inotrope therapy can be due to an acquired catecholamine resistance. This is most commonly a problem in overwhelming sepsis or in the chronically hypoxically stressed or failing myocardium. Dopamine and Dobutamine will not work well in this situation. Early use of epinephrine is advised. For protracted hypotension following adequate fluid-volume neither replacement nor epinephrine is indicated.

Newer Therapies for Shock

Shock due to sepsis, even if treated appropriately with vigorous monitoring and aggressive therapeutic measures results in a mortality rate of 90% even in the best of centers. Newer therapies are being explored to improve this dismal outcome of septic shock.

Corticosteroids: Hydrocortisone in the dose of 1 mg/kg/dose can be used for hypotension refractory to volume expansion and vasopressor. If there is response, it should be repeated 12 hourly for 2-3 days. Massive doses of 2-6 mg/kg of dexamethasone or 30 mg/kg of methyl prednisolone is used for septic shock. It should be given intravenously as early as possible but definitely within 4 hours of occurrence of shock. Delayed initiation of therapy does not offset the complement mediated enzymatic chain of tissue destruction. A maximum of four doses may be used at 12 hourly intervals.

Naloxone: Naloxone in a dose of 0.3 mg/kg intravenously or as continuous infusion of 0.05-0.1 mg/kg/hour has been used successfully in fulminant gram negative septicemia with shock without any adverse effect. It acts by opposing the action of endogenous opiates like endorphins released in septic shock.

ECMO therapy for refractory Shock: Newborns with refractory shock must be suspected to have unrecognized morbidities, including pericardial effusion, pneumothorax, ongoing blood loss, hypoadrenalism, hypothyroidism, inborn errors of metabolism, or cyanotic or obstructive heart disease. When these causes have been excluded, ECMO becomes an important therapy to consider. The expected ECMO survival rate for newborn septic shock is currently 80%. Most centers accept refractory shock or a PaO_2 <40 mm Hg after maximal therapy to be sufficient indication for ECMO support.

Newer modalities of treatment: Still under evaluation.

Pentoxyphyllin: inhibits TNF induced neutrophil activation and endothelial injury (5 mg/kg/hr iv over 6 hr for 5 days). Monoclonal antibody against endotoxins, bacterial lipopolysaccharide and growth factors.

Surgical Care

Structural heart disease or arrhythmias often require specific pharmacologic or surgical therapy. The liver and bowel may be damaged by shock, leading to gastrointestinal bleeding and increasing the risk for necrotizing enterocolitis, particularly in the premature infant.

Diet

Infants in shock should not be fed and feedings should not be resumed until gastrointestinal function has recovered. Total parenteral nutrition should be initiated as soon as possible.

Further Inpatient Care

Infants recovering from neonatal shock are at risk for multiple sequelae and should be intensively screened for neurodevelopment abnormalities, using brain imaging and brainstem audiometric evoked responses. Other tests are determined by the clinical course and complications.

SUGGESTED READINGS

1. Manual of Neonatal care 5th Ed. Edited by Cloherty John P, Eichwald E.C, Stark AR: 181-84.
2. Nelson's textbook of Pediatrics, 17th Ed. Edited by-Behrman R.E., Kliegman RM, Jenson HB: 296-301.
3. Principles of Pediatric and Neonatal Emergencies, 2nd Ed: Edited by Sachdev HPS, Choudhury P, Bagga A, Chugh K, Ramji S, Puri RK. 493-500.
4. "Shock and hypotension in newborn", Sinha Sunil K, Steven M Donn: 2004 (e-medicine, internet).
5. "Neonatal Handbook: Shock": Bowman E, Fraser S: updated on 30th Nov 2004. (NETS Victoria, internet)
6. Carcillo JA, Fields AI. "Clinical practice parameters for hemodynamic support of pediatric and neonatal patients in septic shock". Crit Care Med 2002 Jun; 30(6): 1365-78.(internet).
7. Shock: Schwarz A; last updated Oct 04, 2005 (e-medicine, internet).
8. Care of the Newborn, 6th Ed; Edited by: Singh M: 299-301.
9. Protocols in Neonatology, PGIMER; Mukhopadhyay K, Narang A: 2003;142-46.
10. Advanced Pediatric Life Support. The Practical Approach: 3rd edn. Edited by Jones K.M., Molyneax E, Phillip B, Wieteska S: 90-101.
11. Neonatal Shock; National Neonatology Forum. Manual of Neonatal Care, 1st edn; Ramji S: 238-245.

3 Persistent Pulmonary Hypertension in Newborn

J.N. Sharma

Persistent pulmonary hypertension of the newborn (PPHN) is the result of elevated pulmonary vascular resistance to the point that venous blood is diverted to some degree through fetal channels (i.e. the ductus arteriosus and foramen ovale) into the systemic circulation and by-passing the lungs, resulting in systemic arterial hypoxemia.

CHANGES IN THE PULMONARY CIRCULATION AT BIRTH

Fetal Development and Characteristics

Very little blood flows into the fetal lungs prior to birth because pulmonary vascular resistance is very high compared to systemic vascular resistance. The placenta, the fetal gas exchange organ, is a very low resistance outlet for fetal systemic blood flow. With the loss of the placenta at the time of birth, systemic vascular resistance increases.

Several factors are thought to play a role in maintaining high fetal pulmonary vascular resistance:

1. Hypoxia is a potent vasoconstrictor especially at PaO_2 below 40-45 torr. Fetal PaO_2 averages 20-25 torr, so that persistent hypoxemia exists pro-

ducing persistent active pulmonary vasoconstriction.

2. Because the lungs are not fully expanded in utero, an element of mechanical compression of the vessels exists. During lung expansion, the arteries straighten out and become less resistant to blood flow.
3. Carbon dioxide appears to play a minor role in maintaining vasoconstriction. However, hypocapnia ($PaCO_2$ less than 30 torr) is known to blunt hypoxic vasoconstriction.

Because of the high pulmonary vascular resistance, blood is diverted away from the lungs through the foramen ovale and the patent ductus arteriosus into the low resistance systemic and placental circuit. The ductus arteriosus is also oxygen sensitive and remains patent when hypoxia persists. It remains anatomically patent for several weeks to months after birth, but because the neonate is so much better oxygenated than the fetus, the ductus becomes functionally closed in the full-term infant by 24-36 hours after birth.

Transition at Birth

With birth the following sequence occurs:

1. The placental circulation is removed and systemic vascular resistance increases. This in turn, increases pressures in the left ventricle and left atrium. The foramen will tend to close when pulmonary blood flow increases as increased pulmonary flow will increase the blood volume entering the left atrium and in so doing, increase left atrial pressure. Increased left atrial pressure (more than right atrial pressure) results in functional closure of the foramen ovale.
2. With the onset of ventilation, the oxygen tension in the alveolus and in arterial blood increases. As alveolar PaO_2 increases, pulmonary vasoconstriction relaxes

and pulmonary vascular resistance becomes less than systemic vascular resistance. Increased oxygenation also results in constriction of the ductus arteriosus.

3. The onset of ventilation also represents the onset of lung expansion resulting in the straightening out of mechanically compressed vessels.
4. The end result of these changes is a closure of the fetal conduits that carried blood.
5. In addition, even with the conduits open, the balance of vascular resistance shifts so that increased systemic vascular resistance directs blood flow into the low-resistance pulmonary bed.

With the redirection of blood into the lungs and the complete transition of the lung into an air-filled structure, neonatal cardiopulmonary adaptation is complete.

Pathophysiology

Persistent pulmonary hypertension of the newborn is a pathophysiologic syndrome that results when the pulmonary vascular resistance fails to decrease after birth, despite improved alveolar oxygenation and lung expansion. Although systemic vascular resistance has increased (with the loss of the placenta), pulmonary vascular resistance remains equal to or greater than systemic vascular resistance. This results in blood continuing to flow through the foramen ovale and ductus arteriosus. Subsequently, with the loss of placental gas exchange and the inability to increase pulmonary blood flow, arterial oxygen tension falls to very low levels. If this situation is not reversed, it may result in severe hypoxemia.

Since both the pulmonary and systemic resistances are high, a large mechanical load is placed on the heart (especially the right heart) to continue to pump blood to both pulmonary and systemic vascular beds. With high vascular resistance and the subsequent hypoxemia, myocardial performance may become extremely compromised resulting in right heart dilatation, tricuspid insufficiency, and right heart failure.

This condition is most often associated with perinatal asphyxia in 50-70% of reported cases. Other conditions associated with this syndrome include hypoglycemia, hypocalcemia, hyperviscosity syndrome and sepsis.

The specific abnormality which produces persistent pulmonary hypertension is not known. Possible pathogenetic mechanisms include:

1. Repeated intrauterine closure of the ductus with redirection of blood flow into the high-resistance fetal pulmonary vasculature. This may occur in mothers who take high dose aspirin near term. In studies in fetal lambs, other prostaglandin inhibitors have been found to close the ductus in utero resulting most often in stillbirths. The survivors often have a clinical picture of PPHN. Similar findings have been reported in human infants.
2. Abnormal responsiveness of the pulmonary vasculature to hypoxia with an inability to relax after the stimulus for vasoconstriction is removed, i.e. birth asphyxia.
3. Repeated intrauterine hypoxia stimulates the hypertrophy of medial smooth muscle which surrounds pulmonary arterioles, enabling vessels to constrict to an extreme degree for long periods of time. There is pathologic evidence that babies with PPHN have greater thickness of medial muscle in pulmonary arteries than in normal full-term infants.
4. Regional alveolar hypoxia due to poor ventilation even though other parts of the lung are ventilating normally. This is not apparent radiographically.

5. Undergrowth of the pulmonary vascular tree is frequently the cause in infants with congenital diaphragmatic hernia or other causes of pulmonary hypoplasia.
6. The role of alterations in vasoactive mediator levels is suggested. It is clear that a variety of vasoactive mediators participate in the changes in pulmonary vasomotor activity during transition from fetal to neonatal circulation. Nitric oxide, eicosanoids, and endothelin, all play a role in transitional circulation. Other mediators such as leukotrienes, tumor necrosis factor, and platelet activating factor may participate in active pulmonary vasoconstriction with its resultant hypoxemia.
7. Thrombocytopenia and pathological evidence of platelet-fibrin microthromboembolism has been reported in infants succumbing to persistent pulmonary hypertension of the Newborn. Microthrombi formation in the pulmonary vascular bed and accompanying released mediators may induce pulmonary hypertension.

Classification

Persistant pulmonary hypertension can be classified into three forms depending on the likely etiology of the pulmonary hypertension:

1. **PPHN associated with pulmonary parenchymal disease**, such as hyaline membrane disease, meconium aspiration, or transient tachypnea of the newborn as the cause of alveolar hypoxia. It is also known as secondary PPHN or appropriate PPHN. Here alveolar oxygen tension appears to be the major determinant of pulmonary artery vasoconstriction.
2. **PPHN with radiographically normal lungs** and no evidence of parenchymal disease. It is frequently

called Persistent Fetal Circulation (PFC), or primary or inappropriate PPHN

3. **PPHN associated with hypoplasia of the lungs** most often in the form of diaphragmatic hernia associated with an anatomic reduction in capillary number.

Diagnosis

1. This syndrome is usually noted in term or post-term infants.
2. The baby presents clinically with cyanosis and respiratory distress, with tachypnea, but with minimal retractions during the first day of life. The physical examination is generally less remarkable for PPHN. When a hypoxic perinatal insult precedes PPHN, the cardiac examination is notable for a prominent precordial impulse, a single or a narrowly split and accentuated second heart sound, and/or a systolic murmur consistent with tricuspid regurgitation.
3. A gradient in oxygenation between simultaneous preductal (right upper limb or head) and post ductal (lower limb or abdomen) ABG values or trans-cutaneous oxygen saturation measurements documents the presence of a ductus arteriosus right to left hemodynamic shunt. A 10 % or greater pre/ post ductal difference in oxygen saturation in the absence of structural heart disease suggests PPHN. However, this gradient may not be present if substantial shunting is present at the level of the foramen ovale. A subset of infants with PPHN has shunting only at the level of foramen ovale. Therefore an absence of this gradient does not exclude PPHN.
4. The infant's chest radiograph may be normal (as noted in infants with primary PPHN, i.e. PFC) or demonstrate various abnormalities compatible with

aspiration, pneumonia, diaphragmatic hernia, or hyaline membrane disease.

5. The ECG study commonly shows right ventricular predominance that is within the normal range for age. Less commonly, the ECG may reveal signs of myocardial ischemia or infarction or findings consistent with structural heart disease.
6. The diagnosis is confirmed by echocardiography. It should be performed in all infants of suspected PPHN to evaluate hemodynamic shunting, ventricular function and to exclude cyanotic congenital heart disease. A colour doppler study is useful to assess the presence of intracardiac or ductal shunting. Additional echo findings may be a flattened or left bowed septum suggesting pulmonary hypertension. Estimation of pulmonary arterial pressure can be done by continuous wave Doppler sampling of the velocity of the tricuspid regurgitation jet.

Differential Diagnosis

A number of disorders, some of which are associated with secondary pulmonary hypertension may be confused with PPHN and should be excluded. These conditions include:

1. *Congenital cyanotic heart disease*: Signs favouring cyanotic congenital heart disease over PPHN include: cardiomegaly, weak pulses, active precordium, pulse differential between upper and lower extremities, pulmonary edema, grade III $^{+}$ murmur, persistant arterial oxygen tension (PaO_2) at or below 40 mmHg.
2. *Conditions resulting in right or left ventricular dysfunction associated with right to left ventricular shunting*. Left ventricular dysfunction due to ischemia or obstruction caused by myopathic left ventricular disease or left ventricular out flow obstruction may sometimes present with right to left ductal shunt.

Right ventricular dysfunction may be associated with right to left atrial shunting as a result of decreased diastolic compliance and elevated end diastolic pressure. These conditions must be differentiated from PPHN caused by vascular abnormalities.

Treatment Modalities

The most appropriate treatment of Persistent Pulmonary Hypertension of the Newborn still remains unclear. Substantial variation in clinical practice exists worldwide. However, basic treatment goals do exist. In order of increasing aggressiveness and invasiveness, the modalities of treatment are measures to:

1. Improve alveolar oxygenation.
2. Minimize inappropriate pulmonary vasoconstriction.
3. Considering extracorporeal membrane oxygenation support.

Improving alveolar oxygenation with supplemental oxygen (FiO_2).

Hypoxemia is one of the most powerful pulmonary vasoconstrictors. Therefore, the use of supplemental oxygen to achieve normal or elevated oxygen tension is the most important therapy used to reduce abnormally elevated pulmonary vascular resistance. This is especially important when pulmonary parenchymal disease exists, as improvement in alveolar oxygenation will often result in a normal relaxation of the pulmonary arteries and improved pulmonary blood flow.

Minimize "Inappropriate" Pulmonary Vasoconstriction

By overventilating an infant and producing hypocapnia, hypoxic vasoconstriction can be blunted allowing pulmonary blood flow to increase. This may result in improvement in oxygenation. Since vasoconstriction appears related to intracellular pH rather than pCO_2 levels, use of alkalinizing agents such as sodium bicarbonate has become common place. Controlled trials of alkalosis do suggest a positive benefit in some infants, but not all.

Maintenance of systemic arterial blood pressure and, by inference, pulmonary perfusion, appears to have some benefit. Theoretically, increasing systemic arterial pressure may result in decreased right-to-left shunt flow across a patent ductus arteriosus, increased pulmonary blood flow, and hopefully, improved oxygenation. Dopamine and dobutamine are frequently utilized to improve cardiac output and systemic blood pressure.

Vasodilators have been reported to be effective in a certain proportion of infants. However, these agents are nonspecific and frequently result in vasodilatation of both the pulmonary and systemic vascular beds. Most commonly used is tolazoline. The complete mechanism of action of tolazoline is not clear although it appears to be an alpha-sympathetic blocker. By blocking this effect, tolazoline might produce vasodilation. Other works suggests that tolazoline's effect is mediated by histamine. When histamine receptors in the lung are blocked chemically (experimentally), tolazoline becomes a vasoconstrictor. Endotracheally administered tolazoline has been reported to be helpful.

Inhaled nitric oxide has been studied intensively as therapy for Persistent Pulmonary Hypertension of the Newborn. This gaseous free-radical compound was previously known as endothelial-derived-relaxation-factor. Inhaled nitric oxide directly activates soluble guanylate cyclase resulting in increased levels of cyclic-GMP in vascular smooth muscle cells. This results in vascular relaxation by prohibiting myosin protein cross-bridge formation in smooth muscle. Multiple controlled trials have demonstrated that inhaled nitric oxide improves oxygenation in many infants with PPHN.

Prostaglandin I_2 is a complex molecule made from arachadonic acid and is one of the major endogenous vasodilators in the lung. It is normally produced by the lung when lung vessels are in a constricted state, thereby relaxing them. Whether PPHN is the result of faulty PGI_2 production is not known. Administration of pharmacologic doses of PGI_2 to babies with persistent pulmonary hypertension has proven successful even when tolazoline failed.

Other therapies proposed as beneficial in Persistent Pulmonary Hypertension of the Newborn include magnesium sulphate and arginine infusion and the use of perflourocarbon liquid ventilation. At this point, these therapies are experimental.

When circulatory collapse has occurred, the use of an inotropic agent such as dopamine can increase systemic resistance and improved perfusion. Use of both dopamine and tolazoline together has been tried in desperation with occasional beneficial results.

Extra Corporeal Membrane Oxygen Support

When other therapies have failed to result in patient improvement, Extracorporeal Membrane Oxygenation (ECMO) support has been used with good success.

Management

PPHN is a medical emergency. Immediate and appropriate intervention is aimed to reverse hypoxemia and restore normal oxygenation which is critical to avoid or minimize hypoxic ischemic end organ injury.

1. ***Supplemental oxygen***: This is the first step in the treatment of PPHN. The aim is to achieve a normal or elevated arterial oxygen tension and thereby

reduce elevated pulmonary vascular resistance. In the presence of hypoxemia, 100% oxygen should be administered by hood and continuous non invasive monitoring should be done to detect response and rapid changes of oxygenation. If this is not successful, intubation plus continuous positive airway pressure (CPAP) at 2 to 10 cm of water may be effective.

2. ***Mechanical ventilation***: Respiratory support is instituted with *Conventional ventilation* using a fractional inspired oxygen (FiO_2) concentration of 1.0 if hypoxemia persists despite maximal oxygen administration or PaO_2 is borderline despite supplementation with 100% oxygen. The aim of mechanical ventilation is to maintain adequate oxygenation and mild hyperventilation. When relative normoxemia has been achieved for 12-24 hours, careful weaning can be begun. *High frequency oscillatory ventilation (HFOV)* is often useful in treating infants with PPHN associated with severe pulmonary parenchymal disease. *Extracorporeal membrane oxygenation (ECMO)* has been shown to be effective in the management of selected cases of severe PPHN not responding to the treatment described above. However, some centers report successful treatment of PPHN without use of mechanical ventilation, inhaled nitric oxide or ECMO.
3. ***Metabolic alkalosis***: Correction of acidosis is second in importance to oxygenation in the treatment of PPHN. Alkalosis can be achieved by gentle hyperventilation, optimizing blood pressure and perfusion and/or therapy with sodium bicarbonate. In infants with PPHN a pH of 7.35-7.45 is recommended to be maintained. Sodium bicarbonate can be given as bolus dose of 2-3 meq/kg/dose. If unable to maintain the alkalotic state in this manner,

continuous infusion at 1-2 mEq/kg/hour can be tried. Frequent monitoring of serum sodium levels is indicated.

4. ***Sedation and analgesia***: A narcotic analgesic viz. morphine sulphate in the dose of 0.1 mg/kg every 2-4 hours or fentanyl 3-8 micro gram/kg per hour is a useful adjunct therapy. Fentanyl is a potent short acting narcotic that reduces pain and discomfort and minimizes sympathetic nervous system activity. In rare instances, neuromuscular blockade with pancuronium in the dose of 0.1 mg/kg/dose, every 1-3 hours may have to be used to accomplish muscle relaxation to completely synchronize the infant's breathing with mechanical breathing.
5. ***Optimization of systemic blood pressure:*** Many infants with PPHN have a pulmonary vascular resistance that is at or near normal systemic blood pressure. To maximize tissue oxygenation and mixed venous oxygen content an adequate cardiac out put is necessary. A systemic blood pressure over riding the pulmonary vascular resistance helps in temporarily reducing or eliminating the right to left shunt. Hence it is reasonable to set initial treatment goals of raising systemic blood pressure to levels of 60-80 mm Hg (systolic) and 50-60 mmHg (diastolic) and maintained at the upper limit of normal for gestation. Dopamine (1-20 mcg/kg/min i.v. infusion) and dobutamine (1-20 mcg/kg/min) are the two inotropes usually used. Adrenaline (0.05-2 mcg/min i.v. infusion) may be used in case of severe hypotension. When cardiac function is very poor, cardiotonic drug viz. milrinone is sometimes useful. In the event of systemic hypotension intravascular volume expansion should be tried with normal saline or packed cell volume 10-20 ml/ kg bolus doses I.V. However,

the effect of repeated boluses of volume expanders is usually likely to be limited and the use of ionotropes should be considered. Dopamine infusion should be started in a low dose (2-4 mcg/kg/min) and depending on the response dose is increased to 5-10 mcg/kg/min) and dobutamine is added e.g. dopamine 5 mcg/kg/min + dobutamine 10 mcg/kg/min.

6. ***Correction of metabolic abnormalities:*** Biochemical abnormalities might contribute to right to left shunt through impaired cardiac output. Correction of hypoglycemia and hypocalcemia is especially important in order to provide sufficient substrate for myocardial function and response to drugs.
7. ***Correction of polycythemia:*** To ensure adequate oxygen carrying capacity, the hematocrit should be maintained above 40 %. If there is polycythemia and hematocrit exceeds 65%, partial exchange transfusion should be done to reduce hematocrit to 50-55%.
8. ***Additional drugs used to treat PPHN:*** The use of vasodilator agents is not recommended at this time because of lack of sufficient data regarding specificity and efficacy. Tolazoline infusion is used. It may be given as a loading dose of 0.5 to 1.0 mg/kg i.v. followed by intravenous infusion of 2-4 mg/kg/hour. Tolazoline is not a specific pulmonary vasodilator, and it lowers systemic vascular resistance as well, resulting in systemic hypotension. The blood pressure should be monitored carefully. Systemic hypotension, if present should be treated with volume expanders and dopamine infusion. Side effects of tolazoline include hypotension, increased gastric secretion, gastro intestinal bleeding, decreased platelet count and decreased urine output. About two third of patients respond with an increase in systemic oxygenation.

9. ***Inhaled nitric oxide (NO)*** is a promising therapy for PPHN. Prolonged low dose nitric oxide therapy has shown to cause sustained improvement in oxygenation, with out systemic hypotension. Randomized trials have shown that inhaled nitric oxide causes a rapid improvement in oxygenation and thereby decreases the need for extracorporeal membrane oxygenation. The response to inhaled nitric oxide has been shown to be augmented when used with high frequency oscillatory ventilation. Use of nitric oxide remains still investigational.

Outcome

Prognosis is generally good for neonates with mild PPHN who respond quickly to therapy. Most of these neonates recover without permanent lung damage or neurologic impairment. Those neonates who require maximal ventilator setting for a prolonged time, the chance of survival is smaller and many survivors develop broncho pulmonary dysplasia.

Survivors of persistant pulmonary hypertension have a 20-40% risk of audiologic, neurodevelopmental or cognitive impairments. An abnormal electroencephalogram (upto 80%) and cerebral infarction (45%) have been reported. The overall mortality is 25-50%.

SUGGESTED READINGS

1. Roberts J D and Shaul PW. Advances in treatment of persistant pulmonary hypertension of newborn. Pediatr. Clin. North Am. 1993, 40: 983-1004.
2. A neonatal vade–mecum edited by Brian Speidel, Peter Fleming, John Henderson *et al.* Third edition, 1998. Published by Oxford University Press, New York.
3. Walsh MC and Stork EK. Persistant pulmonary hypertension of the newborn: Rational therapy based on Pathophysiology. Clin Perinatol 2001;28:609 -627.

4. Linda J. Van Marter. Persistent pulmonary hypertension of the newborn in Manual of neonatal care 5th edition, 2004. Published by Lippincott Williams Wilkins, Philadelphia, USA.

4 The Preterm Neonate

J.N. Sharma

A preterm baby is one, which is born before 37 completed weeks of gestation. In India 30-40% neonates are low birth weight out of which 10-12% is born preterm. Low birth weight tops the list of causes of neonatal mortality.

Problems in Preterm Baby

Immaturity of the organ systems is the basic underlying feature of the preterm baby. The major problems encountered in management of these babies are:

1. Maintenance of temperature.
2. Inability to protect against infection.
3. Feeding problems.
4. Vulnerability to complications viz. Asphyxia, RDS, Apnoea, Intracranial hemorrhage, late metabolic acidosis, Hyperbilirubinemia, Retinopathy of prematurity, Necrotizing Enterocolitis.
5. Congenital malformations.

Term newborn babies maintain body temperature by active metabolism in brown fat stores. The preterm babies lack brown fat and therefore become hypothermic at usual ambient temperature. They lack an efficient humoral, cellular and mucosal immune mechanism. Thus, being immunocompromised hosts, are unable to protect themselves against bacterial infections.

Neonates below 34 weeks of gestation do not have

co-ordinated sucking and swallowing. So direct breast-feeding is not possible. Those less than 30 weeks of gestation may not tolerate enteral feeds initially because of gut immaturity. They are at frequent risk of vomiting, gastric stasis, aspirations, abdominal distension and functional obstruction as a result of immature gastro-intestinal digestive and motor function. Late developing digestive enzymes which can compromise nutrition are lactases and lipases often giving rise to lactose and fat intolerance. Enzymes that regulate synthesis of cys-teine from methionine, taurine from cysteine and catabolism of tyrosine are also immature. Therefore, the small preterm is at risk of developing deficiency of some aminoacids and potentially toxic accumulation of others.

Preterm babies, especially those less than 34 weeks of gestation have immature lungs which donot expand well at birth and are unable to perform the function of gas exchange efficiently. They develop respiratory dis-tress syndrome. These babies also have a tendency for apnoeic spells as a result of immature respiratory control mechanism.

Spontaneous bleeding into one or both lateral ventricles of the brain is a characteristic complication of a preterm baby. It may be associated with hyaline mem-brane disease or may develop without lung diseases. This is the result of an immature vascular bed around the brain ventricles. The microvasculature of the germinal layer in the preterm consist of an extensive arrangement of fine capillaries and also of large irregular thin walled vessels which form short connecting channels between arterial and venous trees. These vessels readily rupture when exposed to sudden surges in pressure which can be provoked by both hypoxemia and hypercapnia. The germinal layer involutes from 32 weeks gestation and it is presumed that IVH in later gestations arises in the choroids plexus. IVH is common in newborns below 32 weeks gestation but can occur thereafter.

Immature metabolic pathways predispose preterm babies to develop hypoglycemia, metabolic acidosis, and hyperbilirubinemia. Gluconeogenesis is less effective in preterms; therefore glucose administration is rapidly required to prevent significant hypoglycemia.

Preterm infants given excess oxygen may develop retinopathy of prematurity resulting in blindness because of damage to the immature retina. Main pathology of all these different problems is summarized below:

1. Respiratory problem
- Immature lungs (specially <34 weeks).
- Deficiency of surfactant (HMD).
- Immature respiratory control (Apnea)
- Pulmonary aspiration and atelectasis.

2. Temperature regulation
- Larger surface area.
- Poor insulation.
- Lack of brown fat.
- Decreased thermic response.

3. Feeding difficulty
- Lack of coordinated sucking and swallowing.
- Immaturity of gastrointestinal system.
- Frequent risk of vomiting, aspiration, stasis.

4. Hypoglycemia
- Inadequate store of glycogen.
- Gluconeogenesis is not fully developed.

5. Intraventricular hemorrhage
- Immature vascular bed around ventricles.
- Periventricular capillaries are deficient in smooth-muscle, collagen.
- Increase sensitivity of vessel rupture.

6. Hyperbilirubinemia
- Lifespan of fetal RBC is less.
- Defective uptake from plasma.

- Defective conjugation.
- Decreased excretion.

7. **Necrotizing enterocolitis**
   - Perinatal distress factors.
   - Gut immaturity.
   - Nosocomial infection.

MANAGEMENT

Delivery of Preterm

Every effort should be made to avoid the delivery of a preterm baby at home because in every premature labour, the full resources of a hospital are desirable. None the less, the preterm infant will at times have to be delivered at home. The strategies to increase salvage of the preterm babies include:

1. *Identification of mothers at risk and early referral* Mothers at risk of preterm delivery should be identified and referred to a centre with adequate facilities for newborn care. Transport of the baby in utero should be preferred to transport of the newborn preterm, because mother's womb is considered as the best incubator. The following mothers are considered to be at risk of preterm delivery:
   - Young and unmarried mother.
   - Previous history of preterm delivery.
   - Multiple pregnancies.
   - Complications during antenatal period viz—PET, PIH, Threatened abortion, APH, Cervical incompetence.
2. *Early identification and classification*: If delivery has already taken place, the survival of the preterm baby can be ensured to an extent by early identification and classification of the neonate on the basis of period of gestation and birth weight and suggestion of appropriate level care. Table 4.1 shows the

classification and suggested level of care of preterm babies:

Table 4.1

Wt (gms)	*Gestation (weeks)*	*Care*	*Incidence*
Above 2000	Above 34	Level-I	80%
2000-1500	34-32	Level-II	10-15%
Below 1500	Below 32	Level-III	3-5%

3. *Place of delivery:* Hospital delivery is always preferred. Delivery should always be conducted by trained health professionals, at least one of them should be well trained with the art of neonatal resuscitation. Baby must be provided warmth from the moment of birth. The temperature in the room, where delivery is conducted, should be maintained at 25 degree centigrade, with the help of a heat source like a room heater. The baby should be received in pre warmed cloth (at home) or a pre warmed resuscitation unit with an overhead radiant warmer. In absence of a warmer, a table lamp with 200 watt bulb can be used. This should be kept at a distance of 45 cm over the baby well wrapped from head to foot.
   When induction of preterm labour before 34 weeks is planned in a hospital, betamethasone or dexamethasone IM in a dose of 6 mg every 12 hours for four doses or 12 mg every 24 hours for 2 doses should be administered to the mother before delivery. Maternal glucocorticoid therapy lowers the incidence of HMD, bronchopulmonary dysplasia, PDA and intraventricular hemorrhage. If possible, analysis of the amniotic fluid should be done for determination of phosphatidylglycerol level and L/S ratio. Irrespective of delivery in a hospital or home, the preterms requiring hospitalization and special care include:
   i. Gestation less than 34 weeks.
   ii. Birth weight less than 1800 grams.

iii. The preterm with complication.
iv. Presence of feeding difficulties, irrespective of period of gestation.

Transportation of a Preterm Neonate

Proper care during transport of the baby is very essential since it may determine its ultimate survival. The principles of care during transport include the following:

a. Stabilisation before starting the journey.
b. Provision of warmth.
c. Nutrition.
d. Monitoring of vital signs and cardiorespiratory resuscitation during transport.

Details of neonatal transport are discussed in a separate chapter later on.

Monitoring of a Hospitalized Preterm Neonate

After admission to a special care neonatal nursery (SCNU) or a neonatal intensive care unit (NICU), monitoring of the preterm baby plays an important role in the survival of such babies. The following parameters are to be monitored:

1. *Temperature:*
   - To be checked 1 hourly for first four hours then 4 hourly.
   - Axillary temperature or human touch methods for otherwise well babies.
   - Rectal temperature to be monitored for the sick babies.
   - Nursery temperature to be maintained at 28 ± 2°C.
   - Baby's body temperature should be maintained at 36.5-37.5°C
2. *Respiration:* To be checked 1 hourly for first 6 hours then 4 hourly. Baby should be closely observed for apnea for 1 week.

3. *Blood glucose:* In babies < 35 weeks, < 1500 grams and SFD blood glucose should be monitored at 3, 6, 12, 24 and 72 hours.
4. *Neurological examination:* To look for signs of shock viz. sudden pallor, bulging fontanellae, sudden respiratory arrest.
5. Routine ultrasonography brain to be done in babies < 32 weeks, < 1500 grams on 0-2, 7-10, 21-28 days and close to 40 weeks post conceptional age.

Maintenance of Warmth and Prevention of Hypothermia

The preterm neonate should be nursed in a thermoneutral environment where oxygen consumption is minimal at rest while the body temperature remains normal. Cold stress in the baby wastes energy and oxygen in trying to maintain temperature. Hypothermia can lead to complications like hypoglycemia, bleeding diathesis, pulmonary hemorrhage, acidosis, apnoea, shock and even death in a preterm baby.

At home the baby should be kept effectively dressed in 2-3 layers of non-restrictrive and heat retaining prewarmed clothes. The low birth weight baby's scalp constitutes a fairly large part of the total surface area thus heat loss can be minimized by putting a cap or covering with cloth. In summer months, though no extra effort is required to maintain the room temperature but in winter months a room heater or a fire place may be required. Room temperature must not fall below 21°C. The baby should lie near the mother to receive maternal warmth. If a baby is maintaining normal body temperature, the trunk feels warm and soles and palm are pink and warm. In early stages of hypothermia (cold stress), the trunk is warm but soles and palms are cold to touch. This is a useful method of monitoring body temperature at home.

In the nursery, when under a servo control radiant warmer, the baby should be naked except for the napkin. In order to achieve a thermoneutral environment the nursery temperature should be maintained at 28 ± 2°C and baby's body temperature 36 -37°C. Regular monitoring of axillary/ rectal temperature (sick babies) should be carried out as soon as the baby is admitted in nursery, then hourly for 4 hours, then 4 hourly.

Prevention of Infection

Prevention of infection in the newborn should start in the antenatal period with 2 doses of tetanus toxoid to the pregnant women. This will not only prevent tetanus in the mother but also neonatal tetanus. During conducting a delivery all health professionals should follow the five clean practices viz. clean hands, clean surface, clean scissors, clean cord tie and clean cord stump. During the postnatal period the two most important measures to prevent infection are exclusive breast feeding and hand washing. Care of the umbilical cord and avoiding unnecessary interventions viz. intravenous lines, and needle pricks are also important measures to prevent infections during the neonatal period.

Feeding the Preterm

Feeding the preterm is a formidable challenge because of greatly increased demands, poor endogenous stores and immature digestive and other organ system. These babies require high protein and energy intake if they are to gain adequate weight.

The Choice of Milk

Preterm Milk

Preterm mother's milk is the feed of choice. In the preterm, human milk is better tolerated and full enteral feeding is achieved more rapidly than with formula, gastric emptying is quicker and stool frequency is greater. Preterm milk is different from term milk in composition. It has 3 times more concentration of sodium, protein and IgA and a lower water content producing a general increase in the concentration of most constituents but not of calcium and phosphorous.

Fortified Preterm Milk

Although preterm milk contains higher amounts of constituents than term milk, the levels of these nutrients remain below the recommendations for preterm. Moreover these differences persist only for around first 21 days of lactation. The addition of human milk fortifier (HMF) to human milk increases protein, vitamin and mineral contents to levels more appropriate for preterm infants. Hence fortified human milk is considered to be the most nutritionally optimal diet for preterm infants. Human milk fortifier (recently made in India as dry powder) increases the protein content and energy content of preterm milk upto 2.8 gm/100 ml and 82cal/100 ml respectively.

Preterm Formula Milks

An ideal preterm formula should contain more protein (approximately 1.8-2.5 grams/100 ml), more energy 75-90 kcal/100 ml, higher sodium, calcium and phosphorous content; and addition of iron and vitamins (viz. A, D, E and B complex). It should contain carbohydrate mixtures of 40-50% lactose and 50-60% glucose polymers to compensate for relative lactase deficiency and fat mixtures containing approximately 50% medium chain triglycerides to compensate for limited pancreatic lipase secretion and 50% long chain triglycerides to provide a source of essential fatty acids. Preterm formulae work well, growth rates are good, nutritional deficiencies are rare, and long term outcome almost matches that seen with breast milk.

Unprocessed cow's milk and goat milk are unsuitable for preterm milk in the 1st year of life. Term formula is not adequate for growth of the preterm infant. Preterm formula should be given until an infant weighs 2.0-2.5 kg.

It should be emphasized that a decision to feed a preterm baby with milk other than human milk is a major decision, especially in our country, and should not be taken lightly. The preterm infant should be evaluated for supplementary feeding in situations where lactation is inadequate inspite of all efforts. Moreover, supplementary feeding should be reserved essentially for hospitalized infants and resorted for the minimum period.

Calorie Enhanced Milk

The normal calorie density of breast milk is 20 kcal/ 30 ml. The calorie density of breast milk or a preterm formula milk can be increased by concentrating the feeds to 24 kcal/ 30 ml. MCT oil and glucose polymer have proven to be good fortifiers as they increase the caloric density without altering solute load or osmolarity and easily digested by preterm infants. Addition of 0.25 ml MCT oil per 30 ml of milk increases energy content by about 2 kcal/30 ml. An increase in energy content above 4 kcal/ 30 ml will significantly decrease the protein energy ratio, with deleterious effects. Coconut oil (0.25 ml-1ml/feed) or sugar 2-5 gms/30ml can be used as fortifiers. Coconut oil contains more than 60% MCT and is cost effective for use in our country.

Methods of Feeding

The mode of feeding should be individualized on the basis of gestational age, clinical condition and feeding tolerance. Very sick or VLBW infants may not tolerate enteral feeding for a variable period of time. Whenever possible the enteral route is preferred to parenteral nutrition because it is safer, nutritionally more complete and physiological. However, in infants weighing less than 1200 grams at birth should be started on parenteral nutrition shortly after birth.

Breast Feeding

Infants who are 34 weeks and above and have coordinated sucking and swallowing reflex and respiratory rates below 60/minute can be introduced breast feeding. If breast feeding is unsatisfactory, they can be fed combined with cup feeding.

Gavage Feeding
(Intermittent Nasogastric/Orogastric Feeding)

Nasogastric feeding tubes are better to secure; hence preferred to orogastric tube feeding. The candidates for gavage feeding include:

a. Infants less than 34 weeks gestation. Most of these babies do not have the ability to coordinate suck, swallow and breathe patterns.
b. Infants with high respiratory rates (but < 75/minute), may need gavage feeding. However, with rates > 75/minute enteral feeds should be withheld.
c. Infants above 34 weeks, well, but cannot thrive adequately on breast feeding or cup feeding may require gavage feeding in addition.

d. Infants with impaired suck/ swallow coordination due to conditions like encephalopathy, hypotonia and maxillofacial abnormalities.

Steps of Nasogastric Feeding

1. A polythene tube 5 or 6 F size is selected. The distance from the nose to the ear to the xiphoid process is marked on the tube.
2. With the infant's head placed to the side, the tube is passed through the nose. The catheter position is checked by auscultation over the stomach when air is injected. The tube is taped securely to the infant's nose and head.
3. The residual gastric aspirate is checked. The volume is recorded and the aspirate is returned. This will prevent metabolic complications resulting from continued acid and electrolyte removal.
4. The measured amount of milk is poured into a syringe attached to the tube and is allowed to drip in by gravity. The feed should never be injected under pressure.
5. During removal of the tube, it should be pinched closed to avoid dripping of milk into the pharynx and aspiration.
6. After feeding, the infant should be placed in the prone position. This facilitates stomach emptying and reduces gastric residuals.

Continuous Nasogastric Feeding

Continuous nasogastric feeding is reserved for infants who do not tolerate intermittent nasogastric feeding manifested by gastric distension or regurgitation. A number 6 F size tube is placed in the stomach and milk is delivered at a constant slow rate with an infusion pump. The following precautions are to be taken:

a. The milk delivery should be started @ 0.5 to 1 ml/hour. The feeding may be advanced by 0.5-1.0 ml per hour every 8-12 hours, until full volume is attained. The feed can also be given over a 2 hour period based on a 4 hour feeding interval.
b. The indwelling NG tube is changed every 12 to 24 hours. The extension tube from the pump to the NG tube should be changed every 8-12 hours.
c. An amount of fresh milk is to be flushed through the pump and tubing every 3-4 hours.
d. Gastric residuals are checked every 2-4 hours and taken care of as in intermittent NG feeding.

Continuous Transpyloric Feeding

Transpyloric feeding refers to nasoduodenal or nasojejunal feeding. It is indicated in infants who are intolerant to nasogastric feeding and those with GI abnormalities like microgastria. The tube is passed as in NG/orogastric tube for a distance approximately equal to the distance from the tip of infant's nose to the knee. USG guidance is helpful. The position is confirmed by a Ph reading > 5 and by the yellow colour of the aspirate. Radiological confirmation may be sometimes necessary.

The transpyloric feeding should be always continuous. The gastric residuals should be checked every 4 hours. The indwelling tube is not changed routinely. The connecting tube is changed as in continuous NG feeding. The rate and advancement is same as in continuous NG feeding.

Initiation of Feeds

The first feed in an otherwise hemodynamically stable, non-asphyxiated preterm baby, more than 32 weeks gestation and more than 1.5 kg weight, should be started as soon as possible, within 1 hour after birth. Before the first feed and as soon as after birth as possible, the gastric contents be aspirated. This procedure will exclude esophageal atresia and it seems to lessen the tendency to vomiting.

In all infants who weigh less than 1200 grams at birth should be started on parenteral nutrition shortly after birth. For infants with birth weight between 1200 grams and 1500 grams, enteral feeds are withheld for 12-24 hours. In the acutely ill infants, enteral feeds should be started only when clinically stable.

Early minimal enteral feeding (less then or equal to 10 ml/kg/day every 4, 6, 8 hours) can be given soon after birth to medically stable preterm babies even on parenteral nutrition. These feedings, known as trophic feeding are intended to prime the gastrointestinal tract prior to initiation of more substantial enteral nutrition. Trophic feeding has the following advantages:

1. Stimulates and promotes gastrointestinal hormone response.
2. Improves feeding tolerance.
3. Increases weight gain.
4. Decreases hyperbilirubinemia, osteopenia and gastrointestinal residues.

Feeding Schedule

1. An initial volume of 25 to 35 ml/kg of full strength milk (20 kcal/ 30 ml) is given over a 3 hourly (< 1.5 kg)-4 hourly (> 1.5 kg) schedule.
2. For NG feeding, the feeding volume is advanced according to the following guidelines (Table 4.2) which however, have to be individualized.

Table 4.2: Showing tube feeding guidelines

Birth weight	*Initial rate (ml/kg/day)*	*Volume increase (ml/kg/day)*
Below 1200 grams	10-20	10-20
Above 1200-1500 grams	20-30	20-30
Above 1500-2500 grams	30-40	40-50

3. The recommended volume goal is 140 to 160 ml/kg/day.Volume increases can be done more rapidly than recommended, once tolerance of 100 ml/kg/day or more is established. However it should not exceed 30 ml/kg/day in infants weighing < 1500 grams.
4. For cup feeding the increment may be done as follows:

Infant weight	Amount /feed/day
1200-1500 grams	2-10ml
1500-2000 grams	5-25 ml

   Volume may be advanced more rapidly once feedings are well established.
5. For infants with birth weight< 1500 grams, calorie density of milk is advanced from 20 to 24 kcal/ 30 ml at 100 ml/kg of volume. This volume is maintained for around 24 hours before the advancement schedule is resumed. In infants with birth weight > 1500 grams calorie density is advanced after achieving full volume feedings (140-160ml/kg/day).
6. In infants less than 1200 grams and on parenteral nutrition, once tolerance of full feedings of 24 kcal/ 30 ml is established, the density of feedings may be advanced by 2 kcal/ 30 ml per day up to a maximum of 30-32 kcal/ 30 ml.
7. The intravenous fluid and nutrients must be adjusted downward as enteral feeding increases.
   The total fluid requirements can be estimated from

fluid requirements as shown in the Table 4.3.

Table 4.3: Showing fluid requirements

Day of life	*Birth wt. > 1500 grams (ml/kg)*	*Birth weight 1000 -1500 grams (ml/kg)*	*Birth wt < 1000 grams (ml/kg)*
1	60	80	100
2	75	95	115
3	90	110	130
4	105	125	145
5	120	140	160
6	135	155	175
7 onwards	150	170	190

An extra amount of 30 ml/kg/day should be added for babies nursed under radiant warmer and additional 15 ml/kg/day for those receiving phototherapy.

Types of Fluid

Intravenous fluid administration when necessary should be given as 10% Dextrose in the initial 2 days. Thereafter N/5 saline with 1 ml Kcl/100ml fluid generally meets the electrolyte demand.

Monitoring During Feeding

1. Aspiration of first residual is important. If aspirate is more than 20ml, then intestinal obstruction should be suspected. If nasogastric tube does not go beyond 8 cm, tracheo esophageal fistula is suspected.
2. Baseline abdominal girth is noted.
3. Prefeed aspiration 2-3 hourly for intermittent gavage feeding and 4 hourly for continuous gavage feeding should be done.
4. If prefeed aspirate is more than 20% of previous feed, the amount of next feed is reduced by 20%.
5. If prefeed aspirate is more than 50% of previous feed or the abdominal girth is more than 2cm of

baseline, enteral feeding should be stopped and baby monitored on I.V. fluids till abdominal distension is relieved.

6. Stool should be examined for reducing substance daily.
7. Urine should be examined for specific gravity daily.
8. The weight should be measured once daily in infants weighing > 1500 grams and two times daily in those < 1500 grams.
9. When the baby is on cup feeding, the infant should suck on the breast before each feed. Extra fluid if necessary should be replenished with expressed breast milk from milk bank or I.V. fluid.
10. Feeding tolerance is judged by absence of abdominal distension, vomiting, and gastric residue of less than 20% of previous feed, which is nonbilious and non-hemorrhagic.

Vitamin and Mineral Supplements

- All preterm babies should receive intra-muscular Vitamin K (0.5mg) at birth.
- Vitamin A 1000 IU/day, Vitamin D 400 IU/day, Vitamin C 35 mg/day should be supplemented from 2 weeks of age.
- Iron supplementation (2mg/kg/day) should be started at 8 weeks of age (or wt. 2 kg) and continued upto 2 years age.
- A baby below 32 weeks and below 1500gms also needs to be supplemented with calcium (120mg/kg/day) and phosphorus (60 mg/kg/day) from birth upto 37 weeks of gestation.
- Vitamin E 5 IU/day is to be started after 4 weeks and to be continued upto 37 weeks of gestation.
- All babies born below 35 weeks should be given 7.5% sodibicarbonate (0.5 ml/feed) from birth upto 37 weeks to prevent late metabolic acidosis, when nursed on artificial milk.

Adequacy of Nutrition

The weight pattern of the baby is the key measure of optimal feeding. A preterm baby looses 1 to 2% of body weight every day amounting to 10 to 14% cumulative weight loss during first week of life. Birth weight is regained by 10 to 14 days. They start gaining weight by the 2nd week of life at the rate of about 10-20 gm per day.

It is desirable to weigh the baby at 2 weeks (to check regaining of birth weight), at 4 weeks (to ascertain a weight gain of at least 200-300 gms), then every month. Hospitalised babies however, should be weighed every day (> 1500 grams) and two times a day (<1500 grams) on the same weighing machine.

Problems During Feeding

1. Feeding intolerance.
2. Inadequate weight gain.

Feeding Intolerance

The signs of feeding intolerance in the newborn include poor suck, swallowing difficulties, choking, vomiting, abdominal distension, gastric stasis and reducing substances or blood in stool. Persistent or severe feeding intolerance may indicate NEC, sepsis or metabolic abnormalities.

The infant should be kept in prone position with elevation of head by about 30°C. The milk feeds should be given in frequent small volumes. If NEC or sepsis is suspected, it should be investigated and treated.

Inadequate Weight Gain

The infant may not gain weight adequately due to four causes viz. inadequate feeding, anemia, chronic cold stress and sepsis (urinary tract infection). The infant has to be evaluated and cause treated.

Early Detection of Sickness

Anticipation and early detection of complications and sickness is the cornerstone of care of preterm babies. During the neonatal period clinical monitoring of danger signs is the most important and practical method. Danger signs to be monitored include:

Lethargy	Jaundice over palms and soles
Refusal to feed	Abdominal distension
Hypothermia	Cyanosis
RDS	Pallor
Apnea	Bleeding
Abnormal weight gain pattern	Seizure

A baby who shows one or more of the above features should be immediately referred for hospitalization and prompt management.

Care in the Post Neonatal Period

It is worth mentioning that if a preterm baby can be made to survive for two weeks, the baby will survive if protected from infection. However, they are at increased risk throughout infancy, as regards morbidity and mortality. A preterm baby born below 32 weeks of gestation is also at high risk of psychomotor retardation and low school achievements. All preterm babies should be followed up in “at risk” clinics for advice on feeding, vaccination and neurodevelopmental assessment.

Feeding Advice

Exclusive breast feeding should be advised for 6 months. Complementary feeding should be started at completion of 6 months age. All preterm babies should be advised small frequent feeds and this principle should be continued throughout infancy. This is necessary because the growth rate of these babies is faster than the normal birth weight infants.

Vaccination Advice

If the baby is not sick, the vaccination schedule is the same as for term babies. A sick baby however, should receive vaccine immediately on recovery.

Neurodevelopmental Assessment

All preterm babies should undergo neurodevelopmental assessment. Mothers should be made aware of atleast four developmental milestones and their time of achievement (viz. social smile 2 months, head holding 4 months, sitting without support 8 months and standing 12 months). The mothers should be also made aware to use the corrected age for the preterm babies and report immediately to a health professional if any deviation is observed. This will help early detection of neuromotor deficiency.

Early Detection and Treatment of Common Ailments

During the post-neonatal period prompt recognition and treatment of acute diarrhoeal disorders and acute respiratory infection is important since the risk of death from these acute diseases is higher in low birth weight babies.

Care of the Preterm Baby: What Not To Do?

1. Routine administration of oxygen without monitoring.
2. Prophylactic antibiotics.
3. Prolonged use of I.V. lines.
4. Unnecessary blood transfusion.
5. Unnecessary handling.
6. Excessive light and sound in the nursery.

SUGGESTED READINGS

1. Pursley M. DeWayne and Cloherty P. John. Management of Premature Infant in Manual of Neonatal care edited by John P. Cloherty and Ann R. Stark, 4th edition 1997.
2. Ringer A Steven; Care of the extremely low birth weight infant in Manual of Neonatal care edited by John P. Cloherty, Eric C. Eichenwald and Ann R. Stark, 5th edition, 2004. Published by Lippincott Williams Wilkins, Philadelphia,USA.
3. Deirdre Ellard, Irene E. Olsen, and Yao Sun. Nutrition in Manual of Neonatal Care edited by John P. Cloherty, Eric C. Eichenwald and Ann R. Stark, 5th edition, 2004. Published by Lippincott Williams Wilkins, Philadelphia. USA.
4. Practical Paediatric Problems 6th edition, 1986. Edited by James H. Hutchison and Forrester Cockburn. Published by P G Publishing Pte Ltd, New Delhi.
5. Simon Newell. Care of the preterm infant, Special care-enteral nutrition in Forfar Arneil's Textbook of Pediatrics edited by Neil McIntosh, Peter Helms, Rosalind Smyth, 6th edition 2003. Published by Churchill Livingstone.
6. American Academy of Pediatrics, Committee on Nutrition (AAP-CON). Pediatric Nutrition handbook. Elk Grove Village III: American Academy of Pediatrics, 1998.
7. Pandit A and Bhave A. Feeding of LBW babies. Journal of Quarterly medical review July-September, 1997 published Raptakos Brett and Co. Ltd.
8. Ramji S. Nutrition in newborn infant with special reference to the LBW infant. Nutrisearch, 1999.
9. Mathur NB. Ensuring mother's own milk for her very low birth weight infant. N N F bulletin Vol 2, 1997.

5

Parenteral Nutrition

J.N. Sharma

Parenteral nutrition refers to the intravenous delivery of energy and nutrients. Parenteral nutrition is shown to be an essential component of newborn care for effective nutritional support of the preterm and critically ill infants, especially in the early post natal life.

It is realized that the supply of nutrients to the pretem infant, especially the extremely low birth weight infants (ELBW i.e. < 1000 gms weight) is rarely adequate. Studies have documented that 99% of ELBW infants were below the 10th percentile for weight after 10 weeks in the neonatal intensive care unit (NICU). It has also been demonstrated that early aggressive parenteral nutrition combine with early enteral feeding reduced growth failure without an increase incidence of adverse clinical consequences or metabolic derangements.

Improved growth outcomes, therefore will depend upon initiation of parenteral nutrition within the first 24 hours, continuing until enteral nutrition supplies atleast 75% of the total protein and energy requirements, and reinstituting parenteral nutrition quickly whenever enteral feeding is suspended.

Goal of Parenteral Nutrition

The initial goal of parenteral nutrition is to provide sufficient calories and aminoacids to prevent negative energy and nitrogen balance; thereafter promotion of appropriate weight gain and growth, while awaiting the attainment of adequate enteral intake.

Components of Parenteral Nutrition

The infusate for parenteral nutrition should contain adequate amounts of glucose and lipids for energy, synthetic aminoacid, and appropriate quantities of electrolytes, vitamins and trace minerals.

Energy

The aim of parenteral nutrition in the early post natal life is to provide sufficient energy intake in order to preserve body energy stores. A positive energy balance of 20–25 kcal/kg must be achieved to support normal rates of growth. Accordingly preterm infants with birth weight less than 1500 grams requires 90–100 kcal/kg/day and those below 1000 grams requires 105-115 kcal/kg/day. In both the groups however, the intake is started at 40-50 kcal/kg on day 0 and gradually increased so that the full calorie requirement is achieved in the growing period. Most of the parenteral calories are supplied by a balanced amount of carbohydrate and lipids.

Carbohydrate

The source of carbohydrate in the intravenous solution is dextrose (D-Glucose) which has a caloric value of 3.4 kcal/gram. The initial glucose requirement is defined as the amount that is necessary to maintain euglycemia. The preterm infants require higher rates of glucose, as they have a higher brain to body weight ratio and higher total energy needs. Initial glucose infusion rates of 4-8 mg/kg/minute is required to maintain euglycemia. Rarely infants below 1000 grams may remain hyperglycemic despite very low infusion rates. These infants require exogenous insulin beginning at 0.05 unit/kg/hour for a short period to maintain normoglycemia. The initial infusion rates of glucose may be advanced, as tolerated, @ 1-2 mg/kg /min daily to a maximum of 11 to 14 mg/kg/min. This may be accomplished by increasing dextrose concentration, by increasing infusion rate or a combination of both.

Infusion rates above 11-14 mg/kg/min is not recommended because it may exceed the infant's oxidative capacity. This in turn may cause the excess glucose to be converted to fat, particularly in the liver. This conversion may also increase oxygen consumption, energy expenditure and carbon dioxide production. Moreover, increase in the concentration to 14-17 mg/kg/min will result in a calorie intake of 45-60 kcal/kg/day which is insufficient by itself to meet the total energy needs. Intravenous lipids are necessary to supply the rest of the calories.

The quantity of dextrose that can be tolerated by a particular infant will depend on the gestational age and post natal age. The signs of glucose intolerance include hyperglycemia and secondary glycosuria with osmotic diuresis.

Glucose infusion should be started minutes after birth. The blood glucose should be maintained above 40 mg/dl and below 150-200 mg/dl. The fluid requirement in infants with birth weight below 1000 grams is usually in excess of 100 ml/kg/day. So it is usually necessary to begin with 5% dextrose to maintain glucose infusion rate of 4–8 mg/kg/hour. In infants with birth weight more than 1000 grams 10% dextrose in water is suitable starting point. To supply appropriate amounts of glucose, a glucose solution concentration of more than 12.5% is rarely required unless infants are fluid restricted.

Lipids

Intravenous lipids are made up of triglycerides, phospholipids to which glycerol is added to achieve isotonicity. Some lipid preparations contain long chain triglycerides whereas others contain medium chain triglycerides. But all available intravenous lipid products have a fatty acid profile substantially different from those present in human milk.

A 10% lipid emulsion provide 1.1 kcal/ ml and a 20% emulsion provide 2.0 kcal/ml. The 20% emulsion is preferred to the 10% emulsion because the higher ratio of phospholipids to triglycerides in the 10% emulsion interferes with plasma triglyceride clearance. 20% emulsion also provides a more concentrated source of energy.

An early initiation of lipids (on day one of life) has been now recommended on the basis of the following conclusions in different studies. Early administration of lipids do not result in acute metabolic derangements or long-term effects like increase incidence of broncho-pulmonary dysplasia or increase mortality. It has been observed that biochemical evidence of essential fatty acid deficiency may be noted in preterm infants within 72 hours of birth and this can be avoided if 0.5-1.0 gram/kg/day of intravenous lipid is provided. By providing nonprotein calories as fat and glucose rather than glucose alone, can prevent fatty acid deficiency, lower endogenous carbon dioxide production and promote protein sparing. Therefore all preterm infants should be started on lipid emulsion within the first 24-48 hours.

The initiating dose for infants < 1000 gms is 0.5-1 grams/kg body weight/day. This rate is advanced by approximately 0.5 grams/kg/day as tolerated upto a target of 3 grams/kg/day. In all infants weighing > 1000 grams at birth, lipids are initiated on 1.0 grams/kg/day and the rate is advanced by 1.0 grams/kg/day as tolerated to a target of 3.0 grams/kg/day. A continuous infusion for 24 hours is preferred as it helps optimum clearance. Blood triglyceride levels should be measured and kept below 150 mg/L.

During periods of suspected and proven sepsis, thrombocytopenia (< 50 x 10^{9}/L), acidosis (pH < 7.2) and hyperbilirubinemia warranting phototherapy, the lipid infusion should be reduced to 0.5-1.0 grams/kg/day or stopped for 24 hours until the infant is stable.

The safety of intravenous lipid in infants with hyperbilirubinemia has been questioned because fatty acids potentially can displace bilirubin from albumin binding sites. It has been shown that with a low infusion rate displacement is not significant. When the serum unconjugated bilirubin level exceeds half the projected exchange transfusion level, the lipid infusion rate should be limited to 1 gm/kg/day.

Protein

Protein losses are significant in all neonates in absence of amino acid intake and these losses are highest in the most immature neonates. The protein loss in a 26 weeks gestation infant is around 1.5 grams /kg/day which is approximately double the protein loss in term infant which is 0.7 grams /kg/day. This high rate of loss results in substantial protein deficits. If extremely preterm infants are not provided exogenous amino acids, they will catabolise over 1.5% of their body protein per day to meet their metabolic needs, when they should be actually accumulating protein at the rate of 2 % per day. There is good evidence that early amino acid intake can compensate for the high rates of protein loss and thus preserve body protein even at low calorie intake.

Crystalline amino acid solution provides the nitrogen source in parenteral nutrition.The energy density of amino acids is 4 kcal/ gram. Standard parenteral solution contains 0.5 to 2.0 grams of amino acids per deciliter.

The parenteral protein requirements in preterm infants below 1000 grams are 3.5-4.0 grams/kg/day. For preterms with birth weights above 1000 grams the requirements are 3.0-3.5 grams/kg /day.

Amino acid infusion is initiated @ 1.5 grams /kg/day immediately after birth in preterms with birth weight < 1200 and within 24-48 hours in infants with birth weight between 1200 and 1500 grams. In infants with birth weight above 1500 grams amino acid infusion is initiated only when indicated depending on the clinical condition and estimated time to achieve significant enteral volumes. The infusion rates are generally advanced by approximately 1 gram/kg/day to a target of 3.5 grams/kg/day for all infants weighing up to 1500 grams and 3.0 grams/kg/day for infants weighing more than 1500 grams at birth.

Electrolytes, Minerals, Trace Elements and Vitamins

Addition of electrolytes is not necessary in the initial 48 hours of life. This is because of the expected free water diuresis. Thereafter, 2-4 meq/kg/day of sodium is usually sufficient to maintain serum sodium in a normal range. The chloride requirement is 2-4 meq/kg/day. Potassium intakes of 2-3 meq/kg/day are usually adequate to maintain normal serum concentration. In infants weighing < 1000 grams, potassium should be started only after the kidney function has clearly established. Sodium and potassium requirements should however, be adjusted on the basis of the individual requirements. An excess of anions in the form of acetate should be provided in the parenteral solution. This can prevent hypercholeremic metabolic acidosis.

The calcium and phosphorous concentrations in the standard parenteral solutions can supply only about one third of the daily requirement putting the preterm infant at risk of metabolic bone disease. To prevent the metabolic bone complications the concentrations of calcium and phosphate should be 50-60 mg/dl and 40-45 mg/dl respectively with calcium to phosphorous ratio of 1.7: 1 for optimum bone mineralization. However, this high concentration of calcium and phosphorous increases the risk of precipitation and administration requires a central venous access. Magnesium is also a necessary nutrient. The requirement of magnesium is 0.3-0.6 mEq/dl.

The recommended parenteral intake of trace elements in preterm infants is as follows:

1. Chromium 0.2 microgram/ kg/day.
2. Copper 20 microgram /kg/day.
3. Iodide 1 microgram /kg/day.
4. Manganese 1 microgram/kg/day.
5. Molybdenum 0.25 microgram/kg/day.
6. Selenium 2 microgram /kg/day.
7. Zinc 250 microgram/kg/day.

The only trace element recommended from day one of life is zinc. The doses of zinc should be reduced to half if the infant requires total parenteral nutrition for longer than 3 months. Other trace elements are probably not needed until after the first two weeks of life. In infants with cholestasis, copper and manganese should be discontinued. Chromium and selenium should be used with caution and in smaller amounts in presence of renal failure. Parenteral iron is recommended only when preterm infants are nourished exclusively by parenteral solutions for the first two months of life.

Both fat soluble and water soluble vitamins should be supplied in parenteral solution in the recommended doses. However, preparations that are available provide higher doses of water soluble and lower doses of fat soluble vitamins even when given in the appropriate doses. The pediatric preparation of MVI, if available should be given in the dose of 1.5 ml/ 100 ml parenteral solution administered at the rate of 150 ml/kg.

Indications of Initiating Parenteral Nutrition

Parenteral nutrition is an expensive and complex way of providing nutrition. It should be preserved for those situations in which enteral feeds are not practicable. Ideally it should be practiced by experienced medical and nursing staff and where adequate biochemical, bacteriological and pharmaceutical services are available.

Parenteral nutrition may provide all the nutritional requirements of the infant (total parenteral nutrition, TPN) or may more usually be supplemented by some enteral nutrition (partial parenteral nutrition, PPN). Trophic nutrition or minimal enteral feeding should be started in all sick newborn infants except those at highest risk of NEC.

The three major indications for parenteral nutrition are:

1. Surgical lesions such as omphalocele or gastroschisis or following extensive bowel resection.
2. Necrotising enterocolitis.
3. Preterm and very preterm infants where enteral feeds cannot be fully established due to gastro intestinal immaturity. This group includes all preterm infants weighing less than 1500 grams. For those infants weighing >1000 grams, initiation is often done in conjunction with slowly advancing enteral nutrition. Infants with birth weight of 1501 - 1800 grams needs parenteral nutrition when enteral nutrition is not expected for more than 3

days and in infants more than 1800 grams when enteral nutrition is not expected for more than 5 days.

Administration

Parenteral nutrition may be administered via peripheral or central venous lines (usually the superior or inferioir venacava). Arterial lines are not suitable for parenteral nutrition. Parenteral solutions given through peripheral veins need to maintain an osmolarity between 300 and 900 mOsm/L. This often hampers adequate growth of extremely low birth weight infants. On the other hand; central veins allow for the use of hypertonic solutions but has more risk of catheter related sepsis. The indications for central vein parenteral nutritions may be warranted under the following circumstances:

1. Use of glucose solution concentration of 12.5%.
2. Parenteral nutrition needed for an extended period (> 7 days).
3. When there is an imminent lack of peripheral venous access.

Procedure for Parenteral Alimentation

1. A peripheral venous line is secured with a plastic catheter/canula (no. 22 or 24 F) or a scalp vein needle (22 or 24 G). For central alimentation, 1.9 F silastic catheters are used for infants weighing less than 1000 grams and no. 2.7 F for larger infants. The catheter can be inserted through the antecubital, saphenous, internal or external jugular or subclavian vein or less frequently, through the umbilical or femoral vein. The catheter should be threaded so that the tip lies at the junction of the right atrium and superior vena cava or inferior vena cava.

2. Dextrose and amino acids can be mixed together but lipid emulsions should be given separately. 10 or 20% lipid emulsions may be used in peripheral venous lines.
3. The infusion line should be connected with a T or Y connector. The glucose aminoacid mixture should be connected to the distal end of an infusion line with a 0.22 micron in-line air eliminating filter. The lipid emulsion is connected with the infusion line beyond the filter through the upper portion of the T or Y connector. Use of infusion pumps is best to maintain a constant rate intravenous fluid administration.
4. No medications should be given in parenteral solutions. The catheter may be flushed with saline and then the medication is infused in a compatible intravenous solution. In case of central venous alimentation, because of the increased risk of infection, medications, blood transfusion etc should be infused by a separate line and heparin should be added to the parenteral solution to heparinise the catheter.
5. All solutions should be ideally prepared under laminar flow hoods.
6. The minerals, vitamins and electrolytes should be added as and when recommended.
7. The entire infusion set including the tubing upto the intravenous needle should be changed every 72 hours. The lipid emulsion tubing should be changed every 24 hours. All parenteral solutions should be changed daily.
8. The use of parenteral solution should be accompanied by the early initiation of enteral feeds within 1-3 days of life. Parenteral nutrition should be continued until enteral feedings are well established and providing approximately 100-110 kcal/kg/day. Early termination may be necessary in case of nonavailability of venous access.

Monitoring

Both clinical and laboratory monitoring is essential for all infants on parenteral nutrition. The parameters to be monitored are as follows:

1. Weight daily once.
2. Length and head circumference weekly once.
3. Inspection of IV sites 1 hourly.
4. Urine 24 hours output, specific gravity, pH, glucose, protein and blood daily.
5. Blood urea nitrogen, creatinine, calcium, phosphorous, magnesium, total protein, albumin, transaminases (ALT, AST), bilirubin, alkaline phosphatase, weekly or every other week.
6. Hematocrit, absolute neutrophil count, C reactive protein, urine for fungal hyphae every week.
7. Blood glucose 4 hourly on the first day, then 8-12 hourly or more frequently as necessary. The glucose infusion should be monitored on the basis of blood glucose level as follows:

Blood glucose level	Action
< 120 mg/ dL	Increase dextrose infusion
120-180 mg/ d L	Maintain same percentage
> 180 mg/dL	Decrease percentage of glucose.

8. Triglycerides on day 1, after 4 hours of each increase of 1 gm/kg/day, then every other week if triglyceride level is > 150 mg/dL. Intravenous lipids are poorly tolerated by very premature infants; hence triglyceride levels must be monitored very closely in these infants. The initiation, decrease and discontinuing of lipid will depend on the serum triglyceride level as follows:

Triglyceride levels	Action
< 150 mg/dL	Increase intralipid infusion.
150-200 mg/dL	Decrease or defer intralipid infusion
> 200 mg/dL	Discontinue intralipid infusion.

9. Ammonia monitoring is indicated if ammonia level is > 150 micromol/L. The adjustment of amino acid solution infusion may be done on the basis of ammonia level as follows:

Ammonia level	Action
< 150 micromol/L	Start or increase amino acid solution infusion
150-200 micromol/L	Decrease or defer
> 200 micromol/L	Discontinue.

Complications

The wide variety of complications reported earlier is now rare with current parenteral solutions. Many of the complications relating to the electrolytes and glucose can be prevented or corrected by manipulating the constituents of the infusate. Currently the primary complications of parenteral nutrition include cholestasis and those related to the infusion catheter. Besides cholestasis, the other infusate related complications include hyperglycemia, hypoglycemia, hyperlipidemia, indirect hyperbilirubinemia, metabolic bone disease and metabolic abnormalities like azotemia, hyperammonemia and hyperchloremic metabolic acidosis. These complications have become uncommon with use of newer infusates. Many of these complications can be prevented or corrected by manipulating the constituents of the infusate.

Cholestasis

The precise cause of cholestasis is not known. At present, the risk appears to be the highest in premature infants receiving exclusive parenteral nutrition for prolonged periods. There is growing evidence that enteral feedings, even at low caloric intake, can reduce the incidence of cholestasis. Another important factor implicated is presence of sepsis.

The clinical manifestations are presence of jaundice and conjugated hyperbilirubinemia. A sensitive but nonspecific early indicator is an increase in gamma-glutamyltransferase (GGT). Elevation of AST and ALT occur later. Cholestasis often resolves spontaneously after discontinuation of parenteral nutrition and initiation of enteral feedings. Rarely irreversible liver failure has been documented. In case an infant requires parenteral nutrition in presence of cholestasis, use of small volume enteral feeding may stabilize or improve hepatic function. Amino acid infusion should be reduced to the lower end of the recommended dose. The glucose infusion should also be decreased. Lipid infusion however can be continued maintaining triglyceride concentrations of 150 mg/dl or less. At present, use of phenobarbitone or ursodeoxycholic acid in parenteral nutrition induced cholestasis is not recommended.

Indirect Hyperbilirubinemia

Indirect hyperbilirubinemia can occur as a result of displacement of bilirubin from albumin binding sites by fatty acids. Lipid infusion at rates upto 3 gm/kg/day however can be used because at this rate bilirubin displacement is unlikely. However, in presence of hyperbilirubinemia requiring exchange transfusion, rates < 3 grams/kg/day should be provided.

Hyperlipidemia

Hyperlipidemia is commonly seen at lower gestational age and at early post natal age. A short term decrease in lipid infusion rate is usually sufficient to normalize serum lipid levels.

Hyperglycemia and Hypoglycemia

Presence of hyperglycemia or hypoglycemia can be

taken care of by decrease or increase of glucose %. In case it is persistent sepsis should be excluded.

Metabolic Bone Disease

Metabolic bone disease is seen in case of prolonged exclusive parenteral nutrition. Early initiation of enteral feeding together with parenteral nutrition with higher calcium and phosphorous ratio and use of central venous access has reduced the incidence.

Azotemia, Hyperammonemia and Hyperchloremic Metabolic Acidosis

These complications have become uncommon after the introduction of use of crystalline amino acid solutions. However, they may be seen in case of amino acid intakes exceeding 4 grams/kg/day.

Sepsis

Sepsis is the major catheter related complication. The incidence of sepsis is higher in lower gestational age and increases with the duration of parenteral nutrition. Sepsis is associated with decreased lipoprotein lipase activity and impaired triglyceride clearance. The two most common bacterial agents implicated are staphylococcus epidermidis and staphylococcus aureus. An association has been reported between the use of lipids and staphylococcus coagulase negative. Fungal infection can also occur

The best way to prevent parenteral nutrition associated infection is by meticulous attention to sterile technique in catheter care and early initiation and advancement of enteral feeding. Prophylactic use of low dose vancomycin may diminish the incidence of sepsis but in view of toxic effects and the potential for antibiotic resistance, it is not recommended.

Besides use of appropriate antibiotics, during an episode of sepsis, the lipid infusion is temporarily limited to approximately 2.0 grams/kg/day if the triglyceride level is > 150 mg/dl.

The other infusion related problems include malposition of the catheter, thrombosis of peripheral lines and hemorrhage from the peripheral lines while introducing or if the line is dislodged or disconnected.

SUGGESTED READINGS

1. Lemons JA, Bauer CR, Oh W *et al*. Very low birth weight outcomes of the National Institute of Child Health and Human Development Neonatal Research Network January 1995 through December 1996. Pediatrics 107: E1, 2001.
2. Wilson DC, Cairns P, Halliday HL *et al*. Randomised controlled trial of an aggressive nutritional regimen in sick very low birth weight infants. Arch Dis Child, Fetal neonatal Ed 177: 4F-11 F, 1997.
3. David Wilson. Practical parenteral nutrition in Forfar and Arneil's Textbook of Pediatrics sixth edition 2003 edited by Neil McIntosh, Peter Helms, Rosalind Smyth. Published Churchill Livingstone.
4. Brenda B. Poindexter and Scott C. Denne. Parenteral Nutrition in Avery's Diseases of the Newborn, 8th edition, 2005 edited by Taeusch, Ballard and Gleason. Saunders. Philadelphia, Pennsylvania.
5. Deirdre Ellard, Irene E. Olsen and Yao Sun. Nutrition in Manual of Neonatal care. 5th edition, 2004. Edited by John P. Cloherty, Eric C. Eichenwald and Ann R. Stark. Published by Lippincott, Williams Wilkins. Philadelphia. USA.
6. Jean B. Crouch and Lewis P. Rubin. Nutrition in Manual of Neonatal Care 3rd edition, 1991. Edited by John P. Cloherty and Ann R. Stark. Little Brown and Company. USA.
7. A Neonatal Vade—Mecum edited by Brian Speidel, Peter Fleming, John Henderson *et al*. 3rd edition, 1998. Oxford University Press, New York.

6 Hypothermia in Newborn

J.N. Sharma

The recognition of importance of thermal control in the present day management of the newborn is essential for improving neonatal survival. A newborn infant is physiologically homeothermic; but this ability to stay warm may be easily overwhelmed by extremes of environmental temperature. Pierre Budin (1900) first drew attention to the high neonatal mortality among babies allowed to remain cold. The recognition of 'Neonatal cold injury syndrome' in 1957 once again reviewed the earlier observation that cooling is detrimental for neonatal survival. Subsequently optimum thermal conditions for neonates with varying birth weight and gestational age were identified by mid 1960's and means of keeping babies warm were devised .

Neonatal hypothermia and cold injury are now rare in developed countries. In developing countries it still continues to occur and is an important cause of neonatal morbidity and mortality.

Physiology of Temperature Regulation

Heat balance in the body is maintained by the law of conservation of energy according to which:

Heat production = Heat loss by convection + radiation + evaporation + conduction.

In the newborn infant, control of body temperature can be achieved only over a narrow range of ambient conditions although they are equipped with a thermostat in the hypothalamus. These thermoregulatory efforts are often insufficient in preterm and low birth weight babies.

Before birth, the baby is warm and well insulated in the aqueous uterine environment. Fetal temperature is slightly higher than maternal temperature with a gradient of the heat flow from the fetus to the mother. After birth, the skin and core temperatures of the body of the neonate fall by 0.3°C and 0.1°C per minute respectively. This fall is faster and greater if the temperature of the delivery room is lower than 25°C.

Heat Production

Non-shivering thermogenesis, which is a result of metabolism of brown fat, is the most important source of heat production in the newborn. The body temperature of the newborn is primarily maintained by this mechanism.

The brown fat is located at the nape of the neck, interscapular region, axillae, groin and around the kidneys and adrenals. It is laid down mostly during the third trimester of pregnancy. It accounts for 4% of the total body fat in a term baby. Brown fat contains more mitochondria; it is more vascular and better innervated.

Mechanism of Heat Production

Prerequisites for effective thermogenesis include integrity of CNS pathways, adequacy of brown fat, and availability of glucose and oxygen. When the baby is exposed to cold environment, impulses through the afferent nerves fibres reach the heat regulating centers located in the pre optic area of anterior hypothalamus near the walls of the third ventricle. Neurogenic efferents, on reaching the brown fat trigger the release of noradrenaline which mediates several important thermal responses as follows:

- Oxidation of triglycerides to glycerol and fatty acids. The fatty acids are locally consumed for the generation of heat. About 30% of non-esterified fatty acids are oxidized to generate heat and 10 % released to the circulation. The areas of brown fat become warm and heat is distributed to various parts of the body through blood stream as brown fat is highly vascular. Approximately 2.5 calories is liberated from 1 gm of brown fat and for this metabolic effort, the body needs extra oxygen and glucose.
- The heart rate rises, delivering more oxygen in order to meet the high metabolic needs of non shivering thermogenesis.
- Peripheral vasoconstriction diverts blood from skin towards the organ that drive thermogenesis.

Thus thermogenesis while warming the infant depletes endogenous substrates because of excessive metabolism. As in older children and adults, muscular activity is not a significant source of heat production in the newborn. The tiny infants cannot shiver to generate heat and are also unable to assume a flexed posture to reduce heat loss. However, during exposure to cold, the baby makes some movements of the limbs but the effort is not sustained. Minimal shivering occurs only when the environmental temperature falls below 25°C.

Mechanism of Heat Loss

After birth, the newborn can loose heat by the following four mechanisms:

- Evaporation.
- Convection.
- Radiation.
- Conduction.

Evaporation

A newborn infant wet with amniotic fluid can loose heat by evaporation as the skin dries. Evaporative heat loss is low in mature infants unless they are sweating in response to heat stress. Preterm infants have high trans-epidermal water loss due to passive diffusion of water vapour through the thin, poorly keratinised immature dermis. Hence loss is high in preterms.

Convection

Heat is lost from the skin surface to the surrounding air by convection. Loss is high if the air is cold, the skin surface is exposed and there is rapid movement of air over the skin. A naked baby in a cold draughty room has a high convective heat loss.

Radiation

Heat is lost from the skin surface to the nearest surface which faces the skin by means of radiation. It varies with the temperatures of that surface and its distance from the skin but is independent of the temperature of the intervening air.

Conduction

A newborn loses heat by conduction when in contact with cold surfaces like cloth, tray etc.

Thermoneutral Environment

It is the temperature range during which the basal metabolic rate of the baby is at a minimum, oxygen utilization is least and the newborn infant thrives well. For each newborn infant, this range of temperature varies depending on the weight and post natal age.

The Special Problems in Preterm Infant in Temperature Maintenance:

The increased susceptibility of the preterm infant to develop hypothermia is due to the presence of certain characteristics like:

- A large body surface area in relation to weight.
- A large head in proportion to the body.
- Decreased subcutaneous fat, with less insulative capacity in low birth weight infants.
- Less developed stores of brown fat in preterm infants.
- Inability to take in enough calories to provide nutrients for thermogenesis and growth in preterm babies.
- Limitation of oxygen consumption in some preterm infants with pulmonary problems.

Recording of Temperature

Low reading thermometers should be available at all health care levels. If not, ordinary mercury thermometer with initial reading less than 35°C may be used.

a. *Axillary temperature* is as good as core temperature provided the thermometer is kept for three minutes. The thermometer should be placed vertically upwards high in the axila so that the mercury bulb is covered by the axilla folds.
b. *Skin temperature* is recorded by a thermister taped to the infant skin on abdomen for continuous monitoring. The range of skin temperature is 35.5 to 36.5°C in term and 36.2 to 37.2°C in preterm babies.
c. *Rectal temperature* recording is used in sick and hypothermic babies. The thermometer should be inserted 3 cm for term and 2 cm for preterm babies. Metal thermometers are preferable to glass ones. If glass rectal thermometers are used it should be

inserted in a backward and downward direction to avoid injury.

d. *Human touch method* is the most useful method for monitoring temperature at any level. In this method, the soles and abdomen are touched with the dorsal surface of the hands to feel the temperature.

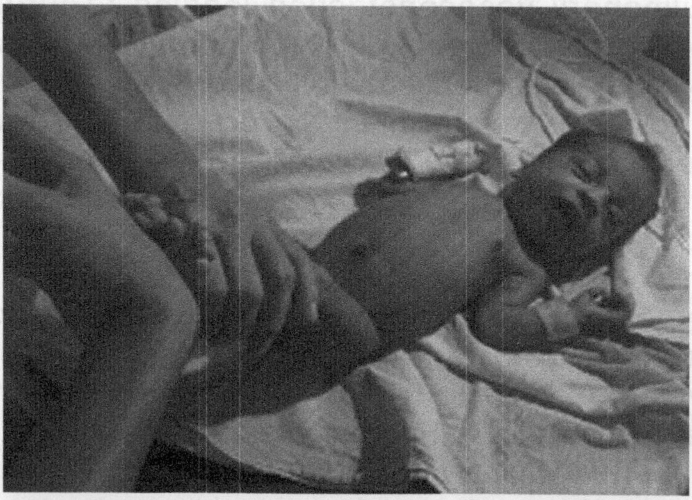

Fig. 6.1: Step 1: Touch sole with dorsum of hand

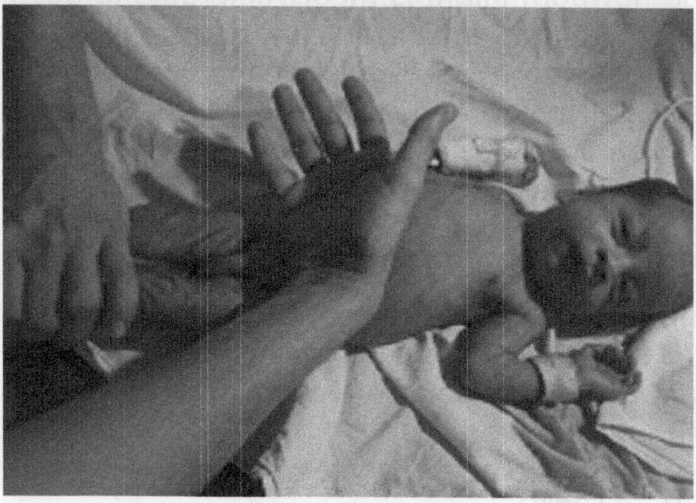

Fig. 6.2: Step 2: Touch abdomen with the dorsum of hand

Effects of Exposure to Cold

1. ***Cold stress:*** The first clinical situation on exposure to cold is called cold stress. A newborn infant, on exposure to cold environment, responds with peripheral vasoconstriction, causing anaerobic metabolism and metabolic acidosis which in turn can cause pulmonary vasoconstriction leading to further hypoxemia, anaerobic metabolism, and acidosis. Hypoxemia further compromises infant's response to cold. The preterm infant is at greater risk of developing hypothermia. However, their more common problem is calorie loss from unrecognized chronic cold stress, resulting in excess oxygen consumption and inability to gain weight.
2. ***Hypothermia:*** It is usually seen in preterm—low birth weight neonates and term infants with nervous system disorders. It is observed more in home deliveries and when inadequate measures are taken to keep the infant warm and prevent heat loss during delivery, in the post natal ward and during transport. The newborn infant is most vulnerable to develop hypothermia during the first few hours after birth but may develop hypothermia at any time during the neonatal period and beyond if exposed to a cold environment. The other risk factors include birth asphyxia, sepsis.

Disorders of Thermoregulation

The normal axillary body temperature of the newborn is 36.5°C to 37.5°C. By human touch method if the trunk feels warm and the soles are warm and pink, the baby is in thermal comfort.

Cold stress: The axillary temperature is between < 36.5°C and 36°C.

Hypothermia: The temperature is below 36°C. Hypothermia is classified into moderate and severe depending on the temperature.

Moderate hypothermia: The temperature is between < 36°C to 32°C.

Severe hypothermia: The temperature is less than 32°C.

Hyperthermia: Elevation of body temperature beyond 37.5°C (99.5°F) is called hyperthermia in the newborn.

Clinical Features

Cold stress is the early stage of hypothermia characterized by pale, cool extremities and a warm trunk. The capillary refill time is prolonged (>3 seconds). The infant fails to gain weight if there is chronic exposure to cold stress.

Continuing exposure to acute cold at this stage makes the infant hypothermic when both the trunk and extremities becomes cold to touch with symptoms and signs of central nervous system depression viz. lethargy, poor feeding, apnoea and bradycardia.

When the core temperature goes below 32°C, the infant has a bright red color. This is a result of failure of oxyhemoglobin to dissociate at low temperature. There may be central pallor or cyanosis. The skin may show edema or sclerema. There is decreased activity, a poor sucking reflex, vomiting, abdominal distension and oliguria. The signs include bradycardia, slow, shallow, irregular respiration, hypotension, and decreased response to stimulus. Hypoglycemia, metabolic acidosis, azotemia and hyperkelemia are present. Sometimes there is tachypnoea, respiratory distress and generalized bleeding, including pulmonary bleeding.

Management

Thermal protection of the newborns is very important

but not difficult. As cooling of the newborn occurs during the first few minutes after birth, it is important to act quickly to prevent heat loss.

The basic principles are same for home as well as institutional delivery. Satisfactory control demands both prevention of heat loss and promotion of heat gain. The warm chain is a set of interlinked procedures to adopt at birth and during the next few days in order to minimize heat loss in all newborns. Failure to implement any one of these procedures will break the chain and put the newborn at risk of hypothermia.

The ten steps of warm chain are as follows:

1. Warm delivery room.
2. Immediate drying.
3. Warm resuscitation.
4. Skin to skin contact between baby and mother.
5. Breast feeding.
6. Postpone bathing and weighing.
7. Appropriate clothing and bedding.
8. Mother and baby together.
9. Warm transportation.
10. Training/awareness raising of heath care providers.

1. *Warm delivery room*: The optimum temperature of the delivery room should be atleast 25°C. It should be clean and free from draught through open window, doors or fans. If the temperature of the room is less than optimal, a room heater or a fire place should be available to warm the room.
2. *Immediate drying*: After delivery, the baby should be immediately dried with a pre-warmed towel from head to feet.
3. *Warm resuscitation*: Throughout the resuscitation process warmth has to be maintained. All the resuscitation equipments including the towels for drying should be prewarmed. It is important to keep the baby warm during resuscitation because asphy-

xiated newborns cannot produce heat efficiently hence are at risk of hypothermia. The newborn infant should be resuscitated under a radiant warmer or under a 200 watt bulb in case of institutional delivery. Under the bulb the infant should be wrapped with prewarmed cloth from head to feet. In case of home delivery, the baby can be wrapped with a warm blanket with only face and upper part of the chest exposed and put on a dry warm surface.

4. *Skin to skin contact* can be achieved by adopting the Kangaroo method. It is an effective method of preventing heat loss in newborn. The mother's chest or abdomen is the ideal surface to receive the newborn as it is clean and has just the right temperature. Kangarooing helps in the following ways:
   - Assists in maintaining temperature of infant.
   - Facilitates breast feeding.
   - Helps to increase duration of breast feeding.
   - Improves infant mother bonding.
5. *Breast feeding*: An early and adequate supply of breast milk is essential to provide the newborn with calories to generate heat.
6. *Bathing* should be postponed. Postponement of bath helps in conservation of heat. A term infant should be preferably given bath on the second day. In low birth weight infants, bathing should be postponed till the baby weighs 2 kg.
7. *Appropriate bedding and clothing*: The bed should be warm and the infant should be wrapped in 4-5 layers of cloth to maintain warmth.
8. *Mother and baby together (bedding in)*: Babies born at home as well as in institution should be kept with mothers in the same bed under the same blanket 24 hours a day in a warm room. The

mother's body warmth will keep the baby warm. Mother is considered as the best incubator.

9. *Warm transportation*: Maintenance of the baby's body as well as environmental temperature during transport is the weakest link in the warm chain. The following are to be maintained during transport:
   - The body temperature of the baby should be stabilized as much as possible before transport.
   - The mother should be encouraged to accompany and the baby carried by kangaroo method.
   - If the mother is unable to accompany, the baby should be carried close to the chest of another adult.
   - The baby should be covered properly from head to feet.
   - If baby passes urine and stool, then it must be ensured that it does not remain wet.
   - Thermocol box, basket padded pouch; polythene covering can be used for ensuring temperature stability during transport.
   - The human touch method for assessing the temperature should be taught to the accompanying person and explained to ensure that baby's trunk as well as the soles and palm are warm to touch.
   - The baby should be transported to the nearest facility, by the shortest route and by using the fastest possible mode of transport.
10. *Training and awareness raising:* All health care providers involved in the process of birth and subsequent care of the newborn need to be adequately trained on the principles and procedures of the warm chain. The family and community need to be made aware of the importance of keeping

newborn infants warm and should be given information on how to do so.

Monitoring of Temperature

A low reading thermometer (recording temperature as low as 30° C) should be preferably used in the newborn.

Axillary temperature is recorded as the standard procedure, because of safety, hygiene and ease. It is as good as the core temperature recorded by rectal temperature in newborn

Rectal temperature is measured only in sick, hypothermic newborn. It is the best guide for core temperature in these infants. In a sick and hypothermic infant, heat production in the body is a result of nonshivering thermogenesis as a result of metabolism of brown fat. Axilla contains a good amount of brown fat. Hence may give false high temperature in hypothermic babies.

At home the newborn temperature can be assessed by human touch method and assessed as follows:

- Cold feet and warm trunk indicates cold stress.
- Both soles and trunk cold indicates hypothermia.
- If soles and trunk are both hot and red, the face is flushed and the baby is restless, the baby could be overheated.

Who Needs Temperature Monitoring?

1. Low birth weight and sick newborn.
2. When there is suspicion that the baby is becoming hypothermic or hyperthermic.
3. When a hypothermic baby is rewarmed or a hyperthermic baby is being cooled down.
4. If a baby needed resuscitation at birth.
5. If it is difficult to maintain the warm chain and provide optimal thermal environment.

Frequency of Monitoring

In healthy newborns, routine temperature monitoring is not necessary. However, to make sure that warm chain is maintained and to identify possible weak links the temperature measurement can be done in early morning hours, when the environmental temperature is its lowest and in the hottest part of the day.

In sick newborns or low birth weight babies the temperature should be initially measured hourly in the first four hours and then 4 hourly or more often if the baby is under the radiant warmer.

During warming of a hypothermic baby, the temperature should be monitored every 15 minutes till the baby is normothermic. If the temperature does not rise within one hour of warming, sepsis has to be suspected, because hypothermia is also a sign of sepsis.

Management Principles

1. Hypothermia should be confirmed by recording actual body temperature.
2. The baby should be rewarmed as soon as possible.
3. The method of warming will depend on the severity of hypothermia, availability of staff and equipment.
4. The methods of warming in use are as follows:
   - Skin to skin contact (Kangarooing), hot packs
   - Overhead lamps and hot water bags.
   - Radiant warmers and incubators.
5. Breast feeding should be continued.

Kangaroo Method

It is a simple method of keeping the baby warm. The naked baby with head covered is to be kept in maximum skin to skin contact with the mother and both covered with blankets or adequate clothing. Low birth weight babies who are stable at birth benefit most by this method.

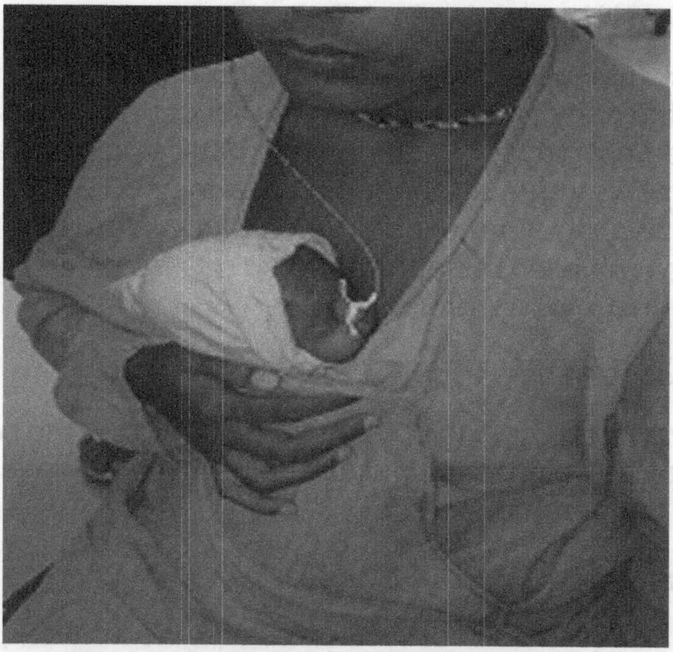

Fig. 6.3: Showing Kangaroo method

Procedure: The baby should put on a cap, mittens and socks. The bare chest should be placed in contact with the bare chest of the mother and wrapped with the same cloth with the mother.

Overhead Lamps and Hot Water Bags

Lamps with a conical shade and a bulb of 200 watts can be used in case a radiant warmer is not available. The lamp should be placed 45 centimeters above the baby. The baby should be well wrapped with clothes from head to feet. It can minimize heat loss from the baby to the environment.

Hot water bags are not safe for use in neonates. If used, sufficient paddings should be used between the baby and the bottles to prevent burns. The other disadvantage is that hot water needs frequent changes.

Radiant Warmers and Incubators

In sick neonates who need continuous observation, placing the baby under a radiant warmer or in an incubator is the best way for keeping such babies warm. Servo control warmers are best because they do not cause over heating. One should be careful while using non servo controlled radiant warmers because of the risk of hyperthermia with prolonged use.

Breast Feeding

It is very important to continue breast feeding the baby to provide calories and fluid. It helps in maintenance of body temperature.

Management of Cold Stress

Cold stress in newborn indicates that the infant needs warming. If not intervened, the infant at any moment may become hypothermic. The steps of management include the measures to prevent heat loss viz.:

1. Cold clothes should be removed, and the baby covered with pre warmed clothes in several layers from head to feet.
2. Heat loss should be reduced from the baby to the environment. This can be achieved by changing the cold bed clothes and replacing with pre warmed clothes. The room should be warmed with the help of a room heater or a smokeless fire place.
3. The baby should be bedded in with the mother in skin to skin contact, under cover of the same blanket.
4. Frequent breast feeding.

Management of Moderate Hypothermia

Moderate hypothermia is an alarming situation. If not taken care of may progress to severe hypothermia. The steps of management include:

1. Measures to prevent heat loss as in case of cold stress.
2. The baby should be provided extra heat till temperature becomes normal. The warming can be done by keeping the baby under a heat source viz. a radiant warmer or a 200 watt bulb. If these are not available, extra heat can be provided with warm packs.
3. Temperature and sucking reflex should be monitored every 15 minutes. If there is no response and hypothermia persist beyond 1 hour after taking adequate measures, sepsis has to be suspected and antibiotics started after sending blood samples for sepsis screen and blood culture.

Management of Severe Hypothermia

Severe hypothermia is a grave situation and should be treated as a medical emergency. The steps of management include:

1. Measures to reduce heat loss as above.
2. The baby should be kept under a radiant warmer. The abdominal skin temperature should be set at 1°C higher than the core temperature for rapid warming. Rapid warming should be done till the temperature reaches 34°C. After that warming should be slowed down but continued till the temperature is normal. For slow warming, the abdominal skin temperature should be set at 36.5°C.
3. Monitoring:
   - Temperature should be monitored every 15-30 minutes.
   - Sucking reflex every 15 to 30 minutes.
   - Blood pressure/Capillary refill time and heart rate.
   - Blood glucose.
4. Additional measures:
   - Vitamin K should be given 1 mg for term and 0.5 mg for preterm babies, intra muscular.

- 10% dextrose 2 ml/kg/dose stat.
- If CRT is > 3 seconds, a bolus dose of 10 ml/kg/ dose of normal saline should be given.
- Oxygen administration.
- Antibiotics should be started to cover both gram positive and gram negative organism if there is slightest suspicion of sepsis after sending blood samples for sepsis screen and culture.

SUGGESTED READINGS

1. Baumgart Stephen. Thermal regulation in the fetus and newborn in Intensive care of fetus and neonate edited by Alan R. Siptzer, 5th edition, 2000. Mosby Publication. St Louis, USA.
2. Rutter N. Thermoregulation in Forfar and Arneil's text book of Pediatrics, edited by Neil McIntosh, Peter J Helius, Rosalind L Smyth, 5th edition, 1998. Churchil Livingstone.
3. Deorari AK. Hypothermia in newborn. NNF teaching aids in newborn care.
4. Resource book for training of PHC Medical officers. Published by WHO collaborating centre for training and research in newborn care. All India Institute of Medical Sciences, New Delhi.
5. Carol A. Miller and Thomas B. Newman. Hypothermia and hyperthermia in Avery's diseases of the newborn, 8th edition, 2005. Edited by Taeusch, Ballard and Gleason. Published by Elsevier, New Delhi.

7 Neonatal Sepsis

A. Saili and S. Nangia

Neonatal sepsis refers to systemic infection of the newborn, often bacterial in origin, which is an important cause of morbidity and mortality in the neonatal period. A high index of suspicion, early and efficient diagnosis and appropriate antibiotic therapy with aggressive supportive care will go a long way in decreasing the morbidity and mortality due to sepsis.

Definition

Neonatal sepsis is a clinical syndrome of bacteremia with systemic signs and symptoms of infection. The national neonatology forum defines neonatal sepsis as follows:

Proven sepsis: Where the baby present with a clinical picture of sepsis with isolation of pathogen from blood, CSF, urine or other body fluids or autopsy evidence of sepsis.

Probable sepsis: Where the newborn present with clinical picture suggestive of sepsis with one or more of the following criteria:

a. Existence of predisposing factors viz. maternal fever or foul smelling liquor or prolonged rupture of membrane (> 12 hours) or gastric polymorph count of more than 6 per high power field.
b. A positive sepsis screen.

Classification of Neonatal Sepsis

Sepsis in newborn is classified into types:

1. Early onset sepsis.
2. Late onset sepsis.

Early onset sepsis: Early onset sepsis usually presents within the first 72 hours of life. Source of infection is maternal genital tract. Clinically neonate usually presents with respiratory distress and pneumonia.

***Late onset sepsis*:** Late onset sepsis usually presents after 72 hours of age. Source of infection is either nosocomial or community acquired. Neonates present with septicemia, pneumonia or meningitis.

Risk Factors for Neonatal Sepsis

The high risk factors associated with early onset sepsis include the following:

- Low birth weight (<2500 gms) or preterm baby.
- Febrile illness in the mother within 2 weeks prior to delivery.
- Foul smelling or Meconium stained liquor amni.
- Prolonged rupture of membranes > 18 hours
- More than 3 vaginal examinations during labour.
- Prolonged and difficult delivery with instrumentation.
- Perinatal asphyxia (Apgar score <4 at 1 minute of age) or difficult resuscitation.

Factors predisposing to nosocomially acquired late onset sepsis:

- NICU admission.
- LBW, prematurity.
- Invasive procedures.
- Parenteral fluid therapy.
- On ventilator.

Factors predisposing to community acquired late onset sepsis:

- Poor hygiene.
- Poor cord care.
- Bottle feeding.
- Pre-lacteal feeds.

Clinical Features

A neonate with sepsis may be asymptomatic or may have non-specific symptoms and signs. The manifestations depend on whether it is early onset or late onset sepsis. Early onset sepsis is usually fulminant whereas late onset is more insidious. The important differences between the two are depicted in Table 7.1.

Table 7.1: Difference between early and late onset sepsis

Features	*Early onset*	*Late onset*
1. Time of onset	<72 hours	>72 hours
2. Complications of pregnancy, delivery	Present	May or may not be present
3. Source of organisms	Mother's genital tract	Nosocomial/Community acquired
4. Usual clinical presentation	Fulminant multisystem	Slowly progressive
5. Mortality	30-50%	15-30%
6. Meningitis	Rare	Common
7. Organisms	E.Coli, Klebsiella, Listeria	Staph. aureus, Coagulase negative staphylococcus

The most common symptoms are lethargy, poor feeding, feed intolerance, regurgitation, abdominal distension, temperature instability (hypo or hyperthermia), hypotonia, depressed neonatal reflexes, seizures, respiratory distress, apnea, cyanotic spells, petechiae, poor perfusion, shock, jaundice or just the sick look of the baby.

Laboratory Diagnosis

The diagnostic work-up for sepsis in all neonates with non-specific clinical manifestations is unnecessary. A complete history, presence of risk factors, physical examination and clinical experience are the best guides in determinating the extent of work-up.

Isolation of microorganisms from blood or central body fluid is the gold standard and most specific method to confirm the diagnosis of neonatal sepsis. The problems with definitive test is that the results are available only after 48-72 hours which means therapy will be delayed by this much duration and most neonates pending initiation of therapy would either die (septicemic) or will be normal (high risk but not infected). Moreover in a substantial number of blood cultures (40%) no bacteria are isolated despite strong clinical suspicion of sepsis.

Non-specific diagnostic septic screening test: The difficulties in accurate diagnosis of neonatal sepsis have prompted investigators to evaluate certain bedside or side-laboratory tests which will indicate infection without identifying the infecting organisms. Such babies can be treated with the first line antibiotics as per unit's antibiotic policy for sepsis. This is essentially based on the profile of organisms isolated in blood cultures in the previous 3-6 months and their sensitivity pattern.

The non-specific tests must be very sensitive so as to pick all cases of sepsis (no case is missed) but at the same time they should be highly specific (so that no case is treated unnecessarily when there is no infection). With a very high negative predictive value no single test can achieve both these accuracy. A practical sepsis screen is given in a tabular form below:

Components	Abnormal values
Total leukocyte count	< 5000/cmm or > 20,000/cumm
Absolute Neutrophil count	< 1800/cmm
Immature /Total Neutrophil	> 0.2
Micro-ESR	> 15 mm AEFH
CRP	> 6 mg /dl

If two parameters are abnormal, it should be considered as a positive sepsis screen.

Other Investigations

1. *Lumbar puncture:* In early onset sepsis a lumbar puncture (LP) is indicated in presence of positive blood culture and in presence of clinical feature of septicemia. In late onset sepsis LP is indicated in all infants with signs and symptoms of sepsis prior to starting antibiotics. CSF characteristics are unique in the newborn period and normal CSF values in neonates are given below:

CSF components	*Normal values*	
	Term	*Preterm*
Cells/ cumm (WBC)	8.2 (0-32)	9 (0-29)
PMN	61.3%	57.2 %
Protein (mg %)	90 (20-170)	115 (65-150)
Glucose (mg %)	52 (34-119)	50 (24-63)
CSF/ blood glucose (%)	81 (44-248)	74 (55-105)

Source: J. Pediatr. 88: 473, 1976

2. *Chest X-ray:* Indicated in presence of respiratory distress or apnea.
3. *Abdominal X-ray:* Indicated in presence of abdominal signs (vomiting, feed intolerance, and abdominal distension) and/or suspicion of NEC.
4. *Ultrasonography Head and CT Scan (Brain):* It should be done in all patients diagnosed to have meningitis.

Management

I. *Supportive therapy*

In addition to anti-microbial therapy, supportive and symptomatic care is of paramount importance to ensure intact survival. This includes temperature regulation, careful fluid and electrolyte therapy, maintenance of normoglycemia, normal pH and normo oxemia.

- It is important to maintain thermoneutral environment and avoid hypo/hyperthermia.
- Intravenous line should be established.
- Neonate should be first stabilized by infusion of 10% dextrose 2ml/kg stat. CRT checked. If CRT >3 secs—Normal saline should be infused 10ml/kg over 5-10 minutes. Same dose can be repeated 1-2 times over the next 30-45 minutes, if perfusion continues to be poor.
- Vit-K 1 mg intramuscularly should be given.
- Oxygen saturation should be maintained.
- Enteral feed is avoided till baby is hemodynamically stable.
- Anemia and bleeding diathesis is managed by packed cells and fresh frozen plasma.
- Seizures should be treated promptly and effectively.
- Vitals to be monitored every 2 hourly initially.

II. *Antimicrobial therapy*

A symptomatic neonate with suspected or probable sepsis should be immediately started on antibiotics based on unit's policy or Ampicillin and gentamycin after sending the sepsis screen and blood culture. A CSF culture (when signs of CNS involvement are present) and a chest X-ray are done when indicated. If the mother has received some pre treatment for infection, the baby should be given full treatment for the existing condition viz. pneumonia, septicemia or meningitis. If the mother did not have pretreatment and the sepsis and blood culture are negative, the antibiotics can be stopped after 72 hours. If the tests are positive, the baby should be given full treatment.

If an asymptomatic neonate has a low risk of sepsis (presence of 1-2 risk factors), then the baby should be observed for 48 hours and a sepsis screen performed. If negative, the baby is not treated but if the screen is positive or the baby becomes symptomatic, then antibiotics are started. If an asymptomatic neonate has high risk of sepsis (> 3 risk factors) then a sepsis screen is done and a blood culture is taken and antibiotics are started. If the screen and culture are negative, the antibiotics are stopped after 72 hours. If the tests are positive, therapy is continued for the duration determined by the clinical state.

Indications for starting antibiotics in early onset sepsis may be summarized as follows:

1. Presence of 3 risk factors for early onset sepsis.
2. Presence of foul smelling liquor.
3. Presence of 2 antenatal risk factors with a positive sepsis screen.
4. Strong clinical suspicion.

Choice of antibiotics is based on unit's policy or empirically ampicillin with gentamycin can be started. If meningitis is suspected chloramphenicol or cefotaxime should be added. Antibiotics once started empirically should be modified according to culture and sensitivity reports.

The indications of starting antibiotics in late onset sepsis are as follows:

- Positive sepsis screen.
- Strong clinical suspicion.

However, when antibiotics are started only on strong clinical suspicion, it is important to send sepsis screen prior to starting antibiotics. If sepsis screen comes to be negative, but suspicion is too strong, then after 12 hours a repeat sepsis screen is usually done; if that comes to be negative, antibiotics can be either stopped at this point or can be continued for 5-7 days in case of strong clinical suspicion. Duration of antibiotic therapy is given in the table below:

Diagnosis	*Duration*
1. Meningitis	21 days
2. Blood culture +ve (no meningitis)	14 days
3. Culture -ve but definite clinical sepsis	10-14 days
4. Culture -ve, clinically probable sepsis, sepsis screen +ve	7-10 days
5. Culture -ve, clinically probable sepsis, sepsis screen -ve	5-7 days

Newer Modalities in the Treatment of Neonatal Sepsis

A neonate is an immuno-compromised host with numerous defects in cellular and humoral immunity. The newer approach mainly focuses on boosting the immunity or on strategies to counter the effects of systemic organ failure caused by septic shock. Some of these newer modalities are intravenous immunoglobulin (IVIG), white blood cell transfusion, growth factors infusion like G-CSF and GM-CSF, exchange transfusion, plasma exchange, endo/exotoxin blockade and inflammatory mediator cascade blockade to minimize tissue damage.

IVIG: IVIG has been used both for prophylaxis and treatment of neonatal sepsis with no constant benefit hence IVIG is not currently recommended for prevention or treatment of neonatal sepsis. This may however be used in a sick preterm with overwhelming sepsis or in a preterm with low IgG levels and recurrent infections. The dose is 500-1000 mg/kg/dose repeated two weekly till improvement.

WBC transfusion: This modality is still considered experimental (even though granulocyte transfusion isolated by continuous flow centrifugation method does decrease mortality in septic and neutropenic neonates) because of a high cost, highly sophisticated set up to isolate granulocytes, risk of transmitting viral infection, risk of graft versus host disease and its effectiveness only if used very early in the course of the disease. Buffy coat isolated granulocyte transfusions have not been found to be effective.

G-CSF and GM-CSF: Experimental animal studies and some human trials have shown promising results but larger multicentric placebo controlled randomized trials are needed before this can be adjunct to antimicrobial therapy.

Exchange transfusion: Though exchange transfusion has been reported to decrease mortality in neonatal sepsis, its effectiveness has not been properly evaluated. It improves oxygen carrying capacity, perfusion, removes toxins and bacteria and provides opsonins but has the potential to introduce transmissible viral infections and graft vs host disease. On line plasma exchange filtration is still in the experimental stage.

Immunomodulatory techniques to treat septic shock: These are monoclonal antibodies to TNF-L and interleukin-I, pentoxiphyllin a phosphodiesterase inhibitor which decrease TNF-L production and nitric oxide. The role of prostaglandins and ketokonazole is being evaluated for this purpose.

Prevention

Prevention of neonatal sepsis requires a multiprolonged

effort. All types of infection in pregnant mothers should be diagnosed early and treated vigorously. Strict asepsis and clean practices should be followed in the labour room and operation theatres. The nursery environment should be clean and strict hand washing should be ensured by all the personnel. Disinfectants like 2% glutaraldehyde (cidex) can be used for cleaning walls, floors and trolleys. An abundant supply of disposable should be ensured. All these will go a long way in preventing sepsis in the neonate.

SUGGESTED READINGS

1. Baley J, Fanaroff A. Neonatal infections II. Specific infectious diseases and therapies in Effective care of newborn babies' editor Sinclair J. Bracken M. Oxford University Press, 1992.
2. Ainbender E, Cabatu EE, Guzman DM *et al*. Serum C reactive protein and problems of newborn infants. J. Pediatr 1982;10:438.
3. Adler SM, Denton RL. The erythrocyte sedimentation rate in newborn period. J. Pediatr, 1975; 86:942.
4. Weishman L , Cruess D, Fischer G. Standard versus hyper immune intravenous immunoglobulin preventing or treating neonatal bacterial infections. Clin. Perinatol. 1993;20:211-24.
5. Perez M Ednardo, Weisman LE. Novel approach to the prevention and therapy on neonatal bacterial sepsis. Clin Perinatol. 1997;24:213.
6. Gillian E, Christensen R, Suen Y *et al*. A randomized placebo controlled trial of recombinant human granulocyte colony stimulating factor administration in newborn infants with presumed sepsis. Significant induction of peripheral and bone marrow neutrophilia. Blood 1994;84:1427.
7. Cairo M, Christensen R, Sender L *et al*. Results of phase I/II trial of recombinant human granulocyte macrophage colony stimulating factor in very low birth weight neonates. Significant induction of circulatory neutrophils. Blood, 1995;86:2509.

8 Respiratory Distress in the Newborn—Approach to Diagnosis

D.K. Patgiri

Respiratory distress, the most common neonatal emergency in the delivery room and nursery, is a symptom complex secondary to many etiological factors. The most striking difference between the foetal and neonatal respiration is that in fetus the gas exchange is entirely dependent on maternal mechanism controlling the placental circulation. The fetal lung is a fluid filled organ, receive 10-15% of cardiac output, and ventilatory movements of the fetus bear no relationship to gas exchange and correlate minimally with fetal PaO_2 and $PaCO_2$ levels.

In almost all infants, even in immature fetus (26-28 weeks gestation) rhythmic respiratory movements begin immediately, provided the birth process has not resulted in severe hypoxia.

Respiratory problems are the most common cause of neonatal illness and death, and accounts for a major proportion of admission to the nurseries.

Common Causes of Respiratory Distress in Preterm Babies

1. Hyaline membrane disease.
2. Pneumonia.
3. Asphyxia.
4. Transient tachypnoea of newborn.

Table 8.1: Causes of respiratory distress in newborn

Pulmonary

A. Commonly occurring:
   Hyaline membrane disease
   Transient tachypnoea of newborn
   Meconium aspiration
   Primary pulmonary hypertension
   Pneumonia specially Gram –ve or Group B streptococcus.

B. Less common:
   Pulmonary hemorrhage
   Pulmonary air leak
   Chronic lung disease–
   Wilson Mikity syndrome
   Bronchopulmonary dysplasia.

C. Congenital malformations:
   Airway obstruction, e.g. Choanal atresia
   Lung cyst
   Diaphragmatic hernia
   Tracheo-esophageal atresia
   Hypoplasia of lung
   Congenital lobar emphysema.

Extra-pulmonary

A. Heart:
   Congenital heart disease
   Patent ductus arteiosus.

B. Metabolic:
   Metabolic acidosis
   Hypothermia
   Hypoglycemia.

C. Brain:
   Hemorrhage
   Cerebral edema
   Asphyxia
   Drugs
   Trauma.

D. Blood:
   Acute blood loss
   Hypovolemia
   Twin to twin transfusion.

E. Chest wall disorders:
   Myasthenia gravis
   Thoracic dystrophy.

Common Causes of Respiratory Distress in Term Babies

Onset within 24 hours:
- Meconium aspiration syndrome.
- Pneumonia.
- Transient tachypnoea of newborn.
- Congenital malformation e.g. diaphragmatic hernia.
- Asphyxia.
- Pulmonary hypertension (PPHN).

Onset at the end of the first- week or later:
- Pneumonia.
- Aspiration.
- Cardiac disease.

Onset at any time:
- Acidosis.
- Pneumothorax.

Diagnostic Approach

An approach to respiratory distress in the newborn essentially includes the following:
1. Is this respiratory distress and not periodic breathing?
2. The gestation of the baby—whether preterm or term?
3. Is there any associated congenital anomaly?
4. What is the age of onset of the distress?
5. Is the respiratory distress due to pulmonary or non-pulmonary cause?
6. Can it be a surgical cause of respiratory distress?
7. Is this one of the commonly occurring causes or a rare cause requiring special intervention?

   The cardinal signs of respiratory distress are:
   - Tachypnoea (RR> 60 / min).
   - Intercoastal, subcostal retractions.
   - Grunting.
   - Central cyanosis.

The clinical diagnosis of respiratory distress is suspected in the presence of two or more of the above signs.

A. *Initial Evaluation:* The importance of history and physical examination must be emphasized to arrive at an early diagnosis of respiratory distress in newborn.

History: Points to be noted.

1. *Antenatal:* Gestational age, prematurity, IUGR, Maternal disease like—Diabetes, APH, PROM, Multiple pregnancy, Addiction, Analgesic, Anaesthesia, Use of steroid, Previous history of RDS, History of Meconium stained liquor, choking, and aspiration during a feed.
2. *Intranatal:* Nature of delivery, fetal distress, use of analgesic and anaesthesia to the mother, instrumental delivery, details of resuscitation, apgar score, any other difficulty during the process.
3. *Physical examination:*
   a. Monitoring of the vital signs: Temperature, colour, respiration, heart rate, blood pressure, activity.
   b. Quick assessment of gestational age.
   c. Assess the clinical severity of respiratory distress (by Downe's or RDS score) as follows:

Table 8.2

Score	*0*	*1*	*2*
Respiration (rate/min)	< 60	60 -80	>80
Cyanosis	None in room air	No cyanosis in 40% FiO_2	Requiring more than 40% FiO_2
Retraction	None	Mild	Moderate to severe
Grunting	None	Minimal	Obvious
Air-entry	Good	Decreased	Barely audible

Score:>4 =Clinical respiratory distress, arterial blood gases to be monitored.

>8 =Impending respiratory failure.

d. To look for other signs like meconium staining of skin, nails or cord, presence of acidosis, capillary refill time (normal<3 secs), hepatomegaly, neurological status.

e. Few important clues can be gathered from chest auscultation:

   i. Diminished intensity of breath sounds: Alveolar and lobar atelectes in pulmonary hypoplasia, pneumothorax, pneumonia.

   ii. Prolonged expiratory phase of breathing: Brochopulmonary dysplasia.

   iii. Cardiac sounds muffled or shifted to opposite side: Pneumothorax or diaphragmatic hernia.

f. Note the age of onset of respiratory distress (the importance of this from etiological point of view is discussed earlier.

B. *Laboratory Investigations:* History and physical findings should guide the need of selecting the laboratory investigations in a particular patient. Depending upon the diagnostic possibilities following investigations may be undertaken:

Table 8.3

Investigations	*Evaluation of*
a. Radiological studies: X-ray chest PA view, lateral view, lateral view of neck and contrast studies	Respiratory and cardiac abnormalities, any congenital lesion of upper and lower respiratory tract
b. Complete blood count (CBC)	Anemia, Polycythemia, or infection
c. Blood glucose	Hypoglycemia
d. Sepsis screen	
e. Gastric aspirate for polymorph count	Septicemia
f. Blood culture	Sepsis
g. Shake test	HMD
Other investigations which are considered helpful are:	
a. CNS ultrasonography	Intracranial hemorrhage, or edema
b. ECG and Echo	Congenital heart disease
c. Arterial blood gas (ABG)	Oxygen and acid base status

Table 8.4: Differential diagnosis of respiratory distress (Common)

Nature	*RDS*	*PHY*	*GBS*	*TTN*	*MAS*
Gestation	Usually preterm	Often preterm	Preterm of term	More of term	Usually postterm
Perinatal history	APH, IDM, rhesus, immature LS ratio	Asphyxia aspirin in pregnancy	Uterine inertia, Asphyxia, PROM	IDM, C/S asphyxia	Asphyxia IUGR
Clinical features	Grunting prominent, gradual deterioration	Cyanosis prominent, sudden deterioration	Shock prominent, early apnea pulmonary hemorrhage	RR > 60, mild distress	Meconium staining, over inflated chest, progressive
Effect of Oxygen	Improvement	Cyanosis unchanged	May improve	Improvement mild	May improve
Blood gases	Hypoxemia, raised PCO_2, mixed acidosis	Marked hypoxemia, Low or normal PCO_2 metabolic acidosis, radial/ aorta difference	Hypoxemia, metabolic or mixed acidosis	Hypoxemia, low or normal PCO_2 mild metabolic acidosis	Hypoxemia metabolic acidosis
Chest X-ray	Under inflation, reticulo granular Mottling	Over inflation, clear lung field, cardiomegaly	Coarse infiltrates, collapse mimic RDS	Over inflation, streaking pulmonary edema, cardiomegaly	Coarse infiltrates over inflation +/-, pneumothorax
Treatment	CPAP helpful, IPPV	CPAP unhelpful, mechanical ventilation or tolatolazoline	Penicillin, blood transfusion, +/– mechanical ventilation	Oxygen, IPPV rarely	Airway suction at birth may need IPPV
Outcome (mortality)	5%	20%	40%	0%	30%

Abbreviations used: RDS—respiratory distress syndrome, PHY-pulmonary hypertension, GBS—group B streptococcal pneumonia, TTN—transient tachypnea of newborn, MAS—meconium aspiration syndrome, APH—partum haemorrhage, IDM—infant of diabetic mother, PROM—premature rupture of membrane, C/S—cesarean section, IUGR—intra uterine growth retardation, L/S—lecithin/sphingomyelin, RR—respiratory rate.

CONCLUSION

The problem of respiratory distress in newborn is a challenging one, as it accounts for significant morbidity and mortality. 4%-6% of neonates may suffer from mild to severe degree of respiratory distress many of which are preventable. Early recognition and referral are important since the management is usually complicated and needs level II or III care.

SUGGESTED READINGS

1. Ramji S. Respiratory distress in the newborn. NNF bulletin, 13(4);1999.
2. Dynio Honrubia and Ann R. Stark. Respiratory distress syndrome in Mannual of neonatal care 5th. Edition, 2004. Edited by John P Cloherty, Eric C. Eichenwald and Ann R. Stark. Published by Lippincott Williams Wilkins, Philadelphia, USA.
3. Singh M Respiratory distress in the newborn babies in Care of the newborn 5th. Edition 1999. Published by Sagar Publication, New Delhi.
4. Respiratory distress in newborn babies, in medical emergencies in children 1st. edition by Meherban Singh.
5. Respiratory tract disorders in Fetus and newborn in Nelsons Textbook of Pediatrics 16th. edition, SAUNDERS.

9 Prevention and Treatment of Respiratory Distress in Newborn

J.N. Sharma

Respiratory distress constitutes the largest classification of causes of morbidity and mortality in the neonatal period. This is mainly due to the minimal respiratory reserve and transition from intrauterine to extrauterine life. Neonatal respiratory problems may lead to chronic respiratory problems in infancy and first few years of life.

Common Causes of Respiratory Distress

The common causes according to the onset of respiratory distress are as follows:

Table 9.1: Showing causes of respiratory distress on the basis of onset of distress

Onset of respiratory distress	*Causes*
At birth	Transient tachypnoea of newborn, Meconium aspiration syndrome Birth asphyxia Choanal atresia Congenital diaphragmatic hernia Pulmonary hypoplasia.
1-6 hours	Hyaline membrane disease Tracheo esophageal fistula

Contd.

Contd.

1st day	Congenital pneumonia Polycythemia
1st week	Persistent pulmonary hypertension Pulmonary hemorrhage Pneumonia Congenital heart disease Wilson Mikity syndrome
2-3 weeks	Patent ductus arteriosus Chronic lung disease
Variable presentation	Inborn errors of metabolism

Anticipation of Respiratory Distress

A careful antenatal clinical and ultrasonography assessment can help to anticipate respiratory distress in the newborn infant. Anticipation will help in utero referral to an appropriate facility for the care of the newborn.

Table 9.2: Showing history and likely cause of respiratory distress

History	*Likely cause*
Preterm, maternal diabetes, antepartum hemorrhage	Hyaline membrane disease
PROM, maternal infection	Pneumonia
Asphyxia, MSAF	Meconium aspiration syndrome
Hydramnios	Tracheo esophageal fistula
Oligohydramnios	Pulmonary hypoplasia
Traumatic delivery	Intracranial hemorrhage
Delayed cord clamping	Polycythemia
Drugs	CNS depression

Confirmation of Origin of Respiratory Distress

The first and foremost in the management of respiratory distress is to confirm whether the respiratory distress is of pulmonary, cardiac or central nervous system origin. This is possible from clinical parameters.

Table 9.3: Showing the difference between pulmonary, cardiac and CNS respiratory distress

Symptoms/ Signs	*Respiratory*	*Cardiac*	*CNS*
Tachypnea	Moderate to Marked	Moderate	Mild/Apnea
Rhythm of respiration	Regular	Regular	Irregular
Intercostal or Sub-costal Retractions	Marked	Mild	Mild/ absent/ paradoxical
Expiratory grunting	Present	Absent	Absent
Cyanosis	Mild	Severe	Mild
Heart rate	Proportional to respiratory rate	Dispropor- tionately higher than Resp. rate	May be associated with bradycardia
Hepatomegaly	Absent or pushed down	Present in CHF	Absent
Chest auscultation	Pulmonic findings may be present	Cardiac murmur and abnormali- ties of heart sounds	Normal
Seizure	Rare	Absent	Common
Effect of 100% oxygen on PaO_2	Raised	No effect	Raised

Laboratory Investigations

1. A complete blood count, hematocrit, blood glucose and a chest X-ray and arterial blood gases.
2. Sepsis screen and blood culture.
3. Serum bilirubin.
4. An ultrasound examination of the head and an echo-cardiography.

5. Serum electrolytes—Potassium and sodium.

A complete blood count, hematocrit, blood glucose and arterial blood gas should be done in all cases. When the hematocrit is < 40% or hemoglobin is < 13 gm/dl, the infant needs a transfusion. A chest X-ray is instrumental in diagnosing medical causes and differentiating from surgical causes. An arterial blood gas can help to decide the degree of hypoxia and also determine management strategies. Hypoglycemia (blood glucose < 40 mg/dl) may ensue if intravenous glucose supplementation is not started. Blood glucose estimation should be done to rule out hypoglycemia.

With clinical suspicion, a sepsis screen and blood culture should be send before starting an antibiotic. Since preterm infants are prone to develop hyperbilirubinemia and intra cranial hemorrhage, serum bilirubin should be monitored daily for early detection of jaundice. A base line ultrasound examination of the head should be done to exclude intracranial hemorrhage. The USG should be repeated to assess presence, absence or progress of hemorrhage. If present it is useful in prognostication.

An echocardiography is mandatory in suspected cases of congenital heart disease and persistent pulmonary hypertension.

Varying degrees of hyperkalemia (normal level: 3.5 mEq/ L) may occur suggesting ongoing tissue catabolism. Other electrolytes remain within normal limits unless the course is complicated by dehydration (caused by excessive insensible water loss) or over hydration caused by excess fluids or decreased renal function.

Prevention

1. *Prevention of preterm delivery:* What triggers preterm labour leading to preterm delivery is still not clear?

Prevention will be possible when the cause is properly known. However, the antecedents of preterm labour include spontaneous labour, premature rupture of membrane, emergency delivery and elective delivery. Premature rupture of membrane probably reduces the risk of hyaline membrane disease but increases the risk of congenital pneumonia. Pre-eclampsia may also increase the risk of hyaline membrane disease because it increases the incidence of caesarean section prior to onset of labour.

2. *Asepsis during delivery:* Adoption of aseptic measures during labour and care of the newly born infant can prevent sepsis during the neonatal period.
3. *Proper resuscitation for MSAF:* A systematic resuscitation of the infant born through meconium stain amniotic fluid prevents meconium aspiration syndrome, one of the most common cause of respiratory distress in the newborn.
4. *Promotion of fetal lung maturity:* It is the most cost effective of perinatal strategies. Prevention of preterm labour is problematic but prevention of RDS with antenatal steroids is effective. There is 50% reduction of incidence of RDS after administration of antenatal steroids. The reduction in the risk of RDS is accompanied by decreases in periventricular hemorrhage and necrotizing enterocolitis. Inj. betamethasone/dexamethasone, 12 mg IM/24 hours or 6 mg/12 hours if labour starts before 34 weeks of gestation. Optimal effect is seen after 24 hours of initiation and therapeutic effect lasts for 7 days. It can be administered in presence of maternal diabetes and hypertension and prolonged rupture of membrane. No need to repeat the dose after 7 days.
5. *Prophylactic surfactant therapy:* The combination of antenatal steroid treatment and prophylactic surfactant seems to be the most cost effective combination for very premature infants. Prophylactic

surfactant therapy can be advocated for all newly born infants of gestational age < 31 weeks (weight <1250 grams).

6. *Immediate referral on anticipation:* All mothers at risk of preterm delivery should be identified and referred to an institution with facilities for management of preterm labour and adequate care of the preterm baby. An in utero transfer is preferred because the mother is the best transport incubator.

Management

The principal problem in infants with respiratory distress is poor oxygenation and increasing respiratory difficulty. The therapeutic goals, therefore, include provision of sufficient oxygen to maintain arterial PO_2 values within an acceptable range. The second aspect of management is supportive therapy with an aim to minimize work of breathing, heat loss and to provide adequate fluid and calories. In addition, anemia and jaundice, the problems usually associated with preterm babies should be properly managed in the usual lines.

Care in the Delivery Room

When respiratory problems are anticipated, care of these infants should be started in the delivery room. Care in the delivery room include:

- Prompt and effective resuscitation.
- Routine intubation for babies < 30 weeks of gestation electively in the delivery room prior to transfer to the neonatal intensive care unit.
- Prophylactic surfactant therapy. True prophylactic administration of surfactant is done in the delivery room prior to the first breath. Surfactant can be also given as early treatment which involves instillation within 30 to 60 minutes after birth. Early surfactant

treatment may be given in the neonatal intensive care unit after stabilization of the infant. Early or prophylactic surfactant therapy is advocated in all babies of gestational age < 31 weeks (estimated fetal weight < 1250 gram).

Transfer/Referral to NICU

All newly born infants anticipated to have respiratory distress should be transferred to the neonatal intensive care unit (in case of hospital born) or referred to a higher centre (if born at home or a peripheral centre) for further management at the earliest.

Care in the Neonatal Intensive Care Unit

Oxygenation

The major consideration in the management of infants with respiratory problems is to improve oxygenation. Hypoxemia can lead to acidemia, patency of ductus arteriosus, decrease in surfactant synthesis and increased risk of persistent pulmonary hypertension. Administration of oxygen necessitates careful monitoring of inspired oxygen concentration and the oxygen tension in the arterial blood. The oxygen tension should be maintained between 60-90 mmHg and oxygen saturation between 90-95%.

Oxygen Administration by Head Box

Humidified oxygen should be administered via a head box. Initially a transcutaneous oxygen monitor or a pulse oxymeter should be used to assess oxygenation. If the infant needs > 40% oxygen or the respiratory signs persist beyond the age of 4 hours, an arterial line should be inserted into the umbilical or peripheral artery and continuous monitoring of PaO_2 is necessary. The PaO_2,

$PaCO_2$ and pH should be measured every 4-6 hours and 30 minutes after any change in management.

Respiratory Support

When infants continue to exhibit respiratory difficulty (with increasing respiratory rate, retraction and grunting), and require inspired oxygen concentration greater than 40% on hood oxygenation, the infant needs support with constant distending pressure (CDP). This can be achieved by application of continuous positive airway pressure (CPAP). In those infants where there is no spontaneous breathing and there is an increasing $PaCO_2$, mechanical ventilation is the therapy of choice. It should be mentioned that CPAP can only be used in infants breathing spontaneously and maintaining normal $PaCO_2$.

The criteria to initiate CPAP include:

1. Clinical or X-ray evidence of hyaline membrane disease.
2. Moderate to severe respiratory distress with PaO_2 < 50 mmHg while patient is breathing 60% oxygen (FiO_2 0.60).
3. Recurrent apnoea.
4. Weaning from ventilation.

The indications of mechanical ventilation are:

1. Respiratory acidosis (pH < 7.25) with a $PaCO_2$ > 55 mmHg or rapidly rising.
2. PaO_2 < 50 mmHg or oxygen saturation < 90% with an FiO_2 > 0.50.
3. Intractable apnea.

Supportive Therapy

Thermo Neutral Environment

The skin temperature of 36.5°C to 37.5°C and a humidity of above 60% should be maintained. A too high or low temperature increases the metabolic demands. The infant should be nursed in an incubator or a radiant warmer to maintain the temperature.

Minimal Handling

Handling of the baby should be minimum. Disturbance of a sick infant may cause apnea or fall in PaO_2. Hence electronic monitors and non invasive oxygen monitors are preferable for monitoring the infant.

Maintenance of Blood Pressure and Perfusion

The circulation is assessed by monitoring the heart rate, blood pressure, peripheral perfusion and acid base status. The peripheral perfusion can be clinically assessed by skin color, capillary refill time and core– peripheral temperature. As a working guide, mean arterial blood pressure in mmHg = gestational age in weeks. Continuous intra-arterial monitoring is more reliable than oscillometric blood pressure monitors because the latter over read in sick and very low birth weight babies. Hypotension may be missed in these cases.

In presence of hypotension, judicious use of crystalloids, blood and pressors may be used to maintain circulation. Pressor drugs are preferred to crystalloid in infants with respiratory distress to avoid capillary leak of fluid into the lung parenchyma and excess administration of sodium from repeated boluses of normal saline. Dopamine, in the appropriate doses (starting at 5 micrograms/kg/minute), can maintain adequate blood pressure and cardiac output to ensure improved tissue perfusion and urine output and avoid metabolic acidosis. However, after the first 12-24 hours, hypotension and poor perfusion may result from a large left to right shunt through a PDA. The infant should be assessed for this.

The volume of blood drawn from the infant should be monitored and packed red cell should be transfused if the hematocrit falls below 35-40%.

Exclusion/treatment of a Possible Infection

Pneumonia can coexist and exaggerate the respiratory distress. Radiological findings of hyaline membrane disease may be similar with pneumonia. In all infants with respiratory distress, total leucocytic count, a differential leucocytic count and a blood culture should be obtained and a broad spectrum antibiotic (according to nursery protocol) should be started to cover both gram positive and negative organisms and continued for atleast 48 hours. Further treatment will depend on the investigation results.

Fluids and Nutrition

Enteral feeding has to be delayed in all cases of respiratory distress. Intravenous fluid, 10% dextrose should be started in the appropriate amount depending on the weight of the infant. Electrolytes viz. sodium (2 meq/kg/day) and potassium (1 meq/kg/day and calcium (100-200 mg/kg/day) should be added to the fluid after 24-48 hours. If it seems unlikely that adequate enteral feeds will not be possible within few days, total parenteral nutrition should be started from the first or second day.

Monitoring

1. Observations of vital signs, FiO_2, ventilator settings.
2. ABG every 4 hours and 30 minutes after any change of management.
3. Blood sugar 4-6 hourly.
4. Urea, electrolytes and creatinine daily.

5. Full blood count every 2-3 days.
6. Record of blood taken from the baby for investigation.

Steps of Management of Respiratory Distress in Newborn

In the labour room:

1. Put Infant under a radiant warmer/in incubator to maintain warmth.
2. Establish airway by position, suction.
3. Prophylactic intubation and surfactant therapy in ELBW infants.
4. Provide adequate oxygen.
5. Establish arterial line. Start IV fluids.
6. Assess oxygenation by change in colour, heart rate, activity and ABG.
7. Administer volume expander, pressor drugs if necessary to maintain blood pressure and perfusion.
8. Administer sodium bicarbonate if there is acidosis.
9. Obtain chest X-ray.
10. Transfer to NICU.

In the NICU:

1. Continue oxygenation.
2. Monitor ABG.
3. Start CPAP as indicated.
4. Start mechanical ventilation as indicated.

SUGGESTED READINGS

1. Halliday Henry. Prevention and management of respiratory distress syndrome in Practical perinatal care 1st edition, 1999, edited by Gill Levitt, David Harvey and Richard Cooke. Published by Butterworth Heineman, Oxford.
2. Vidyasagar D. Respiratory distress syndrome of the newborn in Textbook of Neonatology 1st edition, 1987. Published by Interprint, New Delhi.

3. Saili Arvind. Approach to respiratory distress in newborns. Indian Journal of Practical Pediatrics, 2005; 7: 187-191.
4. Thopmas N. Hansen, Anthony Corbet, Alfred L. Gest and Alicia A. Moise. Principles of Respiratory monitoring in Avery's diseases of the newborn 8th edition, 2005. Saunders.
5. Dyio Honrubia and Ann R. Stark. Respiratory distress syndrome in Manual of neonatal care, 5th edition, 2004. Edited by John P. Cloherty, Eric C Eichenwald and Ann R. Stark. Published By Lippincott, Williams and Wilkins, Philadelphia.
6. A Neonatal Vade—Mecum 3rd edition, 1998 edited by Brian Speidel, Peter Fleming, John Henderson *et al.* Published by Arnold, London.
7. Upadhayay Amit and Deorari A K. Continuous Positive Airway pressure—A gentler approach to ventilation. Indian Pediatr 2004;41:459-469.
8. Sahni Rakesh and Wung Jen—Tien CPAP– A gentler, non invasive approach for managing neonatal RDS. Journal of Neonatology; 2002;16:24-36.

10

Neonatal Seizure

J.N. Sharma

A clinical seizure at any age is associated with a paroxysmal burst of electrical activity within the central nervous system.

The newborn is at a particular risk of development of seizures because metabolic, toxic, structural and infectious diseases are more likely to manifest during this period of life. Although it is commonly a manifestation of an acute brain insult or a biochemical abnormality, in about 25% cases no cause may be identified.

The reported incidence of neonatal seizure ranges from 0.15% in term infants to 20.2% in preterm. The national collaborative perinatal project (UK) reported an incidence of 0.5%, preterm and term babies taken together. However, the precise frequency of neonatal seizures cannot be delineated because many subtle seizures go undetected. Regardless of a precise incidence, it needs mention that seizures are more common in the newborn period than at any other time in life and the tendency towards recurrent seizures and status epilepticus is far greater in the newborn.

Identification of Seizures in Newborn

It is often difficult to decide whether a neonate has had a seizure or not. It may be impossible to diagnose without witnessing the episode oneself and sometimes even then it may be difficult. This is because unlike older infants, newborn rarely have well organized generalized tonic clonic seizure, preterms have even less well organized spells than term neonates.

Types of Seizures

In the newborn period at least 5 essential seizure types have been recognized. They are subtle, focal or generalized tonic, multifocal clonic, focal and myoclonic seizures.

1. *Subtle seizures:* Constitute 50% of seizures in newborn and often occurs in association with other seizure types. Subtle seizures are most difficult to identify, usually not associated with EEG abnormalities and respond poorly to anticonvulsant. Example of subtle seizures include:
   a. Tonic horizontal deviation of eyes or sustained eye opening with ocular fixation or cycled fluttering.
   b. Repetitive blinking or fluttering of eyelids.
   c. Oral-facial-lingual movements viz. chewing, tongue-thrusting, lip-smacking, drooling, yawning.
   d. Limb movements-Cycling, paddling, boxing jabs.
   e. Autonomic phenomenon—Tachycardia or bradycardia.
   f. Apnea may be a rare manifestation of seizure. Apnea due to seizure activity has an accelerated or normal heart rate when evaluated 20 seconds after onset.
2. *Tonic seizures*: May resemble decerebrate or decorticate posturing, often associated with eye deviation and occasionally preceded by clonic movements or apnea. Most often EEG shows severe abnormalities and prognosis is generally poor.
3. *Multifocal clonic seizures*: They are characterized by random clonic movements of limbs similar to those

seen in normal babies less than 34 weeks of gestation. The EEG most often is multifocally abnormal.

4. *Focal clonic seizures*: In this type movements involve weak localized clonic jerking without loss of consciousness. The EEG is unifocally abnormal.
5. *Myoclonic seizures*: Manifestations include synchronous single or multiple slow jerks of upper or lower limbs or both.

Neonatal Seizure: Why Poorly Expressed?

The poor expression of seizure in the neonatal period is primarily due to immaturity of cortical organization of neonatal brain. The arborisation of axonal and dendritic synaptic contacts as well as myelination of cortical pathway is incomplete.

Neonatal seizures tend to be brief because immature neurons are unable to sustain repetitive activity for a long period. They are focal or multifocal because the pathway connecting different cortical regions are poorly myelinated and hence seizure discharge cannot readily be propagated throughout the neonatal brain to produce a generalized seizure. Further, the predominance of oral and buccal phenomena as well as ocular motor abnormalities and apnea may relate to the advanced development of limbic structures and their connection to the brain-stem and diencephalons as compared to other forebrain structures.

In the immature brain, certain changes are observed at the cellular level, which is responsible for the decreased seizure threshold in the newborn. There is a transient overexpression in the density of the excitat`ory amino acid (primarily glutamate) receptors and a relative paucity of glutamate reuptake transporters. This results in prolonged and intense contact of glutamate with postsynaptic receptors. These immature glutamate receptors are far more permissive of cationic influx, facilitating membrane depolarization and seizure activation. Further, the inhibitory Gama amino butyric acid (GABA) ion channels are relatively under expressed in the immature brain. In fact, in certain areas of the developing brain these immature GABA may be depolarizing (i.e. excitatory) rather than hyperpolarizing (i.e. inhibitory). In short, the newborn has a transient over development of the excitatory systems compared to inhibitory systems.

Movements that are not Seizures

Certain movements occur in a newborn, although not seizures may look like and has to be differentiated.

A. Normal movements seen more commonly in preterms:
   a. Benign neonatal sleep myoclonus: Occur during REM sleep in preterm.
   b. Fragmentary myoclonic jerks.
   c. Eye-movements: Roving or dysconjugate eye-movements with occasional non-sustained nystagmoid jerks.

B. Neonate in active REM sleeps with:
   a. Rhythmic eye jerks with irregular respiration.
   b. Sucking movements.
   c. Body movements.
   d. Twitches of face or limb.

   These movements will disappear upon arousing the infant.

C. Agitation and tremulousness when hungry will occur associated with crying and disappear when the baby is given a feed.

D. Jitteriness: May be confused with seizures but distinction can be readily made if the following points are remembered:

a. Jitteriness is not accompanied by abnormalities of gaze or extra ocular movement. Seizures usually are.
b. Jitteriness is provoked by stimulus. Seizures occur spontaneously.
c. Jitteriness is characterized by rhythmic alternating movements, of equal amplitude at a rate of 5-6/sec. The dominant movement in seizure is clonic jerking i.e. movements have a fast and slow component at a slow rate of 2-3/sec.
d. Movement of jitteriness can be stopped by flexion of the affected limb. Seizure movement will not stop by this manoeuver.
e. Jitteriness is not accompanied by increased blood pressure, tachycardia or bradycardia.

Etiology

The causes of neonatal seizures are diverse. Majority are, however secondary to relatively few etiologies. It needs emphasis that determination of etiology is highly critical because it helps one to treat specifically and also to make a meaningful prognostic statement. The causes are given in Table 10.1.

Diagnostic Work-Up

A search for an etiologic diagnosis should proceed simultaneously with management of the seizure episode. Evaluation of the patient should begin with a careful history, physical examination with emphasis on the following points, because not infrequently the clue for an etiologic diagnosis may become obvious from such pursuits.

	Features	Suspected diagnosis
1.	H/O fetal distress, instru-instrumentation, need for resuscitation in labour room with low apgar score (<3 at 5 min)	Perinatal asphyxia
2.	Full term baby with history of trauma, difficult delivery, and bruise	Contusion, Intra cranial hemorrhage
3.	Preterm baby with pallor, Hypotonia, bulging fontanelle, lowering hematocrit	Intraventricular hemorrhage.
4.	Small for date baby with history of maternal diabetes, PET, LFD or SFD	Hypoglycemia, Early Hypocalcemia
5.	Premature rupture of membrane more than 18 hours	Sepsis
6.	History of excess fluid administration during labour to mother	Hyponatremia
7.	History of excess and rapid I.V. administration of Sodibicarb or sodium chloride	Hypernatremia
8.	Hyperemesis gravidarum with vitamin B6 therapy	Pyridoxine deficiency
9.	Family H/O seizure or mental retardation and recurrence of seizure in sibship or unexplained early neonatal death with features of lethargy, vomiting, jaundice etc.	Metabolic disorder
10.	Dysmorphic facies, Microcephaly	Developmental CNS anomaly
11.	Hepatosplenomegaly	I.U. infection
12.	Cutaneous manifestation	Neurocutaneous syndrome
13.	Top feeding with cow's milk	Late onset hypocalcemia

Table 10.1: Showing causes of neonatal seizures

A. Common causes
   1. Perinatal complications
      a. Neonatal encephalopathy
      b. Hypoxic ischemic encephalopathy
      c. Intracranial hemorrhage
      d. Contusion
   2. Bacterial meningitis
   3. Hypoglycemia
   4. Early hypocalcemia
   5. Idiopathic

B. Less common causes
   1. Developmental defect
   2. Subarachnoid hemorrhage
   3. Late hypocalcemia

C. Rare causes
   1. Accidental injection of local anesthetic
   2. Hypo and hypernatremia
   3. Pyridoxine dependency
   4. Other inborn errors of metabolism
   5. Hyperbilirubinemia

The etiology can be suspected also from the day of onset of the seizure as shown below:

Day of onset	*Cause of seizure*
1. 0-3 days	Perinatal complications, hypoglycemia
2. 0-10 days	Hypocalcemia and developmental defects
3. 4-10 days	Infection

Laboratory Investigations

Initial Investigations

The initial laboratory tests should be directed towards the most dangerous but readily treatable diseases and therefore should include:

1. Estimation of blood sugar, serum calcium, magnesium, sepsis screen, ABG, anion-gap.
2. An ECG to rule out symptomatic hypocalcemia.
3. Lumbar puncture: CSF examination should be done in all cases with the slightest suspicion of meningitis or intra cranial hemorrhage, except in severe cardiorespiratory compromise of neonates. It should not be omitted even if another etiology (e.g. Hypoglycemia) is present because meningitis may co-exist.

Specific Investigations: To be picked up as and when necessary:

1. Serum bilirubin (if jaundice is present).
2. Serum sodium, potassium, blood urea nitrogen (BUN), liver function tests to rule out causes and plan fluid therapy.
3. Screen for congenital infections (TORCH) and metabolic screen for inborn errors of metabolism viz. urine pH, blood pH, blood ammonia, anion gap, urine and serum amino acidogram, serum and CSF lactate/pyruvate ratio.
4. An EEG should be done in the interictal period in selected cases. It has both diagnostic and prognostic role in seizure. The value of neonatal EEG has increased with establishment of age related normal and abnormal back grounds. It has now become unquestionable in the modern management of neonatal seizure. But neither diagnostic procedures nor therapy need to be postponed for an EEG. EEG helps in:

a. Recognition of subtle seizures.
b. Recognition of electrical seizures in paralysed and ventilated newborns.
c. Prevent over interpretation of abnormal movement and thereby resultant overtreatment.
d. Prognosticate eventual sequels.

In case of a suspected seizure, ideally an EEG should be done as soon as possible within 24 hours. Whenever possible, the suspected event should be captured on the EEG to confirm the true epileptic nature. If the first EEG is normal, then subsequent EEG is indicated only when there is a recurrence of the clinical spell. The absence of EEG changes during several episodes especially when the interictal EEG background is normal is suggestive of a nonepileptic process.

5. Neurodiagnostic studies viz. Ultrasonography and CT scan of brain should be considered depending on the specific clinical features. Ultrasonography would help identify acute lesions like intracranial hemorrhage and also followup hydrocephalus. CT scan can also delineate small calcification, developmental defects, infarcts etc.

Treatment

There is lack of a single, highly effective anticonvulsant regimen in the newborn. This has led to the proposition of different approaches. It needs mention that basically seizures in newborn are less responsive to conventional anticonvulsant than in older children. Secondly, they may be a result of treatable conditions—metabolic or infective.

The initial steps therefore consists of stabilization of vital functions, exclusion and prompt treatment of rapidly correctable conditions viz. hypoglycemia and hypocalcemia, establishment of diagnosis of other treatable conditions (e.g. meningitis, narcotic withdrawal) and institution of specific treatment.

The Initial General Measures

1. The first step in successful management of seizure is to nurse the baby in the thermoneutral environment and ensure airway, breathing and circulation (TABC).
2. An I.V. access should be secured using a peripheral vein or umbilical vein and oxygen should be started.
3. Dextrostix examination and blood should be collected for the initial investigations.
4. A brief relevant history and quick clinical examination should be done.

Treatment of Rapidly Correctable Causes

1. If glucostix shows hypoglycemia or if there is no facility to test blood sugar immediately, 2 ml/kg of 10% dextrose should be given by bolus followed by maintenance infusion of 6-8 mg/kg/min. In newborn with seizures, the target goal for blood glucose should be 70-120 mg/dL. New observations from experimental studies have indicated that brain tissue levels of glucose may fall during seizures even when blood glucose is normal and hyperglycemia may be neuroprotective.
2. An ECG should be done to look for signs of hypocalcemia (QT interval more than 0.2 seconds in the preterm and more than 0.19 seconds in term babies). A sample for ionized calcium and serum magnesium should be withdrawn and 2 ml/kg of 10% Cal. Gluconate should be given I.V. under strict cardiac monitoring over 10 minutes. Hypomagnesemia is treated with an intramuscular dose of 50% magnesium sulphate at 0.2 ml/kg. Infants treated for hypocalcemia

should be given magnesium because calcium administration increases renal magnesium excretion and magnesium administration increases calcium. It should be noted that an ECG can be a better alternative to rule out hypocalcemia. It should be noted that even if hypocalcemic seizures respond to anticonvulsant drugs, the low calcium level should be corrected.

Anticonvulsant Therapy

1. If seizure persists, even after correction of hypoglycemia/hypocalcemia, anti-epileptic drugs (AED) should be started. Phenobarbitone is the drug of choice. It is given in a loading dose of 20 mg/kg/dose IV very slowly over 20 minutes (not faster than 1mg/kg/min). If seizures persist after completion of this loading dose, repeat dose of phenobarbitone 10 mg/kg/dose may be used every 20-30 minutes till a dose of 40 mg/kg/day has been given.
2. Phenytoin is indicated, if the maximal dose of phenobarbitone (40 mg/kg) fails to resolve seizures or earlier, if adverse effects like respiratory depression, hypotension or bradycardia ensues with phenobarbitone administration. It is given in a loading dose of 20 mg/kg I.V. at a rate of not more than 1 mg/kg/min under cardiac monitoring. A repeat dose of 10 mg/kg may be tried if seizures still persist.
3. Very occasionally in 10-15% of newborns with seizures that donot respond to phenobarbitone and phenytoin, benjodiazepines may be required. Benzodiazepines available are diazepam, lorazepam, and midazolam. Diazepam is generally avoided due to its short duration of action, narrow therapeutic index, and presence of sodium benzoate as a preservative. Lorazepam is preferred over diazepam due to its longer duration of action, less cardiovascular adverse

effects and wider therapeutic index. Midazolam is faster acting but requires strict monitoring for respiratory depression, apnea and bradycardia. Equipment for resuscitation and assisted ventilation should be available at the bedside of all neonates given multiple doses of AED.

Doses:

- Diazepam—0.25 mg/kg I.V. bolus (0.5 mg/kg rectal); may be repeated 1-2 times.
- Lorazepam—0.05 mg/kg I.V. bolus over 2-5 minutes; may be repeated 1-2 times.
- Midazolam—0.15 mg/kg I.V. bolus followed by infusion of 0.1-0.4 mg/kg/hour.

Refractory Seizures

Seizures refractory to aforementioned therapy may be due to:

- Cortical dysgenesis, cerebral infarction.
- Severe HIE.
- Intraventricular hemorrhage.
- Inborn error of metabolism, intrauterine infection.
- Pyridoxine dependency/deficiency.
- Narcotic withdrawal.

These cases should undergo investigations in search of a diagnosis and then treated. The anticonvulsant drugs that may be tried in such circumstances are:

- *Therapeutic trial with pyridoxine:* Pyridoxine deficiency/dependency are treated with 25-50 mg of pyridoxine I.V. under EEG guidance. Control is followed by a maintenance dose of 10-100 mg/day P.O. (dependency) and 5 mg P.O./day (deficiency). If history suggests deficiency of pyridoxine then it can be given prior to anticonvulsant therapy.

- *Lidocaine:* Start with 4mg/kg/hour I.V. on first day, reduce by 1 mg/kg/hour on each subsequent day. It should not be administered with phenytoin.
- *Paraldehyde:* A dose of 0.1- 0.2 ml /kg/dose may be used IM or 0.3 ml/kg/dose mixed with coconut oil in 3:1 ratio may be used by per rectal route.
- *Valproic acid:* Dose is 20-25 mg /kg/day (PO/PR) followed by 5-10 mg/kg every 12 hours.

Treatment During Interictal Period

If a neonate is brought after the seizure is over by itself, baby should be subjected to investigations. If dextrostix detects hypoglycemia it should be treated. If normal, other laboratory tests are carried out to find the cause. The baby is to be kept under observation for recurrence or any abnormality on tests.

Maintenance

Maintenance after response is to be started after 12 hours of bolus:

- Phenobarbitone:3-5 mg/kg/day in 1-2 divided doses PO/IV.
- Phenytoin: 3-8 mg/kg/day in 1-2 divided doses IV.

Recurrence of Seizure During Maintenance

Only life threatening seizures are to be treated with a loading dose of the drug of which the maximum dose has not been used previously, in the same manner as the first seizure. Maintenance has to be started after 12 hours.

When to Stop Anticonvulsant?

It is still controversial. The following guidelines may be followed:

1. Single seizure treated with one drug: No maintenance required.
2. Single seizure treated with more than one drug: Stop all drugs if the baby do not have convulsion for 3-4 days or at discharge. If cause of convulsion is HIE continue anticonvulsant for 10 days and then stop. It has been observed that seizures due to HIE tends to subside by itself by 7-10 days.
3. With multiple seizures, treated with more than one drug, baby is reviewed at discharge. If the baby is neurologically normal, all drugs can be stopped, irrespective of the etiology and EEG. If the baby is neurologically abnormal, phenytoin is stopped at discharge and phenobarbitone is continued for 1 month and baby is reassessed after 1 month. If the baby is neurologically normal at 1 month and is seizure free, phenobarbitone is discontinued over 2 weeks. If neurological assessment is not normal, an EEG is done. If EEG is not overtly abnormal, AED is tapered and stopped. If EEG is overtly abnormal, phenobarbitone is continued and the infant is reassessed in the same manner at 3 months and then 3 monthly till 1 year of age.
4. In most children with neonatal seizures, the seizure rarely recurs during the first 2 years of life. Older infants who present with specific syndromes like infantile spasm will not respond to the conventional anti epileptic drugs prescribed in the neonatal period. Adverse effects of anti epileptic drugs on the morphology and metabolism have been reported. Hence emphasis is on the need to consider early discontinuation of the anti-epileptic drugs.

Prognosis: The overall prognosis of neonatal seizure is as follows:

Lower the gestational age higher the mortality. Good recovery occurs in 55%, about 15% die during the first two postnatal weeks and 30% survive with neurological deficits like mental retardation, persistent seizure and cerebral palsy.

The results of the National Collaborative perinatal project (UK) found that the early predictors of death/ neurological sequelae following neonatal seizure are:

1. Apgar score of 6 or less at 5 min.
2. Need for 5 min of positive pressure ventilation following birth.
3. Early onset of seizure.
4. Seizure duration more than 30 min.
5. 3 or more days with uncontrolled seizures.
6. Hypotonia at 5 min following birth.

CONCLUSION

Treatment of seizure in new born should be vigorous. However, over treatment should be avoided. Detection of specific cause is more important than treatment of spells because most serious error to be made is to delay or miss the diagnosis and treatment of correctable disturbances like hypoglycemia, hypocalcemia or bacterial meningitis.

SUGGESTED READINGS

1. Adre J. du Plessis. Neonatal seizures in Manual of neonatal care, edited by John P Cloherty, Eric C. Eichenwald and Ann R. Stark, Fifth edition (2004), published by Lippincott Williams and Wilkins, Philadelphia.
2. Singhal PK, Mathur GP, Gupta Arun. Neonatal seizures in Seizure disorders in childhood, first edition (1992), published by Nazia Printers, Rodgram Lal Quan, Delhi.
3. Naidu S, Claudine Amiel Tyson. Neonatal seizures. Textbook on neonatology edited by D. Vidyasagar. First edition (1987) published by Imprint, New Delhi.

4. Scher S. Mark. Neonatal seizures in Avery's Diseases of the Newborn, 8th edition, 2005. Published by Saunders Philadelphia, Pennsylvania.
5. Scarpa P, Chierici R, Tamisisari L *et al.* Criteria for discontinuing neonatal seizure therapy: A long term appraisal. Brain Dev. 1983;5:541.
6. Gamstop J, Sedin G. Neonatal convulsion treated with continuous I.V. infusion of diazepam. Ups J Med Science 1982;87:143.
7. Bergman I, Painter MJ. Hirsch RP *et al.* Outcome in neonates with convulsions treated in an intensive care unit. Ann Neurol 1983;14:542.
8. Sharma JN Neonatal seizure. NER Pediatrics 1988; 3:1.
9. Das S and Das A. Neonatal seizures: Diagnosis and management. NER Pediatrics 1993;8:95.

11 Apnea in Neonate

Ajoy Kumar Sarma

DEFINITION

Apnea has been described as cessation of breathing for 20 seconds, often associated with bradycardia, cyanosis or both. However, most of the recent publications have taken a respiratory pause of greater than 10-15 seconds as diagnostic of apnea.

What is Periodic Breathing?

Periodic breathing is a series of respiratory pauses of about 10 seconds duration alternating with periods of hyperventilation of upto 15 seconds and occurring at least three times per minute. It is not associated with cyanosis and bradycardia and may be a physiological response of immature cardio-respiratory system in a pre-term baby. Periodic breathing does not occur during the first 2 days of life and is more frequent during active sleep.

Sequelae of Apnea

- Apnea can cause reduction of cerebral blood flow, resulting in ischemia, neuronal death and eventually leukomalacia.
- Recurrent apnea is associated with spastic diplegia and delayed development.

- During apnea, to protect cerebral blood flow, cardiac output is diverted away from the somatic circulation resulting in intestinal ischemia, possibly necrotizing enterocolitis (NEC).
- Whether apnea of prematurity is a precursor or predictor of subsequent Sudden Infant Death Syndrome (SIDS) is unclear.
- Because of therapy especially from oxygen inhalation, there may be associated problems of oxygen toxicity like brocho-pulmonary dysplasia, retinopathy of prematurity etc.

Etiology

From the etiological point of view, apnea can be divided into primary and secondary.

A. Primary Apnea

Also known as apnea of prematurity. It is not associated with any pathologic condition and characteristically develops within 3-5 days of life in 25% pre-term infants weighing 1800 grams or less, or born before 34 weeks of gestation. Diagnosis is generally made by exclusion of other factors.

B. Secondary Apnea

The causes of secondary apnoea are as follows:

Infection: Sepsis especially in the first day of life, nosocomial infections, necrotizing enterocolitis in the first week of life, meningitis.

Neurological: Intraventricular hemorrhage, ICH, seizure, hypoxic injury, neuromuscular disorder or any pathology, which could lead to, raised intracranial pressure.

Cardiovascular: Impairment of oxygenation from congestive heart failure and pulmonary edema (PDA,

Coarctation of aorta) or from shunting (congenital heart disease).

Pulmonary: Impairment of oxygenation and ventilation from lung disease (Hyaline membrane disease, Pneumonia, Meconium aspiration syndrome, Phrenic nerve paralysis, laryngeal reflex, Obstructive airway disease etc.)

Metabolic: Hypoglycemia, hypocalcemia, hyponatremia and hypernatremia, acidosis etc.

Haematological: Anemia.

Gastrointestinal: Necrotising enterocolitis or gastroesophageal reflux.

Temperature regulation: Hypothermia or hyperthermia.

Drugs: Prenatal exposure with transplacental transfer to the neonate of various drugs (narcotics, beta blockers). Postnatal exposure to sedatives, hypnotic or narcotics.

Pathogenesis

Several mechanisms have been proposed to explain apnea of prematurity; however, the exact cause is still unknown. The various theories are:

1. *Developmental Immaturity:* It is a likely contributing factor. The brain-stem neural function may correlate with the occurrence of apnea, as is the state of sleep. REM sleep predominates in preterm babies, and apneic spells occur more frequently in this state than in quiet sleep.
2. *Chemoreceptor response*: In preterm infants, hypoxia results in transient hyperventilation, followed by hypoventilation and sometimes apnea. In addition, hypoxia makes the premature infant less responsive to increased levels of carbon dioxide.
3. *Reflexes*: Active reflexes invoked by stimulation of the posterior pharynx (for e.g. vigorous use of suction catheters in the pharynx), lung inflation, fluid in the

larynx, or chest wall distortion can precipitate apnea in infants.

4. *Respiratory muscles*: Ineffective ventilation may result from impaired coordination of the inspiratory muscles (diaphragm and intercostal muscles) and muscles of the upper airway (larynx and pharynx). It can result in three types of apnea:

   Central apnea: Here, there is no 'signal to breathe' being transmitted from central nervous system to respiratory muscles. This is due to immaturity of brainstem control of central respiratory drive. The premature infant also manifests an immature response to peripheral vagal stimulation. Stimulation of laryngeal receptors in the premature infant results in apnea. The reflex apnea can be induced by gavage feeds, aggressive pharyngeal suctioning or gastro esophageal reflux.

   Obstructive apnea: Absent airflow in the presence of inspiratory efforts is seen when obstruction of airflow occurs within the upper airway, particularly at the level of pharynx. The pharynx collapses from negative pressure generated during inspiration, because the muscles responsible for keeping the airway open, the genioglossus and geniohyoid are too weak in the premature infants. Once collapsed, mucosal adhesive forces tend to prevent the reopening of the airway during expiration. Neck flexion will worsen this form of apnea. Excessive secretions in the nasopharynx and hypopharynx may also cause obstructive apnea.

   Mixed apnea: It is a combination of both types of apnea, representing as much as 50% of all episodes of apnea in neonates.

Monitoring

All infants born less than 34 weeks of gestation or with a birth weight less than 1800 grams should be monitored for apnea, bradycardia and oxygen saturation. Monitoring should be continued until the infant is at least 34 weeks post-conceptional age or after that time until the infant has been free of bradycardia for 1 week. Heart rate monitors are necessary to monitor because apnea without bradycardia is not significant apnea. Moreover, obstructive apnea with bradycardia is detected reliably with a heart rate monitor and false alarm is infrequent. The principal objections to use of an apnea monitor alone are that it misses obstructive apnea and may confuse bradycardia with breathing. It has become common practice now to monitor with pulse-oximetry because of the importance of both oxygen saturation and heart rate. The baby should be applied a heart rate monitor, apnoea monitor and a pulsoximeter. An alarm should be sound if respiration ceases for more than 20 seconds or if the heart rate drops below 100 beats per minute.

Management

After the first apneic spell, the infant should be evaluated for a possible underlying cause. Evaluation should include a history and physical examination, arterial blood gas measurement with continuous transcutaneous oxygen saturation monitoring, complete blood count, measurement of blood glucose, calcium and electrolyte levels and sepsis screen if sepsis is suspected. Specific therapy should be directed at an underlying cause if one is identified.

Most apneic spells in premature infants respond to tactile stimulation. The use of oscillation waterbeds has been helpful sometimes. It is reasonable to maintain the patient in prone position and in thermoneutral environment. Because diaphragmatic fatigue has been implicated, it is essential to maintain the circulation and a general state of nutrition. Infants who fail to respond to stimulation and general measures should be ventilated during the spell with bag and mask, generally with a FiO_2 of under 0.40 or equal to FiO_2 prior to the spell. It is important to insure that the oxygen concentration remains stable and is not increased. Pulse oximeter reading is maintained in the range of 92% to 96% saturation.

When spells of apnea are repeated and prolonged (i.e. more than two to three times per hour) or when they require frequent bag and mask ventilation, treatment should be initiated in order of increasing invasiveness and risk.

A. If intermittent hypoxia is identified by oxygen saturation monitoring, oxygen supplementation is essential. A nasal cannula is preferred to administer oxygen at a flow rate of 1 to 2 L/min to maintain the pulse oximeter reading in the range of 92-96% saturation.
B. Care should be taken to avoid reflexes that may trigger apnea. Oral feedings should be avoided. Swings in environmental temperature and extreme flexion or extension of the neck should be avoided.
C. The hematocrit level has to be checked. The role of blood transfusion is controversial. However, a transfusion of packed RBC can be given if hematocrit is less than 30% and the infant is having recurrent apnea.
D. The other mainstay of treatment is nasal CPAP. Although the effect of 5 cm H_2O should be tried, frequently as much as 8 to 10 cm is necessary for satisfactory control. Infants may be fed by continuous gastric infusion during this procedure. The chest-radiographs should be reviewed periodically to avoid overextending the lungs. CPAP is effective in treating both obstructive and mixed apnea but not central apnea. CPAP acts via following mechanism: (i) by alteration of Hering-

Breuer reflex, (ii) by stabilization of chest wall musculature, (iii) by splinting the upper-air-way with positive pressure during both inspiration and expiration thereby preventing pharyngeal collapse.

E. Drug therapy can be tried for repeated apneic spells if the above procedure fails to do so. Drugs commonly used are methyl xanthines (theophylline and caffeine) and doxapram.

A loading dose of theophylline, 5 to 7 mg/kg I.V. is followed by a maintenance dose of I.V. aminophylline or theophylline at a dose of 1.5 to 2 mg/kg every 6 to 8 hours. It should be always infused slowly over a period of minimum 20 minutes. A rapid push has been associated with sudden death from cardiac arrhythmias. Dose adjustments are made if a therapeutic effect is not achieved or toxicity is observed. Theophylline is generally discontinued at 34-36 weeks post-conceptual age if no apneic spells occur for 5 to 7 days. Mechanism by which theophylline may decrease apnea include:

1. Stimulation of the respiratory center.
2. Antagonism of adenosine, and
3. Improvement of diaphragmatic contractility.

Toxicity of theophylline usually begins with tachycardia, followed by jitteriness, irritability, and signs of GIT dysfunction. Seizures may occur at extremely high drug levels. No long-term sequelae have been demonstrated following xanthine treatment in infants:

A loading dose of 20 mg of caffeine citrate (10 mg caffeine base) per kilogram orally or I.V. followed by maintenance doses of 2.5 to 5 mg/kg daily (caffeine base) in one dose beginning 24 hours after the loading dose. Caffeine serum levels are maintained at 5-20 micro-gram/ml. Caffeine may be less toxic than theophylline.

Doxapram should be reserved for infants failing to respond to optimal xanthine and CPAP therapy, in which mechanical ventilation would be the next step. Methylxanthine therapy should be continued during doxapram infusion. In addition, doxapram should not be used in the 1st week of life or if serum bilirubin level is high. The drug may be started at 1.0 mg/kg per hour for a few hours to load the patient but then may be decreased to 0.5 mg/kg per hour. Higher doses are associated with side effects such as abdominal distension, increased gastric residuals, hyperglycemia, seizures etc.

F. *Mechanical ventilation:* If all the previously mentioned interventions fail, mechanical ventilation may be required.

Prognosis

Though it is quite a frustrating job for nurses and treating physician, but with proper monitoring and newer modalities of treatment the results of apnea of prematurity is encouraging, but for those with secondary apnea, prognosis depends on the underlying cause.

SUGGESTED READINGS

1. Edward F. Bell and Jeffrey Segar. Management of neonatal apnoea, IOWA Neonatology handbook, 1995.
2. Bhandari V and Narang A. Apnea, Bradycardia and periodic breathing: Are they always pathological? Indian Pediatr 1992, volume 29.
3. Merchant R H and Irani AJ. Pharmacotherapy of apnea. Indian Pediatr 1991; volume 28.

4. Thomus G Keens, Sally L, Davidsonward L. Apnea spells, sudden death and the role of Apnea monitor. The Pediatric clinics North America, 1993, volume 40.
5. Ann R. Stark Apnea in Manual of neonatal care 4th edition, 2004. Edited by John Cloherty, Eric C. Eichenwald and Ann R. Stark. Published by Lippincott Williams and Wilkins, Philadelphia.

12 Neonatal Necrotizing Enterocolitis

A.K. Dutta and Sriparna Basu

Neonatal Necrotizing Enterocolitis (NNEC) is a serious medical and surgical problem in newborn infants, especially those born before term. Because this is a disease that often affects growing pre-mature infants — those who have survived the early neonatal period — it is particularly poignant for both physicians and families. It is characterized by varying degrees of mucosal or trans mural necrosis of the intestine. Despite over a century of clinical and research interests in this disease, its pathogenesis remains unproven, preventive strategies are controversial and morbidity and mortality are still important problems.

Epidemiology

The incidence of NEC varies considerably among different centers. The overall incidence varies between 1-2/1000 live births or 2-5% of admission to NICU.

Prematurity is the single greatest risk factor. The mean gestational age of infants with NEC is 30-32 weeks, and the infants are generally appropriate for age. However, 10% of NEC occurs in full-term infants.

Excluding cocaine exposure, no maternal or neonatal factors other than prematurity are known to increase the risk of NEC. This suggests that the immaturity of the gastrointestinal tract is the greatest risk factor.

Pathogenesis

The causes of NEC are not well defined. Its pathogenesis however is probably complex and multi-factorial.

- *Prematurity* is the only consistent risk factor for NEC. Proposed factors in the premature gut predisposing to NEC include: (i) Lack of immunologic factors such as decreased IgA secretion (ii) Immaturity of the intestinal barrie, (iii) Luminal factors such as less acid output and low enzyme activity (iv) Decreased motility of gut which impairs clearance of potentially pathogenic microbes and toxins.
- *Hypoxia and ischemia*: The physiological explanation for the link of hypoxia and necrotising enterocolitis is the shunting of blood away from the gut at times of hypoxia (diving reflex) leading to ischaemic changes of the gut. The various predisposing factors leading to abnormal blood flow to the gut mucosa are-birth asphyxia, PDA, severe IUGR, umbilical vessel catheterization, hyperviscosity etc.
- *Enteral Feedings*: Factors that have been considered responsible to increase the risk of NEC include: (i) hyperosmolality of formula feeds, (ii) too early initiation of oral feeds except mother's milk, (iii) rapid increase in volume or concentration of oral feeds, (iv) lack of immunoprotective factors in the formula. Breast milk is associated with a lower risk as compared to formula milk.
- *Microorganism*: Various bacterial and viral agents have been implicated such as gram-negative rods, clostridium difficile, staphylococcus epidermis, rotavirus etc. Release of endotoxin and cytokines by proliferation of colonizing bacteria and bacterial fermentation with gaseous distension may play a role.
- *Inflammatory mediators*: Increasing evidence supports a critical role of inflammatory mediators in the pathogenesis of NEC. The mediators are part of a

final common pathway causing intestinal injury and development of necrotising enterocolitis:

1. Platelet activating factor (PAF): Necrotising enterocolitis is associated with increased levels of PAF. Human milk contains PAF antagonist. Hence breast milk is protective.
2. Imbalance between protective and pro-inflammatory cytokines seems to be an important determinant of necrotising enterocolitis. Several factors may promote (e.g. leukotrienes, oxygen radicals, tumour necrosis factor) or inhibit (e.g. steroids, nitric oxide, and prostacycline) PAF induced intestinal injury.
3. Gut trophic factors and growth factors seem to play a role. Epidermal growth factor that promotes mucosal barrier function has been shown to be deficient in premature infants with necrotising enterocolitis. Erythropoietin has been shown to protect against apoptosis, as does intestinal trefoil factor secreted by goblet cells, which protects against microbial invasion.

Clinical Presentation

Infants with NEC have a variety of signs and symptoms. The age of onset is inversely related to gestational age with a mean age of 3-4 days for term and 3-4 weeks for infants born less than 28 weeks gestation. Initial symptoms of NEC are often non-specific and subtle. Functional intestinal obstruction as evidenced by abdominal distension and retention of milk in stomach in a sick looking LBW baby is the earliest marker of the disease. The most common signs and symptoms associated with NEC (gastrointestinal and systemic) are listed in Table 12.1.

Table 12.1: Signs and symptoms associated with NEC

Gastrointestinal	*Systemic*
Abdominal distension	Lethargy
Abdominal tenderness	Apnea/respiratory distress
Feeding intolerance	Temperature instability
Delayed gastric emptying	Not doing well
Vomiting	Acidosis (Metabolic and/or respiratory)
Occult / gross blood in stool	Glucose instability
Change in stool pattern	Poor perfusion / shock
Diarrhoea	DIC
Abdominal mass	Oliguria
Erythema of abdominal wall	
Ascites	

Investigations

The diagnosis of NEC is suspected from clinical presentation and must be confirmed by diagnostic radiographs, surgery or autopsy.

1. Abdominal X-ray: AP/Cross table lateral view may reveal:
   - Bowel wall edema.
   - Dilated bowel loops.
   - Fixed bowel loops on serial X-ray.
   - Pneumatosis intestinalis-pathognomic of NEC.
   - Portal or hepatic venous air, pneumoperitoneum.
2. Hematocrit, platelet count, coagulation profile-Thrombocytopenia is commonly seen.
3. Sepsis screen and blood culture.
4. Stool for occult blood and reducing substance.
5. Serum electrolytes and renal function-Refractory hyponatremia has been observed.
6. Arterial blood gases (ABG)-detects persistent metabolic acidosis.
7. Abdominal paracentesis-for gram-stain and cultures where perforation and ascites is suspected.

8. Contrast studies with metrizamide-to detect gaseous blebs in upper GIT and ultrasonographic picture of microbubbles of gas in the portal vein may aid in early detection.

Staging of NEC (Table 12.2):

Table 12.2: Modified Bell's staging criteria for NEC

Stage	*Systemic signs*	*Intestinal signs*	*Radiological signs*	*Treatment*
IA-Suspected NEC	Temperature instability, Apnea, Lethargy	Abdominal distension, elevated pre-feed residuals	Normal or mild illeus	Nill orally, antibiotics for 3 days pending culture
IB-Suspected NEC	Same as above	Bright red Blood per rectum	Same as above	Same as above
IIA-Definite NEC	Same as above	Same as above + absent bowel sounds	Pneumatosis intestinalis	Nill per oral, antibiotics for 7-10 days
IIB-Definite NEC	Same as above + thrombocytopenia	Same as above + abdominal cellulitis+ tenderness	Same as IIA +portal vein gas	Nill per oral, antibiotics for 14 days
IIIA-Advanced NEC	Same as above + acidosis, DIC, neutropenia	Same as above + signs of peritonitis	Same as above + ascites	Same as above + paracentesis+ ionotropic agents+ ventilation therapy
IIIB- Advanced NEC	Same as IIIA	Same as IIIA	Same as IIB + pneumoperitoneum	Same as above + Surgical intervention.

Management

Initial management is medical. Medical therapy is directed towards: (i) ablation of suspected inciting and/or exacerbating factors (ii) maintenance of gastrointestinal perfusion (iii) inhibition of invasion and propagation of alimentary microbes (iv) provision of adequate nutrition for metabolism, repair and growth.

1. Enteral feeding is stopped and bowel is decompressed by suctioning through a nasogastric tube.
2. IV fluids: In NEC, there is substantial loss of fluids into third spaces. Liberal fluid volumes of 100 to 150% of predicted maintenance based on the infants continuing needs and response should be given. Urine output should be maintained at levels greater than 1 ml/kg/hr.
3. Antibiotics: Broad-spectrum parenteral antibiotic therapy should be instituted as per predominant NICU flora after sending the blood-culture/peritoneal fluid (if available). Commonly a combination of cefotaxime and amikacin is used. Metronidazole may be added in suspected perforation to treat anaerobic G.I. flora. Antibiotic therapy is typically continued for 7-14 days.
4. Correction or modification of systemic response: Infants with NEC are at high risk for poor perfusion, hypotension, clinical coagulopathy and respiratory failure:
   - *Ventilatory status:* Should be assessed and supplemental O_2 and mechanical ventilatory support should be used where required.
   - *Adequate tissue perfusion:* Plasma or blood transfusion should be given when required. Pharmacological support like dopamine and dobutamine may be required.
   - Metabolic acidosis should be corrected with volume expanders or sodium bicarbonate.

- Hematological parameters are closely monitored. Hematocrit should be kept at 35-45% with blood transfusion. Platelet transfusion, FFP or cryoprecipitate may be used in case there is DIC. Vitamin K should be given immediately and repeated weekly.

5. *Total parental nutrition (TPN):* Once fluid, acid-base and electrolyte status have stabilized, parenteral nutrition is instituted to facilitate recovery of damaged bowel and continuing growth.

Monitoring

Aggressive monitoring forms a corner stone for successful outcome in NEC:

A. *Clinical:*
- Abdominal girth hourly.
- Gastric aspirate-quantity and nature 1-2 hourly.
- Continuous heart rate and SpO_2 monitoring.
- Capillary refill time (CRT) and Blood pressure 1-2 hourly.

B. *Radiological:* Both supine and cross-table lateral view of abdomen 8-12 hourly during the first 48-72 hours, thereafter once daily.

C. *Laboratory:*
- Hematocrit and blood glucose 6-8 hourly.
- Serum electrolytes 12 hourly during first 48-72 hours, once daily thereafter.
- Platelet count and WBC count once initially and then after every 48-72 hours.
- Acid base status 12 hourly during the initial 48-72 hours.

Surgical Intervention

Surgical intervention is indicated in the following situation:

- Gastrointestinal perforation.
- Full thickness necrosis of bowel.
- Peritonitis.

At surgery, the goal is to excise necrotic bowel while preserving as much bowel length as possible.

Convalescent Phase

Medical therapy is gradually weaned once the infant has been stabilized and acute disease regresses. Gradually this is begun after 2 weeks of treatment by stopping naso-gastric decompression. If infants can tolerate their own secretions feeding is started very slowly while parenteral alimentation is gradually tapered.

Complications

1. Intestinal stricture-most commonly in the terminal ileum, can also involve the colon. The occurrence of strictures may complicate feeding plan. Although NEC occurs most commonly in the distal ileum, strictures occur more commonly in the large bowel and 80% are located on the left side. These infants typically develop recurrent abdominal distension 2-3 weeks following recovery.
2. Short gut syndrome-resulting in malabsorption, growth failure, malnutrition.
3. Abscess and fistula formation.
4. Stoma problems.
5. TPN related problems—Cholestasis, infection.
6. Failure to thrive.

Course: In uncomplicated cases of NEC, the long term prognosis may be comparable to that of low birth weight babies. Those with disease with stage II or stage III have a higher incidence of growth delay, especially growth of head circumference. Gastrointestinal sequalae can occur in 25-35% cases with or without surgery.

Prevention

Prevention of NEC is the ultimate goal. Various preventive strategies have been suggested to reduce or eliminate the risk of NEC:

1. *Exclusive breast-feeding.* Own mother's or expressed breast milk should be used.
2. Delaying enteral feeding in susceptible pre-term infants. Aggressive increase in volume of feeds in these infants should be avoided.
3. Antenatal steroids: may help in maturation of gut.
4. Oral immunoglobulins viz. IgA and IgG may have potential benefit.
5. Reduction or antagonism of inflammatory mediators. Since PAF is a potent NEC inducer, trial of oral PAF antagonists may reduce the incidence and severity of NEC.

SUGGESTED READINGS

1. R.G. Faix, M. Nelson; Neonatal necrotizing enterocolitis: Progress, problems, and prospects, Recent advances in pediatrics, Ed: T.J. David, Vol. 16, 1998, 1-23.
2. J. Singh, S. Sinha, Necrotizing enterocolitis—An unconquered disease, Indian pediatrics, 2002, 139: 229-237.
3. K.R. McAlmon, Necrotizing enterocolitis in Manual of neonatal care, edited by J.P. Cloherty and Ann R. Stark, 5th edition, 2004.
4. B.J. Stoll, R.M.Kleigman, Neonatal necrotizing enterocolitis in Nelson Textbook of pediatrics, 16th edition.Vol. 1, 512-513.
5. M. Singh, Necrotizing enterocolitis in care of the newborn, 5th edition 401-405.
6. M.I. Levene, D.I. Tudehope, M.J. Thearle, Necrotizing enterocolitis, Essentials of neonatal medicine, 3rd edition 267-271.
7. A. Narang. Necrotizing enterocolitis in Challenges in neonatology, Edited by A. Saili 1st edition.

13 Meconium Aspiration Syndrome

J.N. Sharma

Meconium stained amniotic fluid (MSAF) occurs in 7-15% of live-births. Of such infants 5%-10% develop Meconium aspiration syndrome (MAS). 30% of these require mechanical ventilation and 5-10% expire. So, meconium aspiration syndrome is a potentially life-threatening condition.

The majority of term babies donot pass meconium in utero because of the following reasons. At the most distal end of gastrointestinal tract, the meconium cap is particularly viscous. Secondly, pronounced peristaltic movements are unusual in fetus and the sphincter tone is greater in utero than what it is post-partum. At the same time, in preterm deliveries especially before 34 weeks of gestation, passage of meconium in utero is very rare. Even with severe asphyxia, the anal sphincter does not usually relax in these babies. If meconium staining does occur in a preterm labour, one should consider an alternative cause such as a congenital infection specially that due to listeriosis. The frequency of MSAF rises with advancing gestational age to an extent that around 35% of babies beyond 41 weeks may pass meconium before delivery. Meconium passage prior to birth is most likely to occur in the following three situations:

1. Post-term babies.
2. Term babies with asphyxia.
3. Babies with IUGR.

Recently intrauterine infection by gram negative organism has been implicated as a cause of meconium passage in utero. The bacterial endotoxin is thought to be a potent bioactive agent that stimulates gastro intestinal peristalsis.

Definition

The diagnosis of MAS is made on the basis of presence of any two of the following features:

1. Meconium staining of liquor or staining of nails/umbilical cord/skin, presence of meconium in oro-pharynx or trachea or both.
2. Respiratory distress having onset soon after birth.
3. Radiological evidences of aspiration pneumonia with areas of atelectasis and hyperinflation.

Mechanism of Meconium Aspiration

The fetus normally swallows the amniotic fluid. Although the fetus exhibits breathing like movements in utero, the fluid does not enter the trachea except during episodes of severe hypoxia. In majority of cases meconium passed during labour and delivery may be initially swallowed into the oropharynx and subsequently aspirated into tracheo-bronchial tree with the first breath only.

Pathophysiology

Passage of thick meconium that is not uniformly mixed with amniotic fluid has the potential of obstructing a large airway. On the other hand, meconium uniformly mixed with amniotic fluid has a uniform distribution and when inspired is spread to the smaller bronchioles.

Meconium aspiration leads to 5 major effects viz. airway obstruction, surfactant dysfunction, chemical pneumonia, sepsis and persistent pulmonary hypertension.

In infants with significant meconium aspiration obstruction of large and small airway can occur. Partial obstruction of airway may lead to activation of ball valve mechanism creating potential for development of emphysema, pneumothorax, pneumomediastinum or pneumopericardium. Complete obstruction leads to atelectasis and ventilation-perfusion mismatch.

Surfactant dysfunction may occur due to cytotoxic effects of meconium on type II pneumocytes and decreased levels of surfactant proteins A and B. There is increased airway resistance and reduced compliance of lungs. Several constituents of meconium especially free fatty acids have a higher minimal surface tension and strip it from the alveolar surface resulting in diffuse atelectasis.

Constituents of meconium (enzymes, bile-salts and fat) also have an irritative and toxic effect on the lining of the airways. There is marked alveolar and parenchymal inflammation and edema with leakage of protein into airways. There is release of inflammatory mediators like cytokines (TNF, IL-1B and IL-8). All these lead to chemical peumonia.

Meconium adversely affects neutrophil function by inhibiting oxidative burst and phagocytosis with increased risk of infection. Further, although meconium per se is sterile it can be a good culture medium for micro-organisms specially E.Coli and Staph. aureus.

Pulmonary vasoconstriction occurs due to release of a large number of mediators (leukotrienes, endothelium 1, PGE2) in the alveoli and blood stream. Right to left (R-L) shunt then occurs both at the pulmonary and cardiac levels. R-L shunt occurs both through foramen ovale and patent ductus arteriosus. This condition is clinically and physiologically similar to persistent fetal circulation and is classified as persistent pulmonary hypertension of newborn (PPHN) secondary to MAS.

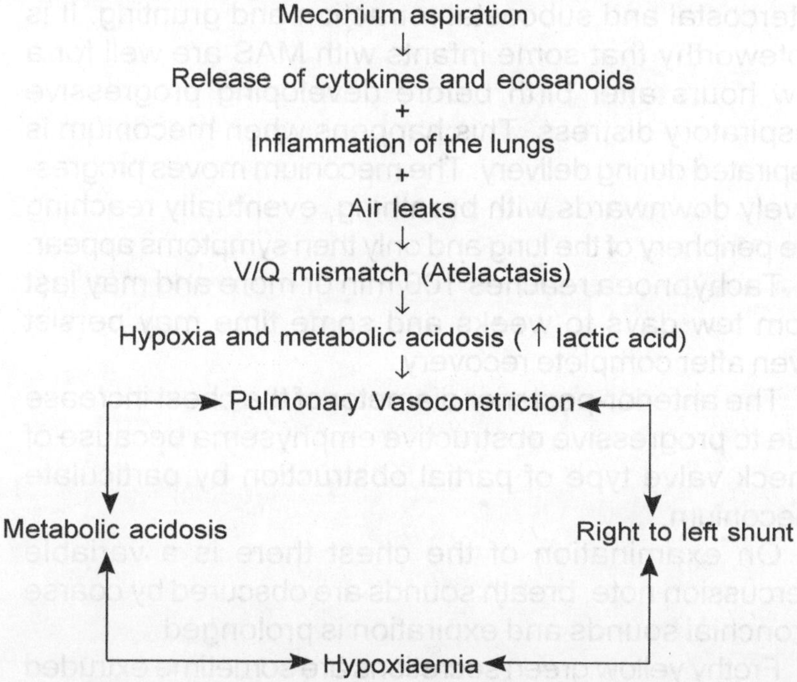

This vicious cycle is often difficult to terminate and results in heart failure, cerebral edema, and bleeding, renal failure and tissue damage. Hypoxemia also causes metabolic abnormalities like hyponatremia due to SIADH as a result of cerebral hypoxia and hypoxic insult of kidney.

Clinical Manifestations

The infant with MAS may be normal term, but are usually post term or small for date. There may be meconium staining of the umbilical cord, nails and skin.

The aspiration of meconium can occur in utero, during the process of birth or after birth. These babies are usually born with severe intra-partum or neonatal asphyxia and needs vigorous resuscitation.

After resuscitation initial apnea is followed by progressive respiratory distress with marked suprasternal, intercostal and subcostal retraction and grunting. It is noteworthy that some infants with MAS are well for a few hours after birth before developing progressive respiratory distress. This happens when meconium is aspirated during delivery. The meconium moves progressively downwards with breathing, eventually reaching the periphery of the lung and only then symptoms appear.

Tachypnoea reaches 100/min or more and may last from few days to weeks and some time may persist even after complete recovery.

The anterior-posterior diameter of the chest increase due to progressive obstructive emphysema because of check valve type of partial obstruction by particulate meconium.

On examination of the chest there is a variable percussion note, breath sounds are obscured by coarse bronchial sounds and expiration is prolonged.

Frothy yellow green secretions are sometime extruded from the mouth.

MAS may exhibit cerebral, cardiac and renal manifestations. Signs of cerebral irritation viz. jitteriness, seizures resulting from cerebral edema, bleeding caused by hypoxia or both may appear soon after birth or later.

Hypotension is found in severely asphyxiated infants. Cardiomegaly, tachypnea, severe cyanosis not responding to adequate ventilation and oxygenation (PPHN) may mimic congenital cyanotic heart disease. The course of the disease is progressive during the initial 48-72 hours.

Laboratory Investigations

1. *Radiological findings:* Abnormal X-rays of chest are found in 50-80% cases. It is notable that endotracheal suction at birth reduces the occurrences of abnormal

X-ray. Moreover, severity of X-ray findings does not always correlate with clinical disease. X-ray of chest taken 1-2 hours after birth (Fig. 13.1) exhibits mechanical effects of meconium aspiration i.e. hyperinflation—hypertranslusance of lungs, flat diaphragm (>7 intercoastal space) horizontal alignment of ribs, and increased cardio-thoracic ratio.

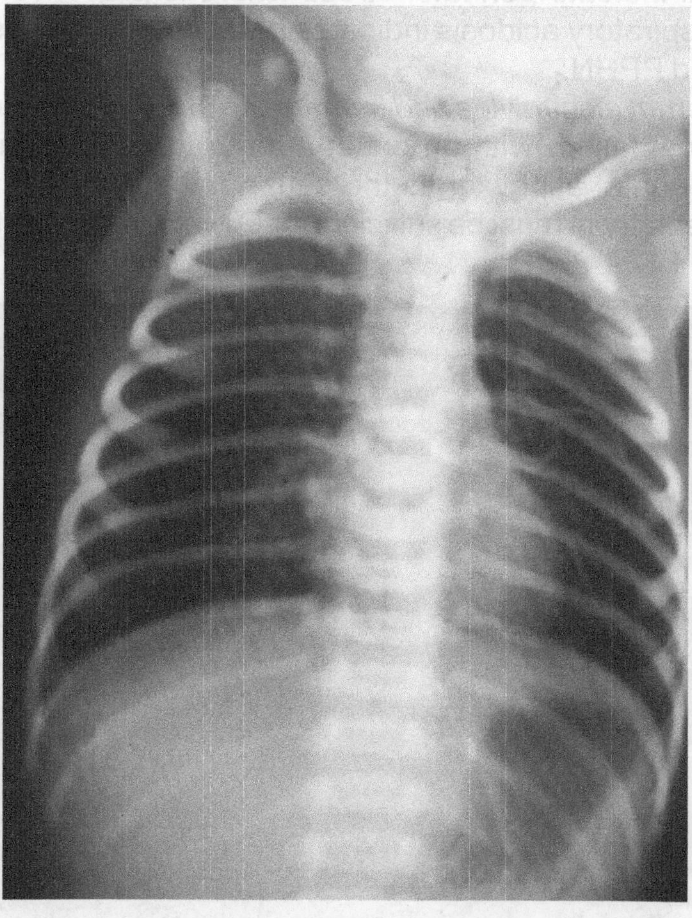

Fig. 13.1

The chemical effects of MAS i.e. consolidation and atelactasis characterized by coarse irregular pattern of increased density throughout the lungs (Fig. 13.2), air-leaks, pleural effusion in the transverse fissure is more prominent after 8-12 hours.

2. *Sepsis screen:* Infection should be excluded because it may be the cause of perinatal stress.
3. *Arterial blood gases:* Presence of metabolic acidosis will indicate perinatal stress whereas presence of respiratory acidosis indicates parenchymal disease and PPHN.
4. *Serum electrolytes and hematocrit:* SIADH and acute renal failure with an onset after 24 hours indicate perinatal asphyxia as the cause rather than MAS. Hematocrit must be sufficient for O_2 carrying capacity.

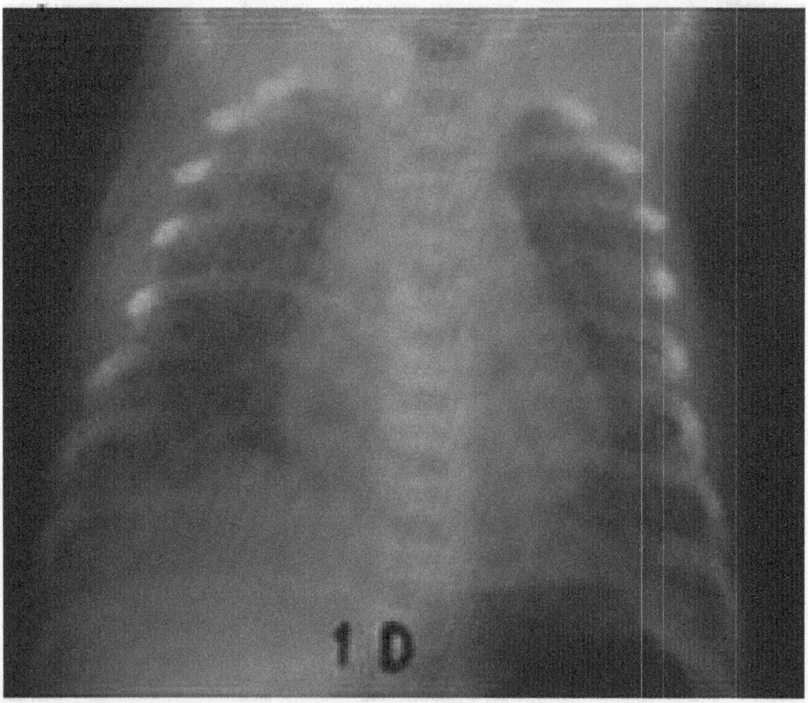

Fig. 13.2

Management

For optimum results in management of MAS, the cooperation of Obstetrician and Pediatrician/ Neonatologist is mandatory. All high-risk pregnancy should be monitored closely. Anticipation as well as prevention of perinatal asphyxia and meconium aspiration and adequate resuscitation at birth is important.

High Risk Pregnancies to be Monitored

Mothers at risk of utero placental insufficiency include the following:

1. Mothers with pre eclamptic toxemia, pregnancy induced hypertension, chronic respiratory and cardiovascular disease.
2. Mothers with poor uterine growth, postmaturity and smoking habit.

Meconium Stained Amniotic Fluid (MSAF) as a Sign of Fetal Distress

That passage of meconium in utero is an independent marker of fetal distress has been questioned. In fact, fetal bradycardia and fetal heart rate deceleration are the recognized signs of fetal distress. Passage of meconium along with fetal arrhythmia is only recognized as true signs of fetal distress and decompensation. MSAF with normal fetal heart rate represents either previous hypoxia or a state of compensated fetal distress until proved otherwise. The view regarding significance of in utero passage of meconium in breech presentation is still inconsistent. It is thought that it occurs due to perinatal stimulation and squeezing of buttocks. However, it should be noted that intrauterine passage of meconium with breech still high at pelvic brim must be given equal importance as with vertex presentation. Fore Meconium (i.e. when present in fore-water) generally represent early decompensation and may be a marker of fetal hypoxia than hind meconium (when meconium is present in hind water).

Prevention of Meconium Aspiration

The risk of meconium aspiration is decreased by the following:

1. Careful monitoring for fetal distress.
2. Amnio-infusion.
3. Suctioning of oropharynx after head is delivered.

Careful Monitoring

Mothers who are at risk of utero-placental insufficiency include those with toxemia or heavy smokers, those with chronic respiratory or cardiovascular disease, those with poor intrauterine growth and those beyond their expected date of confinement. These women should be carefully monitored during pregnancy and fetal heart rate (late deceleration, poor beat to beat variability) should be monitored during labour, with fetal scalp blood pH obtained when indicated.

Amnioinfusion

The use of transcervical amino infusion with warm normal saline solution in women where labour is complicated by thick meconium and oligohydramnios has been extensively studied in the past decade. Although initial reports concerning amnioinfusion were quite promising, the recent publications suggest that amnioinfusion is of little benefit and may actually contribute to mortality.

Suctioning of Oropharynx

Aspiration of meconium before delivery, during birth, or during resuscitation can cause severe aspiration pneumonia. Although some studies suggested that intrapartum suctioning might be effective for decreasing the risk of aspiration, subsequent evidence from a large multicentric randomized trial did not show an effect. Therefore, current recommendation no longer advises routine intrapartum oropharyngeal and nasopharyngeal suctioning for infants born to mothers with meconium staining of amniotic fluid.

Treatment

Infants who are depressed at birth and have had meconium sucked from the trachea are at risk of meconium aspiration syndrome. These neonates:

1. Should be admitted to NICU and observed for respiratory distress.
2. A chest X-ray taken at this stage may help to determine which infants are more likely to have respiratory distress.
3. A sepsis screen should be ordered to exclude infection.
4. Monitoring of O_2 saturation during this period aids assessment of the severity of infant's condition and allows prevention of hypoxemia.

   The treatment plan depends on the severity of MAS:
   - *Mild MAS/Sub clinical MAS:* Majority of babies suffer from mild MAS. The Silverman score is usually less than 3. The neonate can maintain normal arterial oxygen saturation without oxygen therapy. These babies improve within 24-48 hrs. No treatment is required.
   - *Moderate MAS:* The respiratory distress measures between 3 and 6 on Silverman score. Baby may require a FiO_2 of <0.4 to maintain normal arterial oxygen saturation. Clinical improvement takes place within 48-72 hours with adequate oxygen therapy.

- *Severe MAS:* The Silverman score in neonates with severe MAS is usually more than 6. Baby needs high oxygen concentration (FiO2>0.5) to maintain normal arterial blood gas. Artificial ventilation is frequently necessary in these babies.
- *Persistent fetal circulation:* These neonates develop anatomic R-L shunt, severe metabolic acidosis and profound respiratory distress. They usually cannot maintain normal arterial blood gas without mechanical ventilation. (See Table on next Page)

Supportive Care

1. Maintenance of an optimal thermal environment and minimal handling of these babies.
2. Prevention and treatment of hypoglycemia and significant metabolic acidosis.
3. Fluid and electrolyte balance to be monitored and corrected. Perinatal distress and severe respiratory distress preclude feeding. Intravenous fluid therapy should begin with adequate 10% dextrose infusion to prevent hypoglycemia.
4. Monitoring of renal function by maintaining fluid input/ intake and urinary output.
5. Management of hypoxemia:
   - Increasing inspired oxygen by monitoring blood gases.
   - CPAP if FiO_2 requirements exceed 0.40.
   - Mechanical ventilation is indicated when $PaCO_2$ >60 mm Hg and PaO_2 < 50 mm Hg.
6. Newer modalities of treatment:
   - High frequency oscillatory or jet ventilation.
   - Exogenous surfactant therapy.
   - Inhaled nitric oxide.
   - Extra corporeal membrane oxygenation.

Silverman Anderson Score and Its Interpretation

Score	*Upper chest retraction*	*Lower chest retraction*	*Xiphoid retraction*
0	Synchronized	None	None
1	Lag during inspiration	Just visible	Just visib
2	Sea saw	Marked	Marked

None of these modalities have been shown to be superior to conventional ventilation in the treatment of MAS. They may be tried in cases refractory to conventional treatment.

Prognosis

Mortality is high. Residual lung problem are rare but include symptomatic cough, wheezing and persistent hyperinflation for 5-10 years. Ultimate prognosis depends on the extent of central nervous system injury from asphyxia, presence of associated problems with persistent fetal circulation.

SUGGESTED READINGS

1. Wiswell E Thomas and Fuloria Mamta. The Meconium aspiration syndrome: The saga continues. Indian Pediatr 1998;35:1059-1061.
2. Cleayg M and Wiswell TE. Meconium stained amniotic fluid and the meconium aspiration syndrome: An update. Pediatr. Clin. North Am. 1998;45:511-529.
3. Narang A, Nair PM, Bhakoo ON, Vasisth K. Management of Meconium stained amniotic fluid: A team approach. Indian Pediatr 1993;30:9 -13.
4. Finlay RD, Tacusch HW, Walter FJ. Surfactant replacement therapy for meconium aspiration syndrome. Pediatrics 1996;97:48-52.
5. The neonatal inhaled Nitric oxide study group. Inhaled nitric oxide in full term and nearly full term infants with hypoxic respiratory failure. New Engl. J. Med. 1997;336: 597-604.
6. MMA Faridi. Management of Meconium aspiration syndrome in Challenges in neonatology. Editor Arvind Saili. Jaypee Brothers, Medical Publishers (P) Ltd., New Delhi, First Edition, 1997.
7. Eichenwald C. Eric. Meconium aspiration syndrome in Textbook of Neonatology. Editor John P. Cloherty,

Eric C. Eichenwald and Ann R. Stark. 5th edition, 2003. Lippincott-Raven Publishers, Philadelphia, New York.

8. Matsuda H and Vidyasagar D. Meconium aspiration syndrome in Textbook of Neonatology. Editor D.Vidyasagar, 1st Indian edition, 1987. Interprint 16-A Naraina II, New Delhi.

14 Approach to Cyanosis in Newborn

J.N. Sharma

Cyanosis is a bluish discoloration of the skin and mucous membrane resulting from an increased concentration of reduced hemoglobin. The level of hemoglobin greatly influences the occurrence of cyanosis. Normally, about 2 gms/dl of reduced hemoglobin is present in the venules. Clinical cyanosis is evident when the amount of reduced hemoglobin in the cutaneous veins reaches about 5 grams/dl. Cyanosis usually is recognized when arterial oxygen saturation is 85% or lower. Cyanosis is recognized at a higher level of oxygen saturation in patients with polycythemia. Because the hemoglobin level is often high in newborn and the peripheral circulation often sluggish, cyanosis may occur at oxygen saturation as high as 90% in this age group.

Detection of Cyanosis

Early detection of cyanosis in the newborn is crucial. Mild cyanosis may be too subtle for early detection because of polycythemia and excess of fetal hemoglobin in the early neonatal life. Clubbing of fingers and toes, an associated finding, is not usually manifested until late in the first year of life, even in the presence of severe arterial oxygen saturation.

Clinically, one can look for cyanosis in the lips, finger and toe nails, oral mucous membrane, tip of the tongue, conjunctiva and tip of the nose. The tip of the tongue is a good place to look for cyanosis as its colour is not affected by race or ethnic background and the circulation is not sluggish as in peripheral parts of the body. When in doubt, one should obtain the arterial oxygen saturation by a pulse oximeter or arterial pO_2 by blood gas determination to confirm or rule out central cyanosis.

The normal pO_2 in a one day old infant may be as low as 60 mmHg. In certain congenital cyanotic heart disease with increased pulmonary arterial blood flow, the pO_2 may be more than 60 mmHg and usually does not show a large increase with a hyperoxi test. An arterial oxygen saturation of 90% or above does not completely rule out a cyanotic congenital heart defect. An arterial oxygen saturation of 90% can be seen with a pO_2 of 45 to 50 mmHg in newborns because of the normally leftward oxygen hemoglobin dissociation curve.

Central and Peripheral Cyanosis

The critical level of reduced hemoglobin in the cutaneous veins may result from either desaturation of arterial blood or increased extraction of oxygen by peripheral tissues. Cyanosis secondary to desaturation of arterial blood is called *central cyanosis*. Cyanosis with normal saturation is called *peripheral cyanosis*. The latter occurs as a result of sluggish flow of blood. Peripheral cyanosis has no clinical significance except when associated with circulatory shock. Central cyanosis, on the other hand, is a significant clinical finding and may be associated with central nervous system depression, lung disease, or cyanotic congenital heart disease. *Circumoral cyanosis* refers to a bluish skin color around the mouth. It reflects a sluggish capillary blood flow and arterial oxygen saturation is normal. It may be seen in healthy infants with vasoconstriction from exposure to cold. Isolated circumoral cyanosis is of no concern unless it occurs with other signs of low cardiac output. *Differential cyanosis* is a condition where the infant present with a pink upper and a cyanotic lower body with accompanying difference in the oxygen saturation and arterial pO_2. It indicates a right to left ductal shunt and suggest persistent pulmonary hypertension of the newborn or obstructive lesions of the left side of the heart e.g. severe aortic stenosis, coarctation of aorta, interrupted aortic arch with a right to left ductal shunt.

Table 14.1: Causes and clinical features of central cyanosis

1. *Central nervous system depression*
   - Perinatal asphyxia
   - Heavy maternal sedation
   - Intra uterine fetal distress

   Clinical features
   - Shallow irregular respiration
   - Poor muscle tone
   - Cyanosis that disappears on stimulation or oxygen inhalation
   - Increase in pO_2 with oxygen administration
2. *Pulmonary disease*
   - Parenchymal lung disease viz. hyaline membrane disease, atelectasis
   - Pneumothorax, pleural effusion
   - Diaphragmatic hernia
   - Persistent pulmonary hypertension

   Clinical features
   - Tachypnea and respiratory distress with retraction and expiratory grunt
   - Crackles and or decreased breath sounds on auscultation
   - Chest X-ray film may reveal cause
   - Oxygen administration improves or abolishes cyanosis
   - Increase in pO_2 with oxygen administration
3. *Cardiac disease*
   - Congenital heart diseases with right to left shunt

   Clinical features
   - Tachypnoea with mild or no retraction
   - Heart murmur may be present on auscultation
   - Chest X-ray may show an abnormal cardiac silhouette, increased or decreased pulmonary vascular markings.
   - No improvement of cyanosis on oxygen administration

Table 14.2: Clinical findings of central cyanosis

Clinical findings	*CNS depression*	*Pulmonary disease*	*Cardiac disease*
1. Respiration	Shallow irregular	Tachypnoea, retractions, Grunt	Tachypnea without grunt
2. Muscle tone	Poor	Normal	Normal
3. Cyanosis	disappears on Stimulation/ O_2	Improves/ abolishes on O_2 adm.	Not much affected
4. Auscultation	Normal	crackles &/or decreased breath sounds	Murmur may be present
5. CXR	normal	reveal cause in lungs	Abnormal heart/ pulmonary vasculature
6. Hyperoxitest	Increases pO_2	Increases pO_2	Little or no increase in PO_2

Hyperoxitest

The determination of arterial blood gas levels clarifies the type of cyanosis–peripheral or central. Hyperoxitest helps to differentiate cyanosis caused by cardiac disease from that caused by pulmonary disease.

Oxygen Dissociation Curve

It is useful to know the oxygen dissociation curve in the newborn before discussing the hyperoxitest. The position of the oxygen dissociation curve is an expression of the affinity of hemoglobin for oxygen. In the newborn, the curve is shifted to the left. This is a result of high percentage of fetal hemoglobin in the newborn which has a high affinity to oxygen but does not allow release of oxygen to tissues. The adult curve is on the right as adult hemoglobin has less affinity for oxygen and allows release of oxygen to tissues. The newborn curve is replaced by the adult curve by 3 months of age.

Steps of Hyperoxitest

1. The arterial PO_2 is measured.
2. Oxygen should be administered through a plastic hood for atleast 10 minutes so that the alveolar oxygen is replaced completely with 100% oxygen administered.
3. The arterial oxygen is measured again and compared.

Interpretation

1. Arterial oxygen concentration rises above 100 mm Hg: indicates pulmonary disease.
2. Rise in arterial oxygen concentration does not exceed 100 mmHg, and the rise not more than 10-30 mmHg: indicates significant intracardiac right to left shunt.
3. Arterial pO_2 from the right radial artery is 10-15 mm Hg higher than that from an umbilical artery catheter: indicates right to left ductal shunt.

Points to be Noted:

1. The response of pO_2 to 100% oxygen inhalation should be interpreted in the light of clinical picture, especially the degree of pulmonary pathology seen on chest X-ray.
2. Some infants with cyanotic congenital heart defects with a large pulmonary blood flow viz. total anomalous pulmonary venous return may have a rise in arterial pO_2 to 100 mmHg or higher.
3. Conversely, infants with a massive intrapulmonary shunt from lung disease (but with a normal heart) may not show rise in arterial pO_2 to 100 mmHg.
4. Arterial blood samples for measurement of pO_2 should be obtained from the upper part of the body viz. radial, brachial or temporal arteries to avoid false low values caused by a right to left ductal shunt. If a low value is obtained from an umbilical artery line or from a lower

extremity artery, another sample from the right radial, brachial or temporal artery should be obtained and should be compared with a simultaneously obtained sample from an artery of the lower part of the body.

Management of the Cyanotic Newborn

The management of a cyanotic newborn includes the following steps:

1. Confirmation of cyanosis.
2. Confirmation whether peripheral or central cyanosis.
3. Confirm cause: Pulmonary, cardiac or CNS.
4. Laboratory investigations:
   a. An X-ray chest.
   b. ECG.
   c. Arterial blood gas in room air.
   d. Hyperoxitest.

X-ray findings in some common congenital cyanotic heart disease

X-ray findings	*Congenital heart disease*
1. An egg shaped heart with narrow waist	D–TGA
2. Snow man appearance with pulmonary venous congestion	TAPVR
3. Concave pulmonary segment, boot shaped heart, oligemic lung fields	TOF
4. Extreme cardiomegaly	Ebstein anomaly

D-TGA= dextro transposition of great arteries, TAPVR = total anomalous pulmonary venous return, TOF = tetralogy of fallot

Approach to Suspected Congenital Cyanotic Heart Disease

If central cyanosis is present or if the arterial oxygen saturation cannot be raised to a satisfactory level with administration of 100% oxygen, a cardiac consultation, an echo and a doppler examination will reveal the cardiac lesion responsible for central cyanosis. A physical

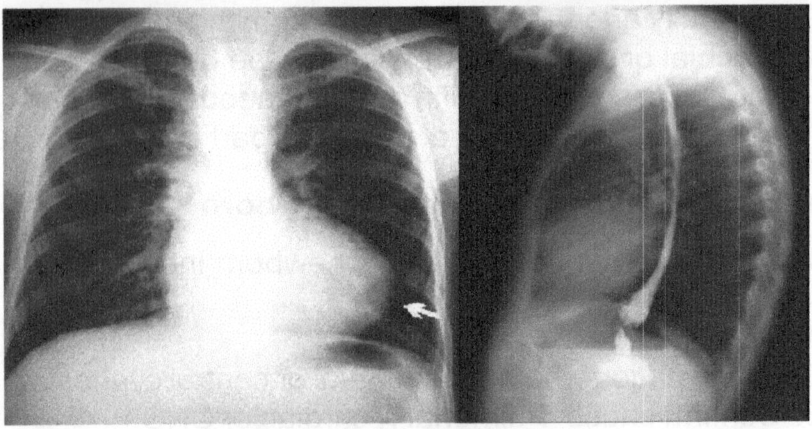

Fig. 14.1: Tetralogy of Fallot

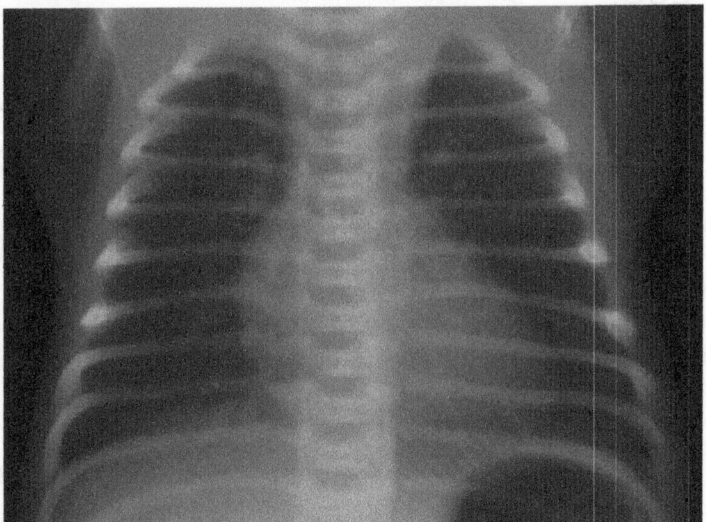

Fig. 14.2: D Transposition of great vessels (D- TGA)

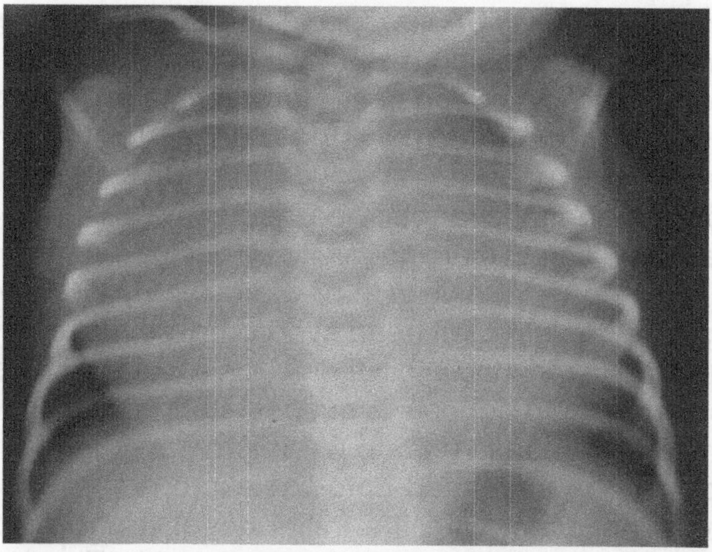

Fig. 14.3: Ebstein anomaly

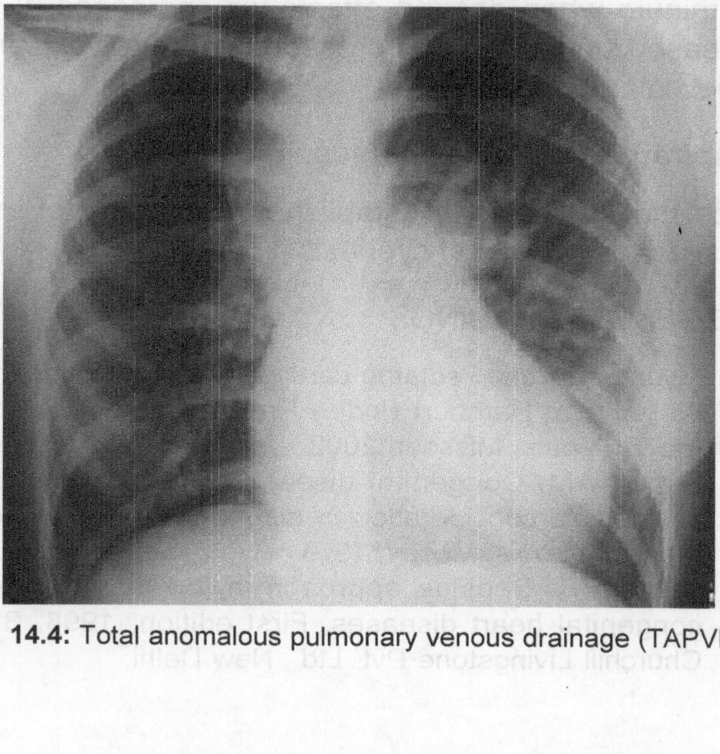

Fig. 14.4: Total anomalous pulmonary venous drainage (TAPVR)

examination, X-ray PA view chest and ECG do not help as much in diagnosing a cyanotic heart disease as in diagnosing a acyanotic defect. However these tools can be sometimes useful, atleast in reducing the possibilities.

If a congenital cyanotic heart defect is suspected, especially a defect that appears to be ductus dependent (e.g. pulmonary atresia with or without VSD, tricuspid atresia, hypoplastic left heart syndrome, severe coarctation of aorta) prostaglandin E_1 infusion should be started as soon as the diagnosis is suspected or established. The starting dose is 0.05 to 0.1 micro gm /kg/ minute which can be increased upto 0.4 micro gm/minute if there is no effect with the initial dose. It should be administered as a continuous intravenous drip. The dose should be reduced step by step to 0.01 micro gm/minute when desired effects viz. increased pO_2, increased systemic blood pressure, improved pH, are achieved.

Respiratory and CNS Causes

Once the diagnosis is established, treatment of the cause leads to relief of cyanosis.

SUGGESTED READINGS

1. Myung K. Park Pediatric cardiology for practitioners, 4th edition, Harcourt (India) Private Limited, Mosby Inc. St. Louis, Missouri 2002.
2. Rudolf AM. Congenital disease of heart: Clinical-physiologic consideration in diagnosis and management, St. Louis, Mosby, 1974
3. Tandon R. Bedside approach in the diagnosis of congenital heart diseases. First edition, 1998. B.I. Churchill Livingstone Pvt. Ltd., New Delhi.

15 Approach to Anemia in Newborn

J.N. Sharma

Anemia in newborn is defined as a hemoglobin level less than 12 gm/dl in the first week, or less than 10 gm/dl after the first week.

Embryonic Hematopoiesis

Embryonic hematopoiesis begins by the 20th day of gestation and is evidenced as blood islands in the yolk sac. In mid gestation, erythropoiesis occurs in the liver and spleen. The bone marrow becomes the predominant site in the last trimester. Fetal hemoglobin increases with advancing gestational age. Hemoglobin concentration increases from 8-10 grams/dl at 12 weeks to 16.5 to 18.0 grams/dl at 40 weeks. At term the cord blood hemoglobin is 16.8 gm/dl (14-20 gm/dl). The hemoglobin levels in VLBW infants are 1-2 gms/dl below those at term.

The Normal Hemoglobin Curve

After birth, hemoglobin levels increase transiently at 6-12 hours. Thereafter, in the term infants, there is a decline of the hemoglobin level to 11 gm/dl at 3-6 months. In the preterm babies, those born before 32 weeks, the hemoglobin levels at birth is 1-2 gms/dl lower than in term and the post natal decline of hemoglobin level is more rapid. At 8-12 weeks, the hemoglobin levels reach their nadir. In infants who receive blood transfusion in the neonatal period have lower nadirs than normal because of their higher percentage of adult hemoglobin. The hemoglobin levels in the newborn period differ on the basis of gestation, birth weight and day of life as follows:

Week	*Hemoglobin level (gm/dl)*		
	Term infants	*Preterm infants (1.2-2.5 kg)*	*Preterm (< 1.2 kg)*
0	17.0	16.4	16.0
1	18.8	16.0	14.8
3	15.9	13.5	13.4
6	12.7	10.7	9.7

Source: Avery's diseases of the newborn, 1991, Philadelphia, Saunders.

Hemoglobin Nadir in Infants

The hemoglobin nadir differs according to the gestation and birth weight of the neonate as follows:

Gestation/ birth weight	*Hemoglobin level at nadir*	*Time of nadir*
Term	9.5-11.0 gm/dl	6-12 weeks
Preterm (1.2-2.5 kg)	8.0-10.0 gm/dl	5-10 weeks
Preterm (< 1.2 kg)	6.5 - 9.0 gm/dl	4-8 weeks

Source: Avery's diseases of newborn, 1991, Philadelphia, Saunders.

Type of Hemoglobin

In the fetus, hemoglobin synthesis in the last two trimesters of pregnancy produces fetal hemoglobin (Hemoglobin F). Synthesis of adult hemoglobin (Hemoglobin A) starts immediately prior to term. Hence, the term infant should have some adult hemoglobin. At birth, fetal hemoglobin represents 60-90% of total hemoglobin. The levels of fetal hemoglobin decline to adult levels of less than 5 grams/dl by 3-4 months of age.

Other Hematological Parameters

The blood volume of the term infant is approximately 85 ml/kg. The placenta and umbilical vessels contain approximately 20-30 ml/kg of additional blood. Hence, delayed clamping of the umbilical cord at birth can transiently increase the blood volume and hemoglobin levels for the first three days of life. Delayed clamping increases the risk of polycythemia, increased pulmonary vascular resistance, hypoxia and hyperbilirubinemia but improves glomerular filtration. Early clamping, on the other hand, may result in anemia, poor peripheral perfusion, but lower pulmonary vascular pressures. To avoid both situations, the cord clamping should be done approximately 30 seconds after birth. Immediately after delivery the infant should be placed below the level of the placenta to avoid feto-placental transfusion. If the infant is kept above the level of the placenta, hydrostatic pressure affects blood transfer between the placenta and the infant at birth resulting in an undesired feto maternal transfusion.

Table 15.1: Showing other RBC values in term and preterm infants

	Hemotocrit (%)	*Reticulocytes (%)*
Term		
Cord blood	45-61	< 7
Day 1	58	< 7
Day 3	55	< 3
Day 7	54	<1
Preterm (birth weight < 1500 grams)		
Cord blood	49	< 10
Day 7	45	< 3

Source: Avery's Diseases of Newborn, 2005, Philadelphia, Saunders.

Etiology

Symptomatic anemia in newborn may be a result of:

1. Blood loss.

2. Decreased red cell production.
3. Hemolysis.

Blood loss may be acute following fetomaternal hemorrhage, rupture of umbilical cord, placenta previa and internal hemorrhage. Chronic blood loss may be due to chronic feto maternal hemorrhage, twin to twin transfusion.

Decreased red cell production due to causes like perinatal congenital infections, Diamond Blackfan syndrome, Osteopetrosis presents with resistant anemia.

Hemolysis due to causes like ABO and Rh hemolytic disease of newborn, red cell enzyme deficiency e.g. G6PD deficiency, RBC membrane defects e.g. Hereditary spherocytosis etc. presents with anemia with associated features.

Table 15.2: Causes of anemia in newborn

	Blood loss	*Decreased production*	*Hemolysis*
Common	Fetal-maternal bleed	Perinatal congenital infections	Rh HDN
	Placenta previa	Anemia of prematurity	ABO HDN
	Abruptio placentae Twin to twin transfusion		Minor gr. HDN
Rare	Vasa previa	Parvo virus infection	RBC enzyme deficiency
	Rupture of cord	Diamond Blackfan syndrome	Hemoglobinopathy
	Hepatic hematoma	Osteopetrosis	RBC membrane defect
	Splenic hematoma	Congenital leukemia	DIC
	Retro peritoneal hemorrhage	Congenital neuro-blastoma Sideroblastic anemia	SLE in mother

Table 15.3: Causes according to onset of anemia

Early anemia (within 7 days)

1. Fetomaternal hemorrhage
2. Twin to twin transfusion
3. Placental causes:
   - Placenta praevia
   - Vasa praevia
   - Abruptio placentae
   - Incision of placenta at caesarean section
4. Fetoplacental transfusion after delivery
5. Hemolysis:
   - Rh and ABO isoimmunization
   - Alpha thalassemia
   - Intrauterine infection specially rubella, parvo virus
   - Bacterial infection

Late anemia (after 7 days)

1. Hemorrhage:
   - Small perinatal bleeding
   - Excessive blood sampling
   - Hemorrhagic disease of newborn
   - Intraventricular hemorrhage
   - Chronic G.I. bleed
2. Hemolysis:
   - Rh and ABO isoimmunization
   - Sepsis and DIC
   - Hemoglobinopathies
   - Congenital spherocytosis
   - Vitamin E deficiency
3. Decreased red cell production:
   - Anemia of prematurity
   - Infection (bacterial/viral)
   - Folic acid deficiency
   - Drugs
   - Diamond blackfan syndrome
   - Congenital leukemia
   - Osteopetrosis

Clinical Manifestation

Anemia at birth can manifest as pallor, congestive cardiac failure or shock depending on the cause and rapidity of blood loss.

Acute blood loss is characterized by pallor, peripheral circulatory collapse and shock. Chronic blood loss presents with marked pallor, heart failure, hepatosplenomegaly with or without hydrops.

Anemia due to decreased red cell production presents at birth with pallor and associated physical signs of the parent disease.

Hemolysis in utero may result in erythroblastosis fetalis or the fetus may be spared and hemolytic disease may appear in the newborn infant. Erythroblastosis fetalis is classically due to Rh blood group incompatibility. ABO blood group incompatibility with sensitization usually do not cause fetal disease except for mild anemia. However, it may produce hemolytic disease of newborn characterized by significant anemia and hyperbilirubinemia. In fact ABO incompatibility is the most common cause of isoimmune hemolysis of the newborn infant.

Table 15.4: Clinical presentations

1. Acute blood loss:
   - Shock
   - No signs of extramedullary hematopoesis, no hepatosplenomegaly
2. Chronic blood loss:
   - Marked pallor
   - Signs of heart failure
   - Hepatosplenomegaly
   - Features of hydrops
3. Decreased Red blood cell production:
   - Pallor at birth
   - Associated physical features of the parent disease
4. Hemolysis:
   - Only pallor
   - Pallor with jaundice
   - Pallor with jaundice and hepatosplenomegaly

Severe Anemia with Shock and Severe Asphyxia

Infants born with acute blood loss during or before delivery are often limp, pale, with shock at birth. They need to be differentiated from severely asphyxiated newborns with peripheral circulatory failure.

Table 15.5: Salient differences between severe asphyxia and anemia with shock

Criteria	*Severe asphyxia*	*Anemia with shock*
1. Antenatal history	H/O fetal distress	H/O blood loss
2. Vitals		
• Respiration	Absent or gasping	Tachypnea, gasping/ Irregular
• Heart rate	Bradycardia	Tachycardia
• Color	May be blue	Pale
• CVP	Normal	Low/high with CCF
3. Response to therapy		
• Intubation and O_2	Dramatic response	No response
• PCV/gasping transfusion	No response	Good response

Laboratory Investigations

Screening tests to be ordered in every case of anemia. The following tests are to be ordered in every case of neonatal anemia which should be followed by specific tests for individual conditions:

1. Hemoglobin, Hematocrit at birth and after 4 hours.
2. Reticulocyte count, MCV, Peripheral blood smear.
3. Blood group and Coombs test.

If blood loss is recent (e.g. at delivery), the hematocrit and reticulocyte count may be normal and the infant may be in shock. The hematocrit will fall later as a result of hemodilution. If the bleeding is chronic, the hematocrit will be low, the reticulocyte increased and the baby is normovolemic.

Other tests to be picked up as necessary:

1. Apt's test to distinguish between fetal and maternal blood.
2. Kleihauer—Betke test of mother's blood to exclude feto-maternal bleed.

3. Serum bilirubin and fractions.
4. Congenital infection screen.
5. Metabolic disease screen.
6. X-ray long bones to exclude osteopetrosis.
7. Sepsis screen and blood culture.
8. Platelet count and coagulation profile.
9. Stool for occult blood.
10. Urine for microscopic examination.
11. Bone marrow.

Tests for Parents

Complete blood count, peripheral smear, RBC indices, RBC enzymes viz. G6PD, pyruvate kinase.

Diagnostic approach to anemia in the newborn

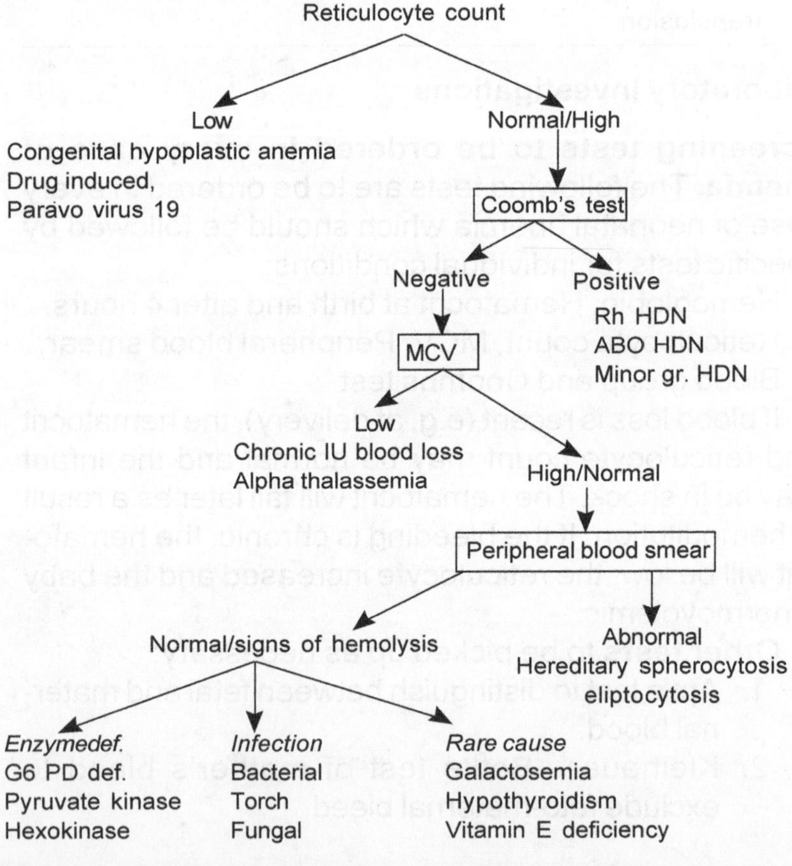

Table 15.6: Laboratory findings and diagnosis

Laboratory findings	*Diagnosis*
1. Presence of fetal hemoglobin in vaginal blood	Fetal hemorrhage
2. Positive Kleihauer-Betke test	Feto-maternal hemorrhage
3. Hematological evidences of iron deficiency anemia	Chronic feto-fetal or feto-maternal hemorrhage
4. Hyperbilirubinemia	Hemolytic anemia Perinatal infection
5. Reticulocytosis	Hemolytic anemia Prematurity Small for date Perinatal asphyxia Chronic feto-maternal hemorrhage

Management

The treatment modality will be different depending on the clinical condition of the child and the cause of anemia. However, a fall of hemoglobin to less than 8 gms/dl (hematocrit < 25%) due to any cause or presence of symptoms viz. poor weight gain, tachypnea, tachycardia, apnea and poor feeding should be treated with transfusion to raise the hemoglobin to 12 gm%. Packed RBCs are usually transfused in the amount 15-20 ml/kg.

Indications of Transfusion

1. *Acute blood loss with signs of peripheral circulatory collapse:* Irrespective of the hemoglobin and hematocrit status these babies will need whole blood transfusion because anemia due to acute blood loss will manifest only after 4-8 hours.

   Type of blood: O Rh negative blood without cross matching.

   Amount: 20-30 ml/kg initially to combat shock.

2. *Infants with severe erythroblastosis:* If the hematocrit is below 30%, a partial exchange transfusion with 50- 80 ml/kg packed red cells (hematocrit 70%) should be performed to raise the hematocrit and increase the oxygen carrying capacity before going for the specific treatment e.g. exchange transfusion in Rh incompatibility.
3. *Transfusion in sick babies:* Infants with significant respiratory disease or congenital heart disease (e.g. large left to right shunt) may need their hematocrit maintained above 40%. Transfusion of adult RBCs provides the added benefit of lowered oxygen affinity, which augments oxygen delivery to tissues.
4. Infants with ABO incompatibility with protracted hemolysis may not require exchange transfusion, but may require a transfusion to correct anemia several weeks after birth.
5. *Preterm babies:* Preterm babies may be comfortable with a hemoglobin level of 6.5 to 7 gm/dl. Sick preterms may need transfusion to increase oxygen carrying capacities. In growing preterms, poor weight gain, apnea, tachypnea, poor feeding indicate need for blood transfusion.
6. *A healthy, asymptomatic newborn* will correct mild anemia on its own if iron intake is adequate.

Blood Component Therapy

Transfusion of other blood components should be advised according to need viz:

- Packed RBC 15-20 ml/kg. Larger volumes need to be given in divided doses.
- Platelet transfusion 1 unit every 12 to 24 hours, for thrombocytopenia.
- FFP, 10-15 ml/kg every 12 to 24 hours in suspected coagulation disorder.

- Both FFP and platelet concentrate every 12 to 24 hours in case of DIC. Fresh blood in small aliquots (10 to 15 ml/kg every 12-24 hours) from a walking donor can be life saving when FFP or platelet concentrate is not available.
- Transfusion of washed platelet packs from mother is the appropriate therapy for replacement of platelet in platelet isoimmunisation.
- Irradiated (5000 rads) or frozen RBCs are recommended in preterm infants weighing less than 1200 grams. Third generation filters helps to deplete leucocyte. Their use reduces the risk of exposure to lymphocytes and cytomegalovirus. For prevention of CMV infection, CMV negative donor blood or blood treated by prestorage leucodestruction can be used.

Drugs

- *Vitamin K:* Vitamin K_1 and K_2 are preferable because synthetic Vitamin K increases the risk of hyperbilirubinemia. A dose 2 mg daily IM should be given in case of hemorrhagic disease of newborn.
- Diuretics (viz. fursemide) for congestive cardiac failure, cardiotonics (viz. dopamine, dobutamine) in case of shock may be used as and when necessary.

SUGGESTED READINGS

1. Helen A. Christou and David H. Rowitch. Anemia in Manual of neonatal care 5th edition, 2003, Editor John P. Cloherty, Eric C. Eichenwald and Ann R Stark. Lippincott Williams and Wilkins. Philadelphia, PA 19106 USA.
2. A Neonatal Vade—Mecum, third edition, 1998, edited by Brian Speidel, Peter Fleming, John Henderson *et al*. Published by Arnold International, London.
3. J.M. Rennie and N.R.C. Roberton. Anemia in neonate in Manual of neonatal intensive care, fourth edition

and first Indian edition 2004, Viva Books Pvt. Ltd, Daryaganj, New Delhi.

4. William C. Mentzer and Bertil E. Glader. Erythrocytic disorders of infancy in Avery's Diseases of newborn, 8th edition, 2005. Philadelphia, Saunders.
5. Gladder B and Nariman JL. Erythrocytic disorders in infancy in Avery's diseases of newborn, 1991. Philadelphia, Saunders.

16 Polycythemia in Newborn

Rukeya Begum

The term polycythemia or erythrocytosis exists when the red cell count, the hemoglobin level and the total RBC volume (hematocrit) all exceeds upper limits of normal. True polycythemia is characterized by increases of both RBC and total blood volume. A decrease in plasma volume can suddenly occur in acute dehydration and burn and result in a high haemoglobin volume value. However, these situations are more accurately designated as hemoconcentration because the RBC mass is not increased and normalization of plasma volume restores the haemoglobin to normal level.

The normal haemoglobin and hematocrit values at different weeks of gestation are as follows:

Weeks of gestation	*Hb gm/dl*	*Hct%*
18-21	11.69 ±1.27	37.3 ± 4.3
22-25	12.2 ±1.6	38.6 ± 3.9
26-29	12.91 ± 1.38	40.9 ± 4.4
>30	13.64 ± 2.21	43.6 ± 7.2
Term	16.5 ± 1.5	51.0 ± 4.5

Physiological Changes in Postnatal Life

Significant changes take place in the hematocrit from cord blood through the first 24 hours of life. The hematocrit peaks at 2 hours of age and a value up to 71% may be normal at this age. It gradually declines to 68% by 6 hours and stabilizes to cord level by 12-24 hours. The initial rise in hematocrit is related to a transudation of fluid from intravascular space.

Definition

Polycythemia in newborn is defined as a venous hematocrit of greater than 65% or a venous hemoglobin concentration more than 22 gm/dl. The hematocrit % is approximately three times the hemoglobin concentration in gm/dl.

Pathophysiology

The primary concern with polycythemia is related to the hemoconcentration and its associated complications. Blood viscosity increases as the hematocrit value rises resulting in abnormal blood flow kinetics. When the hematocrit value increases to more than 60%, hyperviscosity syndrome appears. This manifest as poor flow or sludging of blood. This predisposes the newborn to decrease tissue oxygenation, fall in plasma glucose and a tendency to form micro thrombi. If these events occur in the cerebral cortex, kidneys and adrenal glands, significant damage may result. Hence this condition requires urgent diagnosis and prompt management.

The viscosity of blood is directly proportional to the hematocrit and inversely proportional to the deformability of red blood cell. Newborns have erythrocytes that are less deformable and filterable than the erythrocytes of adults, predisposing to stasis in microcirculation. The relationship between viscosity and hematocrit is almost linear upto a hematocrit of 42%. After that it rises exponentially. In non-polycythemic newborn, the viscosity may result from an increase in plasma proteins especially fibrinogen, platelets, endothelial factor and local blood flow.

Viscosity is measured by Wells-Brookfield cone plate micro viscometer. Since the instruments are not readily available in most neonatal intensive care units, hyperviscosity is usually suspected in the presence of suggestive symptoms and abnormally high hematocrits.

Incidence

The incidence of polycythemia is 1.5-4% of all live births. The incidence is higher among small for gestational age (SGA) and large for gestational age (LGA) infants. The neonates born to mothers at high altitude have a higher incidence of polycythemia. The haemoglobin level increases about 4% for each rise of 1000 metre in altitude. The incidence of polycythemia is 15% among term SGA infants as compared to 2% in term appropriate for gestational age (AGA) infants. The hematocrit is lower with increasing prematurity. So polycythemia is seen less frequently in preterm infants than in term babies. It is unlikely to occur in neonates born at a gestational age less 34 weeks.

Causes of Neonatal Polycythemia

A. *Hyper transfusion:*

1. Delayed cord clamping allows for an increased blood volume to be delivered to the infant. When cord clamping is delayed more than 3 minutes after birth, blood volume increases by 30% as compared to early cord clamping within 30 seconds.
2. Gravity also may be a factor when the delivered baby is hold below the level of the maternal introitus.
3. Twin to twin transfusion syndrome due to a vascular communication occurs in approximately 10% of monozygotic twin pregnancies.

4. Maternal fetal transfusion may occur.
5. As a result of intrapartum asphyxia, the direction of blood flow in the umbilical cord tends to be toward the fetus.
6. Cord strippling i.e. pushing more blood into the infants can cause hyper transfusion.

B. *Placental insufficiency (resulting in increased fetal erythropoiesis secondary to chronic intrauterine hypoxia):*
1. Small for gestational age infants (increased number of nucleated RBC in IUGR babies is a marker of intrauterine hypoxia).
2. Maternal hypertension syndromes (toxemia, renal disease, etc).
3. Post mature infants.
4. Infants born to mothers with chronic hypoxia (heart disease, pulmonary disease).
5. Pregnancy at high altitude—results in hypoxic polycythemia.
6. Maternal smoking.

C. *Other conditions:*
1. Infants of diabetic mothers (increased erythropoiesis correlates with macrosomia).
2. Some large for gestational age (LGA) babies.
3. Endocrine abnormalities secondary to increased oxygen consumption resulting in fetal hypoxia may be due to congenital thyrotoxicosis, congenital adrenal hyperplasia, and Beckwith-Wiedemann syndrome.
4. Genetic disorders (eg, trisomy 18, trisomy 21) also may cause inutero hypoxia.
5. Drugs (maternal use of propranolol).
6. Dehydration of infant.

Clinical Features

Most infants with polycythemia are asymptomatic. The symptomatic neonates may have the following features:

1. *Central nervous system (CNS):* Poor feeding, lethargy, hypotonia, apnea, tremors, seizures, cerebral venous thrombosis.
2. *Cardio respiratory:* Cyanosis, tachypnoea, heart murmurs, congestive heart failure, cardiomegaly, elevated pulmonary vascular resistance, prominent vascular markings on chest X-ray.
3. *Renal:* Decreased glomerular filtration, decreased sodium excretion, renal vein thrombosis, hematuria, proteinuria.
4. *Others:* Thrombosis, thrombocytopenia, increased jaundice, persistent hypoglycemia, hypocalcemia, testicular infarcts, necrotizing enterocolitis, priapism, disseminated intravascular coagulation.

All of these symptoms may be associated with polycythemia/hyperviscosity but may not be caused by it. They are common symptoms in many neonatal disorders.

Screening for Polycythemia

Screening should be done for polycythemia in the following high risk groups:

1. Small for gestational age (SGA).
2. Infants of diabetic mothers (IDM).
3. Large for gestational age (LGA) infants.
4. Monochromic twins especially the larger twin.
5. Morphological features of growth retardation.

The screening of high risk neonates is to be done at 2 hours of age. A normal value at 2 hours of age (hematocrit < 65%) does not merit any further screening unless the infant is symptomatic. Hematocrit value > 65% at 2 hours of age merits repeat screening at 12 and 24 hours. Polycythemia is diagnosed when a hematocrit is > 65%. Any infant found to be symptomatic with clinical features suggestive of polycythemia should be examined for polycythemia.

Capillary versus Venous Hematocrit

The capillary blood or peripheral venous hematocrit should be determined when screening for polycythemia is required. Capillary hematocrit measurement depends on regional blood flow and can vary widely from central venous hematocrit measurement. Depending on local perfusion, the capillary blood hematocrit will be 5-20% higher than the central hematocrit. This difference is more apparent in infants receiving large parenteral transfusion. Warming the heel prior to drawing blood for a capillary hematocrit determination will give a better co-relation with the peripheral venous or central venous hematocrit. If the capillary blood hematocrit is above 65%, the peripheral venous hematocrit should be determined.

Methods of Hematocrit Analysis

Two methods are available:

a. *Automated hematology analyzer:* This calculates the hematocrit from a direct measurement of mean cell volume and the hemoglobin.
b. *Micro centrifuge:* Blood is collected in heparinized micro capillaries (110 mm length and 1-2 mm internal diameter) and centrifuged at 10,000-15,000 rounds per minute (rpm) for 3-5 minutes. Plasma separates and the packed cell volume is measured to give the hematocrit.

An automated analyzer gives lower values as compared to hematocrits measured by centrifugation method. Most of the reported data on polycythemia is on centrifuged hematocrits.

Treatment

Before the diagnosis of polycythemia is considered, it is mandatory to exclude dehydration. If the etiology is dehydration then the infant is to be rehydrated over 6-8 hours. The hematocrit is to be repeated after correction of dehydration. Once the diagnosis of polycythemia is made, associated metabolic problems including hypoglycemia should be excluded. Two modes of therapy have been described for polycythemia.

Conservative Management with Hydration

This is tried in asymptomatic polycythemia. An extra fluid of 20 ml per kg may be added to the daily fluid requirement either by enteral route or the parenteral route (I.V. fluids). The rationality of this therapy is hemodilution and the resultant decrease in viscosity. However, this extra fluid therapy may be associated with problems in pre term babies. Hence this mode of therapy is reserved for hemodynamically stable babies with asymptomatic polycythemia under cardio pulmonary monitoring. Hematocrit and glucose level is to be repeated every 6 hourly. The patient is to be observed for symptoms.

Partial Exchange Transfusion (PET)

Indications of partial exchange transfusion are:

1. Presence of symptoms suggestive of hyperviscosity and a hematocrit > 65%.
2. Hematocrit > 70% in an asymptomatic infant.

The aim is to reduce the central hematocrit to 50-55%. The volume of blood to be exchanged is calculated as follows:

$$\text{Volume to be exchanged} = \frac{^{*}\text{Blood volume} \times (\text{Observed hematocrit} - \text{Desired Hct})}{\text{Observed hematocrit}}$$

* Blood volume is estimated to be 80-90 ml/kg in term babies and 90-100 ml/kg in preterm babies. As a rough guide, the volume of blood to be exchanged is usually 20 ml/kg.

Fluids to be used for PET:

1. *Crystalloids:* Normal saline, ringer lactate.
2. *Colloids:* Fresh frozen plasma, 5% albumin.

Crystalloids are preferred because they are cheap and easily available, produce a similar reduction in hematocrit as colloids, and do not have a risk of transfusion associated infections (e.g. HIV, Hepatitis B, C and CMV). Also adult plasma has been shown to increase the viscosity when mixed with fetal erythrocytes.

Route

A partial exchange transfusion may be carried out via the peripheral route by using a peripheral arterial and venous line. Blood is withdrawn from the arterial line and replaced simultaneously with saline via the venous line. A central route requires umbilical vein cannulation and used for both withdrawal of blood and replacement with saline. Alternatively umbilical venous catheter may be used for withdrawing blood and same amount of saline is replaced through a peripheral vein. Both the peripheral and central routes are equally effective in the treatment of polycythemia. Regardless of method used, the aliquots should not exceed approximately 5 ml/kg delivered or removed over 2-3 minutes.

Algorithm for management of Polycythemia

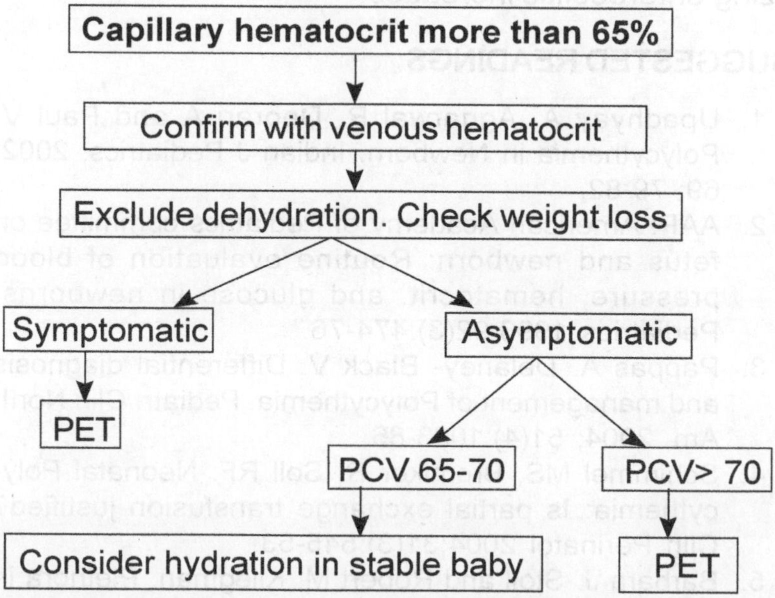

Long Term Outcome with Polycythemia

A partial exchange transfusion reverses the physiological abnormalities associated with polycythemia—hyper viscosity syndrome. It improves capillary perfusion, cerebral blood flow and cardiac function. However there is very little data to suggest that PET improves long term outcome in patients with polycythemia. It is possible that the underlying etiology of polycythemia is a more important determinant of ultimate outcome. Therefore it may be better to do a partial exchange transfusion in this group of neonates since the procedure is safe, quick and is effective in resolving the symptoms.

The long-term prognosis of polycythemic infants is unclear. Reported adverse outcomes include speech deficits, abnormal fine motor control, reduced I.Q., and other neurologic abnormalities. Partial exchange transfusion may reduce the risk of neurologic problems. If performed through an umbilical vein, the risk of necrotizing enterocolitis increases.

SUGGESTED READINGS

1. Upadhyay A, Aggarwal R, Deorari A and Paul V. Polycythemia in Newborn. Indian J Pediatrics, 2002; 69: 79-82.
2. AAP: American Academy of Pediatrics committee on fetus and newborn: Routine evaluation of blood pressure, hematocrit, and glucose in newborns. Pediatrics 1993;92(3):474-76.
3. Pappas A, Delaney- Black V: Differential diagnosis and management of Polycythemia. Pediatr. Clin North Am, 2004; 51(4):1063-86.
4. Schimmel MS, Bromiker R, Soll RF: Neonatal Polycythemia: Is partial exchange transfusion justified? Clin Perinatol 2004;31(3):545-53.
5. Barbara J. Stoll and Robert M. Kliegman. Plethora in newborn (Polycythemia) in Nelson textbook of pediatrics: 17th edition 2004, Saunders, Philadelphia, USA.
6. Goorin M. Allen. Polycythemia in Manual of Neonatal Care, fifth edition, Editors: John P Cloherty, Eric C. Eichenwald, Ann R. Stark. Lippincott Williams and Wilkins, Philadelphia, USA.
7. Teusch William H, Ballard A. Roberta, Gleason CA. Polycythemia in Avery's diseases of newborn, 8th edition, 2005. Saunders, Philadelphia.

17 Congestive Cardiac Failure

Bijan Saha, Rajkumar Kayal

Congestive heart failure is defined as a pathologic condition where heart is unable to pump sufficient blood to meet the metabolic need of the body. Recognition of congestive heart failure in neonatal period is very difficult. Signs and symptoms of congestive heart failure can be subtle and vary in time of presentation. One of the difficult problems is that symptoms often get confused with RDS of pulmonary origin which is very common in clinical practice. Cardiac murmurs may be absent in organic heart disease.

Aetiology

1. *Myocardial dysfunction:*
   - Asphyxia.
   - Sepsis.
   - Hypoglycemia.
   - Hypocalcemia.
   - Myocarditis.
   - Transient myocardial ischemia.
2. *Pressure load:*
   - Aortic stenosis.
   - Coarctation of aorta.
   - Hypoplastic left heart syndrome.
3. *Volume overload:*
   - Great vessels level shunt.

- Patent ductus arteriosus.
- Truncus arteriosus.
- Aorto pulmonary window.

4. *Ventricular level shunt:*
   - Ventricular septal defect.
   - Single ventricle.
   - Atrio ventricular cannal defect.
5. *Tachyarrhythmias:*
   - Supraventricular tachycardia.
   - Atrial flutter.
   - Atrial fibrillation.
6. *Bradyarrhythmias:*
   - Congenital complete heart block.
7. *Hematological:*
   - Severe anemia.
   - Hyperviscosity syndrome.
   - Hydrops fetalis.
8. *Others:*
   - Congenital thyrotoxicosis.
   - Glycogen storage disease.
   - Hypertension.
   - Acute cor pulmonale.

Clinical Features

Age of Onset

The neonate with increased pressure load on the left side of the heart secondary to aortic stenosis or coarctation of aorta become symptomatic in the first week of life. The neonate with right sided lesion is asymptomatic because patent foramen ovale allows the right side to decompress by right to left shunting leading to cyanosis rather than symptoms of congestive heart failure.

As the pulmonary vascular resistance is high in the first few weeks of life, the newborn with left to right shunt do not develop congestive heart failure in the first week or two. Only by the third or fourth week, pulmonary vascular resistance drops sufficiently to cause congestive heart failure.

Symptoms and Signs

1. Feeding difficulties or slow feeding are the most common symptoms in the neonatal period. Neonates take prolonged period for feeding. Nursing is prolonged and associated with significant sweating. The neonate seem to be tired and fall asleep after taking a small feed.
2. Parents often notice excessive perspiration which is out of proportion to the ambient temperature. This results from increased autonomic nervous system activity to improve myocardial performance.
3. On physical examination there is tachycardia (heart rate > 180/ minute) which should be evaluated when the baby is quiet.
4. Respiratory rate more than 60/minute is characteristic. Combination of tachypnea and tachycardia indicates a strong possibility of congestive cardiac failure. There may be cyanosis, cool extremities and low blood pressure.
5. JVP is not appreciated because of the short neck. The elevated systemic venous pressure cause enlargement of liver which is soft and tender. Edema is difficult to elicit because of the presence of abundance of subcutaneous fat. An unexplained rapid weight gain is a sign of fluid retention and an important sign of congestive heart failure.
6. Cardiomegaly, if present is a strong indicator of heart failure. It is not always present.
7. On auscultation there may be a S_3 gallop, muffled heart sound and murmurs. Presence of such findings

favour the possibility of underlying organic heart disease. Occasionally there may be presence of rales and rhonchi over the chest.

Investigation

1. A chest X-ray may demonstrate cardiomegaly (cardio thoracic ratio more than 0.55). Cardiomegaly may not be evident during the first two days. There may be pulmonary oligemia or plethora.
2. The electrocardiogram may reveal increased heart rate, chamber enlargement and nonspecific ST–T changes.
3. An echocardiography may reveal the anatomic abnormality which may be present and responsible for the congestive heart failure.
4. Tests relating to specific cause.

Management

Neonates with congestive heart failure should be taken as emergency and preferably referred to a good center where facilities are available.

General Measures

1. The baby should be kept in propped up position in a cardiac chair or on the mother's lap. Oxygen is to be administered through an oxygen hood (4 – 6 litres/ minute). Temperature and humidity to be controlled. Babies with large left to right shunt sweat profusely. So these babies should be nursed at lower temperature.
2. Fluid is restricted to 75% of normal maintenance requirement. Restriction of sodium is not required if baby is on diuretics. Acidosis needs correction to reduce pulmonary vascular resistance. It also improves myocardial performance. Tube feeding is to be started if baby is tachypneic.

Drugs

1. *Furosemide:* It is given in the dose of 1-2 mg/kg/dose intravenous. It is repeated if necessary 12 hourly. Side effects of furosemide include hypokelemia, hypochloremic alkalosis, hyponatremia, and acute sodium depletion. The risk of furosemide induced ototoxicity has not been clearly assessed in the newborn.
2. *Digoxin:* Digoxin probably has little effect in conditions with large left to right shunt but may be useful if there is any left ventricular dysfunction given in the dose 4 mcg/kg 12 hourly in preterm infants and 5 mcg/kg 12 hourly in term infants. Digoxin should be omitted if the PR interval is more than 0.16 and heart rate falls below 100/minute.
3. *Others:* In presence of systemic hypotension and peripheral hypoperfusion dopamine should be given in the dose of 5 mcg kg/minute. Additional benefit may be obtained by using vasodilators viz captopril and hydrallazine. Prostaglandin (PGE_1) infusion has been successfully tried in cyanotic congenital heart disease to maintain the patency of ductus arteriosus. If the above measures fail, surgical correction should be considered.

Surgery

Surgical intervention is required for congenital structural heart disease with severe congestive heart failure not responding to medical treatment. These patients are likely to die unless palliative surgery is done. Palliative surgery is done in the following situations:

- Patent ductus arteriosus.
- Tetralogy of Fallot.
- Pulmonary stenosis with intact intraventricular septum.

- Complete transposition of great vessels.
- Complete heart block.

SUGGESTED READINGS

1. Donald C Fyler. Congestive cardiac failure in Nadas' Pediatric cardiology 1st Indian edition 1992. Jaypee Brothers, Medical Publishers (P) Ltd., New Delhi.
2. Fernandez A and Mondkar J. Congestive cardiac failure in Manual of neonatal care, 1st edition 1993, Churchill Livingstone, New Delhi.
3. Stephene Burns Wechslers and Gil Wernovsky. Congestive cardiac failure in Manual of neonatal care, fifth edition 2003, edited by John P Cloherty, Eric C. Eichenwald and Ann R.Stark. Lippincott Williams and Wilkins, Philadelphia, USA.
5. Singh M. Congestive heart failure in Care of the newborn, 4th edition 1991. Sagar Publications, New Delhi.
6. A Neonatal Vade-Mecum. Edited by Brian Speidel, Peter Fleming, John Henderson *et al*. Third edition, 1998. Published by Arnold, London.

18 Acute Renal Failure in Newborn

J.N. Sharma

Acute renal failure is characterized by a sudden fall in glomerular filtration rate which leads to disturbances in water and electrolyte balance and acid base homeostasis, and to accumulation of nitrogenous products.

Functional Development of the Kidneys

Placenta is the homeostatic organ in the intrauterine life. After birth, the kidney replaces the placenta as the major homeostatic organ to maintain fluid and electrolyte balance and excretion of waste products. This transition occurs as a result of three changes viz. renal blood flow, glomerular filtration rate and tubular functions.

Renal Blood Flow

The renal blood flow in the fetus accounts for only 2-3% of the cardiac output. At birth, the renal blood flow rapidly increases to 15-18% of the cardiac output. This is a result of: (i) decrease in renal vascular resistance, (ii) an increase in systemic blood pressure, (iii) increase in inner to outer cortical blood flow.

Glomerular Filtration

The pelvicalyceal system is well delineated in the 13th or 14th week of gestation. The nephrons continue to form upto the thirty four weeks of gestation upto the total number of one million nephrons per kidney. Glomerular filtration begins soon after the first nephrons are formed and the glomerular filtration rate (GFR) increases in parallel with body and kidney growth, approximately 1 mL/minute/kg of body weight. Urine is produced by the 12th week. After 34 weeks of gestation, the GFR continues to increase until birth because of decrease in the renal vascular resistance. After birth, the GFR doubles by 2 weeks of age and reaches the adult levels by 1 year of age.

Tubular Function

Although the capacity to reabsorb sodium is developed by 24 weeks of gestation, tubular reabsorption of sodium is low until 34 weeks of gestation with fractional excretion of sodium ranging from 5-10%. After 34 weeks of gestation, 99% of filtered sodium is reabsorbed, resulting in a fractional excretion of sodium of less than 1%. Term neonates can retain sodium when in negative sodium balance. Both term and preterm neonates are limited in their ability to excrete sodium load because of their low GFR.

The newborn infant has a limited ability to concentrate urine. The maximal urine osmolality is 500 mOsm/L in premature infants and 800 mOsm/L in term infants. Both preterm and term infants can dilute their urine with a minimal urine osmolality of 25 to 35 mOsm/L but both have limited ability to handle water loads.

There is a decrease distal tubular secretion of potassium in preterm infants as a result of decreased aldosterone sensitivity and low sodium-potassium ATPase activity and low GFR. This results in limited ability of the preterm to excrete large potassium loads.

In term and preterm infants, acid and bicarbonate handling is limited. It improves as maturation of Na^+- K^+ ATPase and Na^+-H transporter occurs.

The handling of phosphate and calcium is characterized by increased phosphate retention. The cause is not clearly known. Tubular absorption of phosphate however, is altered by gestational age. It increases from 85% at 28 weeks to 93% at 34 weeks and 98% by 40 weeks. Calcium levels in fetus and cord blood are higher than those in the neonate. Calcium levels fall in the first 24 hours. There is relative hypoparathyroidism as a result of the physiologic response to hypercalcemia in the fetus.

The plasma calcium values in premature infants may be as low as 8 mg% but it is usually asymptomatic because the ionized calcium level is usually normal. Factors that favour the normal ionized calcium include low serum albumin and relative metabolic acidosis in the neonate. The urine calcium excretion in the preterm infant varies directly with sodium intake, urinary sodium excretion and inversely with plasma calcium.

Variation in Clinical Presentation

Oliguria is usually the first sign of acute renal failure. However, a normal urine output does not exclude the diagnosis. Moreover, the practical difficulty in measuring the urine output, oliguria may escape observation. Plasma creatinine is a reliable indicator of GFR. A rise of > 20 umol/ 24 hours suggest a fall in GFR. Further, hypercatabolism in sick neonates leads to uremia and hyperkelemia due to protein breakdown despite a normal GFR.

Etiology

Acute renal failure may be secondary to circulatory insufficiency without structural damage (pre-renal), parenchymal damage (intrinsic renal failure) or congenital anomaly, or due to bilateral urinary obstruction (post renal). Pre-renal failure is the most common cause of renal failure in the neonate but if not corrected promptly it may lead to intrinsic failure.

Table 18.1: Causes of acute renal failure

A. Pre-renal failure:
   1. Hypovolemic: Blood loss, fluid loss (diarrhoea and vomiting), insensible loss (phototherapy in VLBW infants), NNEC, congenital heart disease.
   2. Normovolemic (increased renal vascular resistance) Asphyxia, sepsis, polycythemia, drugs (indomethacin, tolazoline).

B. Intrinsic renal failure:
   1. Uncorrected pre-renal failure.
   2. Congenital abnormalities e.g. renal agenesis, polycystic kidney disease.
   3. Acute tubular, medullary or cortical necrosis.
   4. Thromboembolic disease viz. bilateral renal vein or arterial thrombosis.
   5. Nephrotoxins viz. aminoglycosides, radiographic contrast media, maternal drug use (indomethacin, captopril).

C. Post-renal (Obstructive):
   1. Posterior urethral valves, urethral stricture.
   2. Vesico-ureteric obstruction, pelvic-ureteric junction obstruction.
   3. Neurogenic bladder.
   4. Ureterocele, megaloureter syndrome.

Anticipation of Renal Failure

Acute renal failure can be anticipated in presence of the following conditions viz. history of oligohydramnios (in mother), perinatal asphyxia, polycythemia, bleeding disorder, presence of a lower abdominal mass, no passage of urine beyond 48 hours, or maternal drug use.

When to Suspect Renal Failure?

Renal failure should be suspected when urine output is less than 0.5 mL/kg per hour and/or if serum creatinine is elevated 2 standard deviation above the mean value for the gestational age or rising 0.3 mg/dl per day.

Clinical Symptoms and Signs

Symptoms

Symptoms of renal failure include poor feeding, vomiting, seizures, bleeding, and cardiac arrhythmias.

Signs

There may be signs of fluid overload (hypertension, excess weight gain, hepatomegaly, tachypnoea), signs of dehydration (poor peripheral perfusion with prolonged capillary refill time, hypotension), renal abnormality (palpable bladder, kidney), low birth weight.

Investigations

1. Examination of the urine for osmolarity, microscopy, sodium, urea, creatinine and FeNa. The urine sample can be obtained by catheterization. Catherization will also help to rule out lower urinary tract obstruction, measure residual urine and monitor urinary output.
2. Serum electrolytes viz. sodium and potassium, plasma creatinine and urea.
3. An ultrasound examination of genitourinary system.
4. Serum calcium and magnesium, a blood count, blood glucose, acid base status, and coagulation profile as and when indicated.

Differentiation Between Pre-renal, Intrinsic and Post Renal Causes of Renal Failure

It is important to differentiate between the three main causes of acute renal failure as their lines of treatment differ:

1. Obstructive causes can be easily confirmed or excluded on renal ultrasound examination.
2. The pre-renal and intrinsic renal failure are difficult to distinguish more so when the former progresses to the latter. The renal indices are less reliable especially in preterm infants in comparison to older children. In case of doubt an intravenous isotonic fluid challenge, done carefully may help in the diagnosis.

Table 18.2: Renal indices to differentiate pre-renal and intrinsic renal failure

Indices	*Pre-renal*	*Intrinsic*
Urine sodium (mEq/L)	10-50	30-90
Urine/plasma creatinine	29.2 +/- 1.6	9.7 +/- 3.6
FeNa	0.9 +/- 0.6	4.3 +/- 2.2

Fluid Challenge Test

Normal saline 10-20 ml/kg is given over 1 hour if there is no evidence of heart failure or fluid overload followed by administration of Frusemide, 1 mg/kg. No response suggests intrinsic or post renal failure. In such cases, infusion of low dose dopamine should be started to increase renal blood flow and urine output.

Management

Diagnosis and management of acute renal failure should proceed simultaneously to correct the defect as quickly as possible. Early intervention will limit the compromise of kidney.

A. Pre-renal failure is treated by restoration of circulating volume with isotonic saline 10-20 ml/kg I.V. over 30-60 minutes. If there is no sign of fluid depletion but only hypotension an infusion of dopamine started @ 5-10 mcg/kg/minute.
B. Post renal failure can be treated by relief of the obstruction surgically or by a suprapubic or urethral

catheter as appropriate followed by specific treatment.

C. Intrinsic renal failure is treated as follows: After establishment of intrinsic renal failure, immediate attention should be directed towards the management of complications that may be present when the neonate is first seen. These include: (i) hyperkelemia, (ii) pulmonary edema and heart failure, (iii) hypertension, (iv) severe acidosis, (v) severe anemia.

This requires a clinical evaluation which include: (i) measurement of blood pressure, (ii) search for signs of congestive heart failure and fluid overload, (iii) pattern of breathing, and (iv) assessment of severity of anemia.

The immediate investigations should include estimation of hemoglobin, blood urea, serum creatinine, sodium, potassium and bicarbonate. An ECG may be helpful to detect potassium cardio toxicity. An X-ray of the chest should be obtained.

Maintenance of Fluid and Electrolytes

Fluid management is based on the patient's fluid status. It should be limited to replacement of insensible loss (25-40 ml/kg/day) and urine output.

Sodium is restricted and sodium concentration is monitored. Hyponetremia is usually secondary to excess of free water. Phosphorous is restricted by using exclusive breast milk/low phosphorous formula. Oral calcium carbonate can be used as a phosphate binding agent. Calcium supplement is given if ionized calcium is decreased or patient is symptomatic. Conservative measures to lower potassium should be used temporarily until the cause of the renal failure is corrected or dialysis is instituted.

Hyperkelemia is said to be present when the plasma potassium is more than 7 mmol/L. ECG changes include peaked T waves, prolonged PR interval, absent

P waves and arrhythmias. The following temporary measures should be instituted under ECG monitoring:

a. 10% Calcium gluconate I.V., 0.5-1 ml/kg given over 2-4 minutes 6-8 hourly. It is cardio protective for 30-60 minutes.
b. Correction of acidosis with sodium bicarbonate 1-2 mEq/kg, effective for 1-2 hours.
c. Ion exchange resin I gm/ kg/day, orally or rectally.
d. Salbutamol, I.V. 4 mcg/kg by bolus injection. It is as effective as and safer than glucose-insulin infusion.
e. Glucose infusion with insulin: 0.1 unit /kg insulin with 4 ml/kg of 25% dextrose. The blood glucose should be closely monitored. This measure should be used in extreme circumstances.

Metabolic Acidosis

Metabolic acidosis is usually mild unless there is significant tubular dysfunction or increased lactate production due to decreased perfusion due to heart failure or volume loss from hemorrhage. Severe acidosis ($pH < 7.2$) requires correction with sodium bicarbonate 1-2 meq/ kg body weight.

Hypertension

Hypertension is defined as persistent blood pressure greater than 2 standard deviation above the mean. The clinical symptoms and signs may be absent or non-specific. They include cardio respiratory features viz. tachypnoea, cardiomegaly, tachycardia, enlarged soft tender liver and neurological features viz. irritability, lethargy, or seizure. Management of hypertension is directed at correcting the underlying cause when ever possible. Antihypertensive therapy is administered for sustained hypertension not related to fluid overload or medications.

Severe Anemia (hematocrit < 30)

Packed red cells in aliquots of 3-5 ml/kg should be slowly infused. In presence of fluid overload, partial exchange transfusion should be done.

Maintenance of Blood Glucose

The blood glucose should be closely monitored. Hypoglycemia is a common complication during fluid restriction. In contrast, hyperglycemia is common in polyuric renal failure occurring after release of urinary obstruction, especially if the infusion rate is higher than the normal utilization rate (i.e. 5-8 mg/kg/min).

Nutrition

Infants who can take orally can be given breast milk or low phosphate formula. Calorie density is increased to a maximum of 50 Kcal/30 ml with addition of glucose polymers and corn oil. Parenteral nutrition is indicated when oral feeding is not possible.

Use of Drugs

Drugs that are potentially nephrotoxic should be avoided. Dosage of the drugs having renal excretion should be adjusted according to the renal function status of the patient.

Peritoneal Dialysis

Dialysis is indicated when conservative treatment has been unsuccessful in correcting the complications. Urgent indications are:

1. Severe hyperkelemia i.e. Serum Potassium 8.0 mmol/L or more despite conservative measures.
2. Severe fluid overload with or without pulmonary edema.

3. Severe metabolic acidosis (pH< 7.2 with $PaCO_2$ < 40 mmHg).
4. Inadequate nutrition (despite infusions of 10-15% glucose) because of severe fluid restriction in the anuric infant is a relative indication.

SELECTED READINGS

1. A Neonatal Vade-Mecum 3rd edition 1998. Edited by Brian Speidel, Peter Fleming, John Anderson *et al.* Arnold. 338 Euston Road, London NW 1 3 BH.
2. Melanie S. Kim and John T. Herrin. Acute Renal failure in Manual of neonatal care, 5th edition, 2004. Edited by John P Cloherty, Eric C. Eichenwald and Ann R. Stark. Published by Lippincott, Williams and Wilkins, Philadelphia.

19

Bleeding Neonate

Anupama Deka Roy

Bleeding in the neonate is a life-threatening emergency and is most commonly seen in LBW and sick neonates. Neonates have decreased activity of certain clotting factors, impaired platelet functions and sub optimal defence against clot formation. The increased risk of hypothermia, sepsis, acidosis, necrotising enterocolitis and acidosis makes the preterm infant prone to have haemostatic defects. Gestation related lower plasma coagulant levels; low level of anti-thrombin III and hepatic immaturity provide a further handicap. The following are the reasons for which newborn is susceptible to bleeding complications:

1. Physiologic deficiencies of coagulation factors (both quantitative and qualitative).
2. Prenatal influences such as maternal disease and drugs.
3. Immaturity of development of fetal blood vessels and supporting structures.
4. Haemostatic disturbances secondary to underlying diseases (septicemia, preterm, asphyxia).
5. Vulnerability to birth trauma.
6. Platelet defects (quantitative and qualitative).

Etiology

A. ***Deficiency of clotting factors:***

1. *Transitory deficiencies of vitamin K* dependant factors II, VII, IX, X and protein C which may be accentuated by:
   a. Administration of total parenteral alimentation or antibiotics or the lack of administration of vitamin K to preterm infants.
   b. Term infants may develop vitamin K deficiency by day 2 or 3.
   c. Drugs to the mother during pregnancy: Phenytoin, Phenobarbital, salicylates and coumarin compounds.
2. *Disturbances of coagulation* related to associated disease e.g.-DIC.
3. *Inherited abnormalities of clotting factors:*
   a. Sex linked recessive (expressed in males): Hemophilia, Christmas disease.
   b. Autosomal dominant (expressed in both males and females with one parent affected): Von Willebrand's disease, Dysfibrinogenemia, Factor XI deficiency.
   c. Autosomal recessive (occurs in both males and females with parents as carriers): Deficiencies of clotting factors I, II, V, VII, X, XII, XIII, dysprothrombinemia due to abnormal factor II, variants of Von Willebrand's disease.

B. ***Platelet problems:***
   a. *Qualitative disorders* e.g. Glanzmanns disease (thrombosthenia), and disorders resulting from use of aspirin by mothers.
   b. *Quantitative disorders*: Immune disorders, Infective DIC, Intravascular coagulation, leukemia, inherited thrombocytopenia, giant hemangiomas, hyperviscosity, renal vein thrombosis, NEC.

C. ***Other causes of bleeding:*** Intra cranial hemorrhage, pulmonary hemorrhage, A-V malformation and Hemangiomas.

D. ***Miscellaneous problems:***

Trauma viz.

a. Rupture of liver or spleen associated with breech delivery.
b. Retro-peritoneal bleeding or intra peritoneal bleeding.
c. Subdural hematoma, cephalhematoma, subgaleal hemorrhage.

Diagnostic Workup

In determining the cause of bleeding and its management a detailed history and physical examination along with selected laboratory tests provides useful information.

1. *History:*
   a. History of bleeding in previous sibling or other family members (suggestive of clotting factor deficiency).
   b. Maternal illness during pregnancy (Abruptio placentae, PET, Intrauterine infection).
   c. Maternal medications (aspirin, phenytoin, phenobarbitone, diuretics, indomethacin).
   d. Expected date of delivery, actual date of delivery, mode of delivery, any complications during delivery.
   e. Any illness, medications, anomalies, procedure done to the infant.
2. *Examination:*
   a. Weight of the baby, gestational assessment.
   b. Look for the sites and extent of bleeding (bleeding from GIT, umbilical cord and sub-aponeurotic scalp hemorrhage are common in classical HDN while intracranial and pulmonary hemorrhage are usually seen in DIC; mucosal, skin and subcutaneous tissue bleeding in thrombocytopenia and DIC.
   c. Determining whether the baby is sick or healthy.

d. Petechiae, small superficial ecchymosis or mucosal bleeding—suggests a platelet problem.
e. Large bruises—deficiencies of clotting factors, DIC, Platelet consumption, Vit. K deficiency.
f. Generalized bleeding—DIC, platelet consumption, Vitamin K consumption, Vitamin K deficiency and severe liver disease.
g. Enlarged Spleen—IU infection, erythroblastosis.
h. Jaundice—infection, liver disease.
i. Abnormal retinal findings—suggest IU infection.

3. *Laboratory tests:*
   a. *Apt test:* If solely G.I. bleeding is present in the first 48 hours—perform Apt test to rule out swallowed maternal blood. (One part of vomitus is mixed with 5 parts of distilled water and centrifuged. Add 1 ml of 1% NaOH to the pink supernatant and wait for 1-2 minutes. If the solution changes to yellow brown, it favours possibility of swallowed blood (HbA gets denatured by alkali, while HbF stays pink).
   b. *Blood smear:* should be done to determine the number, size and kind of platelets, presence of fragmented cells (DIC) and large platelet or young platelet.
   c. Platelet count should be done in both mother and baby, if infant's platelet count is decreased in PBS.
   d. PT (Prothrombin time) to measure the extrinsic coagulation pathway factors.
   e. PTT (Partial thromboplastin time) to measure the intrinsic pathway factors.
   f. PT and PTT may be performed if the platelet count is low. PT greater than 17 seconds in neonates of any gestational age and PTT greater than 45 to 50 seconds in term infants should be considered abnormal.

g. **Fibrinogen and fibrin split products (FSP):** If PT, APTT and platelets are abnormal then tests for fibrinogen and FSP are performed. If fibrinogen is decreased along with the presence of FSP indicates DIC and liver disease.
h. D-dimer test has replaced the FSP in some laboratories. D-dimmers are formed from the action of plasmin on fibrin clot. Normal levels are less than 0.5 microgram/ml.
i. **Bleeding time** measures platelet's quantity and

Table 19.1: Diagnostic possibilities based on state of the infant, platelet, PT, APTT

Clinical Evaluation	*Platelet count*	*PT*	*APTT*	*Diagnostic possibilities*
Sick	Decreased	Increased	Increased	DIC
	Decreased	Normal	Normal	Platelet consumption (Infection, NEC, Renal vein thrombosis)
	Normal	Increased	Increased	Liver disease
	Normal	Normal	Normal	Altered vascular integrity (hypoxia, acidosis, extreme prematurity
Healthy	Decreased	Normal	Normal	Immune Thrombo-cytopenia occult infection, bone marrow hypoplasia or bone marrow infiltrative disease
	Normal	Increased	Increased	HDN (vitamin K deficiency)
	Normal	Normal	Increased	Hereditary clotting factor deficiencies
	Normal	Normal	Normal	Bleeding from local factors. Swallowed maternal blood Qualitative platelet abnormalities, factor XIII deficiency(rare)

quality and vascular integrity. It is used to diagnose von Willebrand's disease and functional platelet disorder. BT in preterm Baby is 3.4+/-1.3 mins.

j. Clotting time is a very insensitive test for neonates.

k. **If sepsis is suspected:** (a) sepsis screen and (b) blood culture should be done.

Differential diagnosis of clotting disorders

Long PTT + normal PT + normal platelets + normal bleeding time	Factor VIII, IX, XI, XII
Long PTT + normal PT + normal platelets + long bleeding time	von Willebrand's disease
Long PTT + long PT + normal platelets	Vitamin K deficiency
Long PTT + long PT + decreased platelets	DIC or generalized coagulopathy
Normal PTT + long PT	Factor VII
Normal PTT + normal PT + normal platelets + normal bleeding time + bleeding especially umbilicus	Factor XIII
Normal PTT + normal PT + low platelets	ITP, aplasia, leukemia, etc.
Many petechiae and normal platelets	HSP, CMV, etc.

Management

Infant in shock: Baby with cold peripheries, CRT > 3 sec, BP (35 mmHg):

a. Transfuse uncrossmatched O –ve blood 15-20 ml/kg over 15-20 mins or normal saline 10-20 ml/kg over 5-15 min.

b. If still in shock, transfuse a further 15- 20 ml/kg over 15-20 min.

c. Monitor CRT, BP, and CVP: The aim is to achieve BP > 40 mmHg (in term infants) and CVP < 8 cm H_2O.

Infant not in Shock:

a. Infant who was not given Vitamin K at birth should be given Vitamin K 1 mg IV immediately. Infant receiving TPN and antibiotics more than two weeks should be given Vitamin K 0.5 mg IM weekly.
b. All critically ill infants with weight less than 1500 grams should be given I.V. fresh frozen plasma (F.F.P), 10ml/ kg if PT and APTT are more than 2 times normal.
c. If Hb% is less than 10 gm% transfusion with cross matched packed cells 10-15 ml/kg over 2-3 hours with 2mg/kg frusemide I.V. is given.
d. Platelet problems: Platelet transfusion is given when platelet count is less than 20,000/cumm.
   i. *Autoimmune/maternal ITP:*
      - Prednisolone 10-20 mg qid x 10-14 days prior to delivery to mother.
      - IVIG.
      - LSCS in those with fetal scalp platelet count < 50,000/ cumm.
      - Postnatally give platelet, steroid, IVIG, Exchange transfusion.
   ii. *Neonatal alloimmune thrombocytopenia:*
      - *Prenatal*—IVIG, steroid, platelet transfusion to mother. LSCS if fetal scalp platelet < 50,000/ cumm.
      - *Postnatally*—Platelet transfusion, P1A1 (-) ve platelets collected 24 hours prior to delivery and washed prior to transfusion. IVIG 0.4 gm/kg/ day. Prednisolone 2 mg/kg/day with continued low platelet count or continued bleeding.
e. *Coagulation disorders:* Replacement factor with specific concentrates, fresh frozen plasma (FFP), stored plasma or cryoprecipitate are indicated. 10ml/ kg bodyweight FFP is sufficient to stop bleeding. If

higher plasma concentration is desired then factor concentrate or cryoprecipitate should be used to avoid volume overload.

f. *Acquired haemostatic disorder e.g. DIC:*
   i. Underlying cause should be treated.
   ii. Vitamin K 1 mg I.V. should be given.
   iii. Platelet and FFP are given to keep the platelet count > 50,000/ cumm and stop bleeding respectively. FFP can be given 10-15 ml/kg every 12-24 hours.
   iv. If bleeding persists then exchange transfusion with fresh citrated whole blood or packed cell mixed with FFP and administration of cryoprecipitate (10ml/kg). If DIC is associated with thrombosis of great vessels heparin as a bolus 25-35 units/kg then 10-15 unit/kg/hour as a continuous infusion should be given.

g. *Hemorrhagic disease of the newborn:*
   - *Classical HDN:* Healthy infant: bleeding within 2-5 days, vitamin K 1mg I.V. or 10 ml/kg of FFP is given. In severe bleeding Vitamin K 1 mg 4-8 hourly for 2-3 doses I.V. should be given.
   - *Early HDN (<24 hrs):* If mother is treated with Phenytoin, phenobarbitone, INH, Salicylates, delivery should be by C.S. to avoid trauma. Mother should be given Vitamin K Injection 10mg IM 24 hours prior to delivery and baby should be given vitamin K 1 mg at post partum and repeated after 24 hours, FFP if fresh bleeding occurs. Monitor Platelet, PT, APTT.
   - *Delayed hemorrhagic disease (onset 4-12 weeks):* Treat underlying condition and weekly Vitamin K 1 mg IM/orally if available for the first 3 months of life or daily supplementation of 50-100 mcg of Vitamin K.

SUGGESTED READINGS

1. Allen M Goorin and Ellis Neufeld. Bleeding in Manual of neonatal care, Fifth edition, 2003. Edited by John P. Cloherty, Eric C. Eichenwald and Ann R. Stark. Lippincott Williams and Wilkins. Philadelphia, USA.
2. Saili A. Approach to bleeding neonate in Challenges in neonatology, 1st edition, 1997. Jaypee Brothers Medical Publishers Pvt. Ltd., New Delhi.
3. Singh M. Hematological problems. In Care of the newborn, 4th edition 1991. Sagar Publications, New Delhi.
4. Singh M. The bleeding neonate in Medical emergencies in children. 1st edition 1988. Sagar Publications, New Delhi.

20 Neonatal Hyperbilirubinemia

J.N. Sharma

Adults appear jaundiced when the serum bilirubin level is greater than 2 mg/dl. Clinical jaundice, in newborn appears first on the face at a serum bilirubin level of 5 mg/dl. Over 60% of term and 80% of preterm babies develop clinical jaundice and by adult standards almost all newborn babies are jaundiced during the early days of life. Hyperbilirubinemia in newborn may be indirect or unconjugated and direct or conjugated. The rise of bilirubin in newborns is predominantly of indirect type and in the first weeks of life level of total bilirubin is considered as synonymous with indirect bilirubin.

Severe unconjugated hyperbilirubinemia, if untreated is potentially neurotoxic and conjugated hyper bilirubinemia indicates a serious hepatic or systemic illness.

Assessment of Severity of Jaundice

Assessment of jaundice in the newborn infant can be done by clinical assessment, by using an icterometer or a transcutaneous bilimeter.

Clinical assessment has been acclaimed as the best method of assessment of severity worldwide. It utilizes the principle that clinical jaundice has a cephalo caudal progression as it increases in intensity.

Assessment of jaundice should be done in natural light in a white background. The pulp of the finger or thumb is pressed on the baby's skin, preferably on a bony part, till it blanches. The initial assessment should be done over the tip of the nose and over the nasolabial fold. The underlying skin is noted for the yellow color. Extent of jaundice thus detected gives a rough estimate of serum bilirubin.

Table 20.1: Krammer's criteria to estimate clinical jaundice

Area of body	*Range of bilirubin*
Face	4-8 mg/dl
Upper trunk	5-12 mg/dl
Lower trunk and thighs	8-16 mg/dl
Arms and lower legs	11-18 mg/dl
Palms and soles	> 15 mg/dl

By experience and with concerted efforts, the observational skills can be sharpened and the accuracy of clinical assessment can be enhanced to within +/- 2 mg/dl. However, serum bilirubin estimation should be done by laboratory test to document bilirubin levels for proper management. Also, it should be emphasized that after phototherapy the skin gets bleached and clinical assessment of severity becomes unreliable and one has to rely on estimation of the serum bilirubin level.

Icterometer assessment is done by matching the skin color with the color codes depicted on the plastic strip. This method can be used by health workers for screening.

Transcutaneous billimiters work on the principle of computerized spectro-photometry and provide digital display of total bilirubin. The photoprobe is pressed against the forehead or sternum to take the reading. Every hospital should have a normogram to compare.

Laboratory Estimation of Serum Bilirubin

The laboratory estimation of bilirubin is usually done by the Vanden Berg test and with the help of the Bilimeter.

It should be noted that blood samples for bilirubin estimation should be protected from light.

Vanden Berg test is the test carried out in most neonatal unit for estimation of serum bilirubin. Its limitations include large blood sample size, lack of accuracy, reliability etc. The inter laboratory variation in the levels of serum bilirubin range between 10-20% for total bilirubin and upto 25% for conjugated bilirubin.

The bilimeter needs a micro centrifuged sample of blood in a capillary tube and provides an instant digital read out of the total bilirubin. It should be noted that during the first week of life the total bilirubin is by and large equivalent to the unconjugated fraction for practical purposes. It is a convenient and reliable method increasingly becoming popular for use in the neonatal unit.

Prediction of Hyperbilirubinemia

In recent years, efforts have gone in to predict hyperbilirubinemia in healthy term babies. Reliable predictors can identify babies at risk of pathological jaundice indicating close monitoring in such babies and reducing hospital stay in babies at low risk.

1. *Universal newborn screening:* Bhutani et al, has prepared a normogram with percentile values of serum bilirubin at different post natal ages for healthy term babies (Fig. 20.1). They have concluded that if the value of the serum bilirubin estimated at 24-36 hours after birth is plotted on the normogram, subsequent hyperbilirubinemia can be predicted. For example, if the total serum bilirubin level at this age falls in the high risk zone (> 95th percentile) then chances of subsequent hyperbilirubinemia is around 40 %. Whereas, when it falls in the low risk zone (< 40th percentile) there is no measurable risk at all.

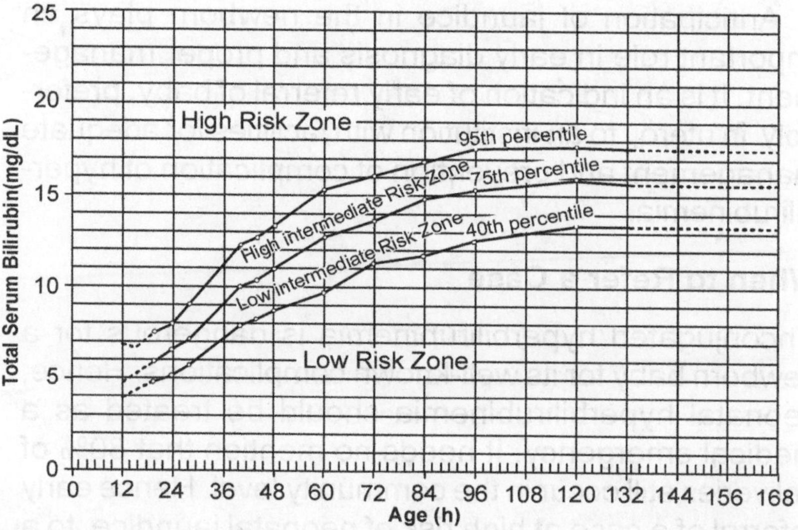

Fig. 20.1: Normogram for risk designation of term and near term well newborns based on their hour specific serum bilirubin levels.

2. *Cord blood bilirubin level:* Raised cord blood bilirubin indicates ongoing in-utero hemolysis. A cord blood bilirubin level > 2.5 mg/dl predicts development of pathological jaundice (defined as bilirubin > 13 mg/dl) with sensitivity of 71% and specificity of 96%.

Anticipation of Hyperbilirubinemia

Hyperbilirubinemia can be anticipated in the following circumstances:

1. Rh negative and O group mothers.
2. Administration of drugs to the mother e.g. large doses of Vitamin K, salicylate, oxytocin etc.
3. Presence of family history of hyperbilirubinemia.
4. History of maternal illness suggestive of IU infection viz. febrile illness within 2 weeks of delivery, fever with rash in the early antenatal period.

Anticipation of jaundice in the newborn plays an important role in early diagnosis and proper management. It is an indication of early referral of baby, preferably in utero, to an institution with facilities for adequate management and prevention of complication of hyperbilirubinemia.

When to Refer a Case

Unconjugated hyperbilirubinemia is dangerous for a newborn baby for its well-known complications. Hence, neonatal hyperbilirubinemia should be treated as a medical emergency. It needs no mention that 80% of deliveries still occur in the community level. Hence early referral of a case at high risk of neonatal jaundice, to a center where facilities for care is available, goes a long way in proper management. The following cases need urgent referral:

- Rh negative mother with previous bad obstetric history.
- History of neonatal jaundice in siblings.
- Appearance of jaundice within first 24 hours of birth.
- When a newborn baby's trunk is distinctly yellow stained with yellow tinge of palms and soles.
- Presence of signs of underlying illness (vomiting, lethargy, poor feeding, temperature instability, apnea, weight loss).
- Persistence of neonatal jaundice beyond 10 days in term and 14 days in preterm baby.

UNCONJUGATED HYPERBILIRUBINEMIA

Unconjugated bilirubin is neurotoxic in certain concentrations and under various conditions. The area of bilirubin toxicity still remains controversial. A level of safe bilirubin is yet to be clearly defined. The clinical manifestation of acute and chronic bilirubin encephalopathy has been relatively clearly defined in term babies. In preterm babies the risk posed is still a matter of controversy.

Is There A Safe Bilirubin Level to Prevent Adverse Neurological Out come?

Studies world wide have shown the following:

1. Bilirubin encephalopathy is unlikely to occur if the bilirubin level is kept < 20 mg/dl in neonates with hemolytic disease. The hemolytic diseases include Rh and ABO incompatibility, G6PD and pyruvate kinase deficiency and hereditary spherocytosis.
2. There is little evidence showing adverse neurological outcome in healthy term babies with non hemolytic unconjugated hyperbilirubinemia if the bilirubin level is kept below 25 mg/dl.
3. In exclusively breast fed babies, during the first 3 days, a bilirubin level upto 18 mg/dl is considered safe as regards neurological out come.
4. In preterm babies maintaining the bilirubin level below 1 mg/dl for every 100 grams weight of the infant is probably safe. The present belief is that kernicterus is uncommon in preterm babies. The low bilirubin kernicterus reported was largely due to factors other than bilirubin alone viz. intra cranial hemorrhage, exposure to drugs that displace bilirubin from albumin, and conditions that can disrupt the blood brain barrier and lead to enhanced deposition of bilirubin in neural tissue. Further, the post mortem findings have shown pathological changes more consistent with nonspecific damage rather than changes of true kernicterus.

Pathogenesis of Bilirubin Toxicities

Entry of bilirubin into the brain occurs as free (unbound) or as bilirubin bound to albumin in the presence of a disrupted blood brain barrier. 1 gm of albumin binds with 8.5 mg of bilirubin. Free fatty acids and drugs interfere with bilirubin binding with albumin. Acidosis affects bilirubin solubility and its deposition into brain tissue. Factors that disrupt blood brain barrier include hyperosmolarity, intra cranial hemorrhage, anoxia, and hypercarbia. Preterms/sick babies are more vulnerable to bilirubin toxicity and low bilirubin kernicterus because:

1. The blood brain barrier is more permeable.
2. The binding capacity is less in preterm and sick babies.
3. Presence of complications which disrupts the blood brain barrier.

Methods for Early Diagnosis of Bilirubin Toxicity

The methods of early diagnosis of bilirubin toxicity are as follows:

1. Monitoring serum bilirubin level.
2. BAER (brain stem auditory evoked response).

Limitations for Rational Management

Although a medical emergency, there are limitations for the rational management of hyperbilirubinemia. Most newborn units lack facilities for round the clock estimation of serum bilirubin. Bedside evaluation of BAER is not possible. The danger levels of serum bilirubin are yet to be identified and there are no uniformly accepted guidelines for management. At present '*we know to treat but not sure when to treat*'. Hence prevention should be given top priority.

Preventive Measures

The following measures can help prevent hyperbilirubinemia to a large extent. This can be practised at all levels of newborn care.

1. Prevention of Rh Isoimmunisation: All unsensitized Rh negative women should receive prophylactic injection of Anti D immunoglobulin in the following situations:
   - After birth of each Rh + ve baby.
   - After abortion of Rh + ve conceptions.
   - The situations with increased risk of fetomaternal hemorrhage e.g. amniocentesis, manual removal of placenta etc.
   - To further enhance its effectivity it has been recommended to administer anti-D immunoglobulin to all unsensitized women at 28-32 weeks gestation.
2. Prevention of birth trauma and perinatal distress factors e.g., asphyxia, hypothermia, hypoglycemia and acidosis all of which aggravates jaundice.
3. Avoidance of drugs which may increase or precipitate hyperbilirubinemia e.g. large dose of vitamin k, salicylates to mother.
4. Institution of early and adequate feeding. It helps in colonization of gut, reduces enterohepatic circulation, cause effective evacuation of meconium and prevent hypoglycemia and maintain hydration.
5. Early diagnosis of sepsis and treatment or referral.
6. Phenobarbitone administration. Rh sensitized mother should be administered phenobarbitone antenatally at a dose 90-120 mg daily for 2 weeks prior to delivery. The postnatal indications for phenobarbitone administration to the neonate include the following:
   - ❑ Cord blood bilirubin > 2.5 mg/dl.
   - ❑ Difficult or instrumental delivery.
   - ❑ Oxytocin induced delivery.
   - ❑ Birth trauma.
   - ❑ G6PD deficiency.

   The dose should be given as 10 mg/kg IM single dose or 5 mg/kg PO two times daily for 3 days in the post natal period.

Management

When to test for serum bilirubin?

A blood sample should be collected for estimation of total serum bilirubin in the following situations:

1. Onset of jaundice before 24 hours.
2. When upper trunk is yellow and the palms and soles yellow tinged.
3. To predict significant hyperbilirubinemia in the post natal period.

Laboratory Investigations to be Done When There is Pathological Hyperbilirubinemia

1. Blood groups Rh and ABO: infant and mother.
2. Direct Coombs test (cord blood or infant's blood).
3. Antibody screen in mother after delivery (Indirect Coombs test).
4. Reticulocyte count, peripheral blood smear and hematocrit.
5. G6PD screen of baby or parents.
6. If baby is unwell: (a) urine for reducing substances (b) Sepsis screen.

Infants of mothers who are Rh negative should have the Rh and ABO grouping and direct Coombs test done at birth. Infants born to O positive mothers should have the grouping and Coombs test if there is significant jaundice, if the infant has to be discharged early or if follow up is not possible. An indirect Coombs test should be done in the mothers during pregnancy and after delivery.

The peripheral smear study and reticulocyte count should be done to detect causes of Coombs' negative hemolytic anemia e.g. hereditary spherocytosis. The hematocrit estimation will detect polycythemia or suggest blood loss from occult hemorrhage. Normal blood values of hemoglobin in newborns range from 13.7

to 20.1 gm /dL with a mean value of 16.8 gm/dL in term newborns. An elevated reticulocyte count of > 6 % accompanied by a hemoglobin level < 13 gm/dL is suggestive of hemolysis.

A G6PD screen should be done in male infants with pathological jaundice when other causes are not present. A G6PD screen of the parents may be helpful in making the diagnosis.

Treatment Modalities

The goal of therapy is to prevent the concentration of unconjugated bilirubin from reaching the levels at which neurotoxicity may occur. Phototherapy and exchange transfusion are the two treatment modalities which have been recommended for this purpose. Besides, simultaneous treatment of the underlying cause, if identified (e.g. antibiotics for sepsis) and the causes which may increase the risk of neurotoxicity should also be taken care off (e.g. acidosis).

Facts About Phototherapy

The use of phototherapy has decreased the need for exchange transfusion in low birth weight babies with or with out hemolytic disease. It has also reduced repeated exchange in infants with hemolytic disease.

It is not known whether phototherapy prevents kernicterus or milder forms of brain injury associated with bilirubin toxicity. Hence, when there is an indication for exchange transfusion, phototherapy should not be used as a substitute.

Phototherapy is indicated only in unconjugated hyperbilirubinemia. It should not be used in infants with liver disease or obstructive jaundice. If indirect bilirubin is high in presence of conjugated hyperbilirubinemia exchange transfusion is the treatment of choice.

Clinical assessment of jaundice from skin color cannot be relied on for evaluating the effectiveness of phototherapy .The skin of babies exposed to light may appear almost without jaundice in the presence of marked hyperbilirubinemia. Consequently bilirubin levels should be measured every 12 hourly during phototherapy.

In infants with hemolytic disease, care must be taken to detect developing anemia, which may require transfusion.

Phototherapy should be given until serum bilirubin comes down to safe level (i.e. below 10mg %) or baby is old enough to handle increased levels of serum bilirubin (i.e.10.7 +/-1.2 mg/dl by 7th day in preterm and 13 +/- 0.7 mg/dl by 4th day in term babies). A bilirubin level is to be checked 12 hours after the lights are stopped.

The baby should be subjected to continuous intensive phototherapy with interruptions only for breast feeding.

To achieve intensive phototherapy, exposure of maximal body surface area and two or more light sources (combination of overheads, spots, biliblankets) is required. The overheads should be placed as close as to the baby as possible without hyperthermia or burn.

In infants with hemolytic disease or those with toxic levels of bilirubin, serum bilirubin & hematocrit should be estimated 6-8 hours after starting phototherapy. There after monitoring every 12 hours suffices. Monitoring should continue for at least 24 hours after cessation of phototherapy in babies with hemolytic disease to detect rebound and plan further management.

Normally bilirubin should decline by 1-2 mg/dl within 4-6 hours of intensive phototherapy and continue to fall and remain below the threshold level for exchange transfusion. Failure of intensive phototherapy is indicated when this normal fall does not occur. Infants under phototherapy should be kept naked except for eye patches and diapers. The infants are turned every 2 hours, if under single surface phototherapy.

Infants should be weighed daily (small infants twice daily). Between 10-20% extra fluid over the usual requirements is required to compensate for the increased insensible water loss.

The Facts About Exchange Transfusion

It is a widely excepted treatment. It may have to be repeated as frequently as necessary to keep serum levels under the safe level for age and gestation.

Hypoxia, acidosis and hypoalbuminemia if present should be corrected prior to exchange transfusion. However these infants should be put under intensive phototherapy while a decision to exchange is made.

Sick infants who are anemic (hematocrit < 35%) should be given a partial exchange transfusion with packed RBCs (25-80 ml/kg) to raise hematocrit to 40 % before further exchange can be performed for hyperbilirubinemia.

After exchange transfusion, intensive phototherapy is continued. The bilirubin level is measured after 30 minutes and then every 4-6 hours. The glucose level has also to be monitored.

A double volume (i.e. 160 ml/kg body weight whole blood) exchange transfusion removes 87% of infant's blood volume and lowers the bilirubin level to about 45-50% of the pre-exchange levels. However, it increases to 60% of the preexchange value within half an hour due to rapid influx of the bilirubin into the vascular space. A larger increase in the bilirubin level reflects newly formed bilirubin due to hemolysis of antibody coated RBCs sequestrated in the bone marrow and spleen, from senescent donor RBCs, and from early labeled bilirubin.

It should be noted that higher the pre-exchange value higher is the rebound.

The indications of exchange transfusion include: (a) failure of phototherapy to prevent rise of serum bilirubin to toxic levels, (b) Correction of anemia and improvement of heart failure in hydropic infants with hemolytic disease, (c) Removal of antibody and sensitized RBCs and stop hemolysis and bilirubin production.

An early exchange transfusion is indicated in presence of: (i) hydrops, (ii) history of previously severely affected infants or (iii) a known sensitized infant. An early exchange transfusion removes sensitized RBCs before hemolysis and removes bilirubin before it is distributed to the extravascular space.

It should be noted that a serum bilirubin approaching a critical level at day 1 or 2 may not be considered so on 4th day in a term baby or on the 7th day in a preterm baby. This is because after this age an imminent fall in bilirubin levels may be anticipated as hepatic conjugating mechanisms become more effective. When taking a decision to perform an exchange one should always take into account the age of the baby.

Blood Used in Exchange Transfusion

- Blood should be whole collected in citrate phosphate dextrose (CPD)
- It should be as fresh as possible (<24 hrs old for hydropic or sick infants and< 72 hrs for all others)
- In Rh HDN, in emergency situation O Rh negative blood can be used without cross matching. When blood is collected in anticipation, O Rh negative blood cross matched against maternal serum can be used. For subsequent exchange O Rh negative blood crossed matched against infant's serum should be used.

- In ABO HDN, the blood should be O Rh negative or Rh compatible with mother and infant cross matched against the mother and infant and have a low titre of naturally occurring anti A and anti B antibodies.
- For non-immune hyperbilirubinemia blood is typed and cross-matched against the plasma and RBC of the infant.
- Exchange transfusion usually involves double the volume of infant's blood and is known as two volume exchange. The infant's blood volume is 80 ml/kg. So a two volume exchange requires 160 ml/kg of blood.

Other Treatment Modalities

Drugs to increase conjugation: The drug used is phenobarbitone in a dose of 5-8 mg /kg every 24 hours. It has been found to be useful in treating indirect hyperbilirubinemia in Crigglar Najjar syndrome type II and direct hyperbilirubinemia associated with parenteral nutrition. It has to be continued on a long-term basis in case of Crigglar Najjar syndrome. Phenobarbitone, given antenatally, can lower bilirubin levels in erythroblastotic infants. However, phenobarbitone does not augment the effects of phototherapy.

Substances blocking bilirubin reabsorption viz. oral agar in a dose of 500 mg / kg can be used to augment the efficacy of phototherapy. It acts by decreasing enterohepatic circulation. It is an economical therapy. It is as effective as phototherapy even when it is used alone, but experience is limited.

Substances inhibiting bilirubin production: Tin (Sn) protoporphyrin has been used as an agent for reduction of bilirubin. It acts by inhibiting the conversion of biliverdin to bilirubin by heme oxygenase. A single intramuscular dose on anticipation of jaundice (e.g. G6PD deficiency) may reduce the need of phototherapy. It can also be given in patients with hyperbilirubinemia but effect is not better than phototherapy. More data about the efficacy and toxic effects is necessary for its recommendation as therapy.

Agents inhibiting hemolysis: Intravenous immunoglobulin, 500-750 mg/kg/dose over a 2-4 hours period given 12 hourly for three doses is shown to be effective in reducing bilirubin in Coomb's positive hemolytic anemia. The mechanism of action is not clearly known. The immunoglobulin could act by occupying the Fc receptors of the RE cells thereby preventing them from taking up and lysing antibody coated RBCs.

Management Guidelines

1. Hemolytic disease of newborn (Rh incompatibility, ABO incompatibility, Hemolytic diseases due to other causes).

General Care, Initial Investigation, Phototherapy

In *Rh hemolytic disease*, if the baby is born with hydrops, the infant should be stabilized with correction of acidosis and partial exchange transfusion to correct circulatory overload. In others, intensive phototherapy should be started immediately after birth and cord blood sent for hemoglobin and serum bilirubin and monitored for necessity of exchange transfusion.

Infants with *ABO incompatibility* are considered to have hemolysis if they have anemia (Hct < 45%), an abnormal blood smear ($3\text{-}4^+$ spherocytes), or if reticulocyte count is 4.5% in first 24 hours, or if reticulocyte count is > 1-2% in the first 1-2 weeks. The screening for early detection of ABO hemolytic disease of newborn babies with A or B group born to O group mothers can be done by the following ways:

1. ABO grouping and direct Coombs' test in cord blood and follow up of the babies on the basis of bilirubin levels.

2. Estimation of serum bilirubin at 12 hours of age in all infants born to Group O mothers.
3. Clinical observation of jaundice.

In term babies with ABO incompatibility with no medical problem, phototherapy should be started when serum bilirubin is 10mg/dl at 12 hours, 12 mg/dl at 18 hours, 14 mg/dl at 24 hours or 15 mg/dl at any time. The serum bilirubin and hemoglobin should be monitored and exchange transfusion done when indicated.

Hemolytic disease due to other causes includes G6PD deficiency, hereditary spherocytosis, minor blood group incompatibility, homozygous alpha thalassanemia, congenital intrauterine infections. As in Rh hemolytic disease, intensive phototherapy should be started immediately after birth and cord blood sent for hemoglobin and serum bilirubin and monitored for necessity of exchange transfusion.

Indications of Exchange Transfusion: Irrespective of the cause of hemolytic disease, the indications for exchange transfusion are as follows:

1. Cord bilirubin level is over 4.5 mg/dl and cord hemoglobin level is under 11 gm/dl.
2. The bilirubin level is rising over 1 mg/dl / hour despite phototherapy.
3. The hemoglobin level is between 11 and 13 gm/dl and the bilirubin level are rising over 0.5 mg/dl/hour.
4. The bilirubin level is 20 mg/dl or if the rate of rise indicates that it will reach 20 mg/dl.
5. Presence of progressive anemia inspite of adequate control of serum bilirubin by phototherapy. Persistent hemolytic anemia (reticulocyte count > 6% accompanied with a hemoglobin level of < 13 gms/dl).

Indications of Repeat Exchange Transfusion: The indications for repeat exchange transfusion are same as the indications for the initial exchange.

2. **Hyperbilirubinemia in healthy term newborn**
Guidelines of management on the basis of serum bilirubin levels is shown in the table below:

Age (hours)	*Phototherapy (Serum bilirubin in mg/dl)*	*Exchange transfusion*
25 – 72	15 or more	20 or more
72 or more	20 or more	25 or more

3. **Hyperbilirubinemia in sick term neonates**
Sick term neonates are those who have hemolysis, sepsis, hypoxemia, acidosis, hypoalbuminemia (< 2.5mg/dl), or any infant requiring intensive care. In sick neonates exchange in lower bilirubin level is recommended if Hct is 35% and/or S.bilirubin increase > 0.5 mg/dl/hr even if the serum bilirubin level is below exchange level. The indications of phototherapy and exchange transfusion are as follows:

Age in hours	*Phototherapy*	*Exchange transfusion*
	(Serum bilirubin in mg/dl)	
25 to 72	10 or more	20 or more
Above 72	12 or more	20 or more

4. **Hyperbilirubinemia in healthy and sick Preterm:**
There are still no consensus guidelines for phototherapy and exchange transfusion in low birth weight babies. The decision to use phototherapy will vary with age of the baby and the judgement as to what the natural history of the rise and fall of the bilirubin level. The current practice for treating jaundiced preterm infants is as follows:

1. *Infants < 1000 grams:* Phototherapy is started within 24 hours. Exchange transfusion is performed at bilirubin levels 10-12 mg/dL.

2. *Infants 1000-1500 grams:* Phototherapy at bilirubin levels 7- 9 mg/dL. Exchange transfusion at levels of 12-15 mg/dL.
3. *Infants 1500-2000 grams:* Phototherapy at bilirubin levels of 10-12 mg/dL. Exchange transfusion at levels of 15-18 mg/dL.
4. *Infants 2000-2500 grams:* Phototherapy at bilirubin levels 13-15 mg/dL. Exchange transfusion at levels of 18-20 mg/dL.

PROLONGED NEONATAL UNCONJUGATED HYPERBILIRUBINEMIA

Definition

Jaundice persisting beyond 14 days in a term baby and 21 days in a preterm is usually considered to be pathologically prolonged.

Causes

1. Breast milk jaundice.
2. Extravasated blood e.g. cephalhematoma.
3. Persistence of hemolysis e.g. Hemolytic disease of newborn.
4. G6PD deficiency.
5. Hypothyroidism.
6. Congenital hypertrophic pyloric stenosis.
7. Functional or organic intestinal stasis.
8. Malaria.
9. Crigler Najjar type II.
10. Sepsis.

Common Causes

1. Breast milk jaundice.
2. Extravasated blood.
3. Persistence of hemolysis.

4. G6PD deficiency.
5. Hypothyroidism.
6. Infection e.g. urinary tract infection, septicemia.

Workup

As per American Academy of Pediatrics practice parameter, babies with prolonged hyperbilirubinemia should be investigated after 3 weeks provided 1) they are not ill 2) there is no abnormal physical examination and 3) no dark urine or light stools.

1. Careful history and clinical examination.
2. Rule out cholestasis on the basis of birth weight, age at onset, stool color.
3. Investigations: Serum bilirubin and fractions
   - PBS, CBC, Hb%, Rh and ABO grouping.
   - Urine RE and culture, reducing substances.
   - Thyroid function test (TSH, T_3, T_4).
   - X-ray knee joint.
   - Sepsis screen.

Management of Some Conditions

1. Breast milk jaundice

Etiology

This condition may manifest as persistence of physiological jaundice or jaundice may appear for the first time at the end of first week. It is seen in term infants. The intensity of jaundice is maximum between 10-14 days. Instead of the usual fall of serum bilirubin by the fourth day, the bilirubin level continues to rise and may reach 20-30 mg/dL by 14 days. If breast feeding is continued, the bilirubin level will stay elevated and then fall slowly by 2 weeks and return to normal by 4-12 weeks. If breast feeding is stopped, the bilirubin will fall rapidly in 48 hours. If breast feeding is started again, the bilirubin level may rise by 2-4 mg/dL but usually will not reach the previous high level. Neonates with breast milk jaundice are well, show adequate weight gain, with normal liver function test results and show no signs of hemolysis. The recurrence rate of breast milk jaundice in future pregnancies is around 70%.

The exact cause is still not known. Breast milk jaundice is thought to result from compromised hepatic conjugation of bilirubin due to presence of 3 alpha 20 beta pregnanediol in breast milk in about 1-2% of women. High concentration of unsaturated fatty acids in the human milk due to over activity of lipase may also inhibit hepatic glucoronyl transferase enzyme and Y acceptor protein. The inhibitory substances in breast milk are excreted for about 4 to 10 weeks. Hence breast milk jaundice may last for upto 10 weeks. In addition, breast fed infants are more likely to have increased entero hepatic circulation because they ingest the beta-glucuronidase present in breast milk. They are slower to be colonized with intestinal bacteria that convert conjugated bilirubin to urobilinoids, and excrete fewer stools.

Diagnostic Features

- Infant in good health, vigorous and feeding well.
- Gaining weight adequately.
- Colourless urine and golden yellow stools.
- Other causes of prolonged jaundice has been excluded.
- Unconjugated hyperbilirubinemia.
- Liver function tests normal.
- No evidence of hemolysis.

Management

- Continue frequent breast feeding.

- Phototherapy if Serum bilirubin is more than 20 mg/dl.
- Reassurance to parents.

2. Aspiration of a Cephalhematoma

Aspiration of cephalhematoma may introduce infection; hence contraindicated. Anemia and hyperbilirubinemia should be treated as needed.

Crigler-Najjar Syndrome

It is a condition characterized by unconjugated hyperbilirubinemia due to congenital deficiency of enzyme glucoronyl transferase. There are two types:

Type I: Is inherited as an autosomal recessive disorder. Parents of affected children have a partial defect in conjugation but their serum bilirubin concentration is normal.

Diagnostic Features

1. Onset of jaundice is during first 3 days, severe in intensity and rapidly progressing to Kernicterus and a fatal outcome.
2. If child survives with treatment, there is persistence of unconjugated hyperbilirubinemia above 20 mg/dl after 1st week without signs of hemolysis.
3. Laboratory test:
   - Bilirubin concentration in bile is < 10 mg/dl (normal 50-100 mg/dl).
   - Absence of bilirubin glucoronide in bile (white bile).
   - Hepatic tissue enzyme assay by closed liver biopsy is confirmatory.

Type II: Is inherited as an autosomal dominant disorder. It is a milder form where onset of jaundice occurs between birth and 10 years.

Diagnostic Features

1. In the neonatal period, onset of jaundice may be in the first 3 days. Serum bilirubin concentration may be in the physiologic range. Kernicterus is unusual.
2. Persistence of unconjugated hyperbilirubinemia beyond 3rd week with bilirubin concentration in the range of 1.5-22 mg/dl.
3. Infants are well.
4. Lab tests:
   - Bile bilirubin is normal.
   - No signs of hemolysis.

Treatment: Oral phenobarbitone, 5 mg/kg/day. Response with a decrease in serum bilirubin concentration to 2-3 mg/dl is shown in 7-10 days. It has to be continued on a long-term basis.

NEONATAL CHOLESTASIS

Definition

A newborn is considered to have predominantly conjugated hyperbilirubinemia when the conjugated fraction is greater than 2 mg/dl or 20 % of total bilirubin.

Neonatal cholestasis is defined as prolonged elevation of serum levels of conjugated bilirubin beyond the first 14 days of life. Cholestasis in newborn may be due to infectious, genetic, metabolic or undefined abnormalities giving rise either to mechanical obstruction of bile flow or to functional impairment of hepatic excretory function and bile secretion. The clinical features of any form of cholestasis are similar.

Neonatal cholestasis constitutes 30% of hepatobiliary disorders. A multicentric study in India reveals the following causes of neonatal cholestasis.

Hepatocellular causes	*Metabolic causes*
1. Idiopathic Neonatal Hepatitis	1. Galactosemia
2. Torchs infection	2. TPN related
3. Sepsis, malaria, UTI	3. Tyrosinemia
4. Varied etiology e.g.	4. Storage disorders
a. Inspissated bile plug syndrome	
b. Recurrent intrahepatic Cholestasis	Obstructive causes:
	1. Biliary atresia
c. Progressive familial cholestasis	2. Choledochal cyst
	3. Ductal paucity
d. Hypothyroidism	

Evaluation

Cholestasis in the neonate may be the initial manifestation of numerous disorders; the clinical manifestations are usually similar and provide very few clues about the etiology. All affected infants have icterus, dark urine, light or acholic stools, and hepatomegaly resulting from decreased bile flow due to either hepatocyte injury or bile duct obstruction. The evaluation of the infant with cholestasis should follow a logical multistep process.

Steps

1. Identification of cholestasis by estimation of serum bilirubin and fractions.
2. Recognition of conditions for which specific therapy is available to prevent further damage and avoid long term complications. These conditions include sepsis, hypothyroidism, panhypopituitarism, metabolic disorders viz. galactosemia, tyrosinemia.
3. Differentiation of neonatal hepatitis and extrahepatic biliary atresia.

Clinical Criteria

The following four clinical criteria should be emphasized before planning the laboratory investigations:

- Birth weight.
- Assessment of color of stool for 10 consecutive days.
- Age of onset of stool pallor and characteristics of progression.
- Clinical characteristics of hepatomegaly.

A normal birth weight, early persistent stool pallor, and a huge hepatomegaly which is firm to hard in consistency favours extrahepatic biliary obstruction.

A low birth weight baby, gradual onset of change of stool color with waxing and waning of colour and a moderate hepatomegaly which is normal to slightly firm in consistency favours intrahepatic cholestasis.

The other clinical features to look for are splenomegaly, petechiae, chorioretinitis and microcephaly.

Investigations

It should be noted that these four clinical criteria, on their own can differentiate between extrahepatic and intrahepatic cholesasis in 82% cases. Liver biopsy together with the clinical findings enables a differential diagnosis to be made in 85% cases. With addition of HIDA Scan, 95% of extrahepatic obstruction can be diagnosed before surgery.

In absence of facilities for liver biopsy and HIDA scan the following laboratory tests may help in differentiating extra and intrahepatic choestasis.

1. **To confirm conjugated hyperbilirubinemia:**
   a. Urine for bilirubin: presence of which indicates conjugated hyperbilirubinemia. At the bed side, foam test can be done to detect bilirubin in urine. It is a simple, qualitative, valid procedure. When normal urine is taken in a test tube and vigorously shaken, the foam is white. In urine containing bilirubin, the foam will be yellow.

b. Estimation of serum bilirubin and direct bilirubin as well as serial estimation of total Serum bilirubin. Initial high levels, often above 10 mg/dl, is found in hepatitis with a tendency towards an irregular decline with time. In biliary atresia, the levels are initially low with gradual increase with time.

2. **To assess the degree of hepatic dysfunction:**
   a. Enzymes SGPT, LDH, S. Alkaline phosphatase, 5, nucleotidase.
   b. Serum cholesterol, serum protein and fractions.
   c. Prothrombin time.

An increase of SGPT in early stages indicates intra hepatic Cholestasis. LDH and 5 nucleotidase are increased in intrahepatic and extrahepatic cholestasis respectively. A 3 fold increase in S. alkaline phosphatase and a serum cholesterol level > 250 mg/dl indicates intrahepatic obstruction.

3. **To rule out definite causes:**
   a. Urine C/S, blood C/S, Sepsis screen.
   b. Serological tests for TORCHS, Hepatitis.
   c. Urine for reducing substances (Galactosemia, fructose intolerance).
   d. Coomb's test.
   e. TSH, T_3, T_4.
   f. Blood, urine, CSF cultures.
4. **To differentiate between idiopathic neonatal hepatitis and bile duct anomalies**, when other known causes have been ruled out.
   a. *USG of hepato biliary system:* USG can assess gall bladder size, detect dilation of biliary tract, and define choledochal cysts. In infants with biliary atresia the gall bladder is usually small or absent and CBD is not visualized.
   b. *Hepatobiliary scans with imido diacetic acid analogs (HIDA):* In hepatitis, uptake is sluggish, excretion to intestine eventually occurs but in

Extrahepatic biliary obstruction, uptake is normal but excretion into intestine is absent. Oral administration of phenobarbitone, 5 mg/kg/day for 5 days prior to the study enhances biliary excretion of the isotope in neonatal hepatitis.

c. A less sensitive but simple method for demonstration of biliary patency is aspiration of duodenal contents. Gall bladder contraction is stimulated by administration of fluid and the aspirate is examined for bile. A positive result (i.e. presence of bile in the duodenal contents) rules out biliary atresia. A negative result indicates severe cholestasis consistent with but not pathognomonic of biliary atresia.

d. Liver biopsy provides a precise histological diagnosis. It also helps in enzyme analysis to detect inborn errors of metabolism.

e. An operative cholangiography is indicated in infants in whom the HIDA and liver biopsy indicate extrahepatic obstruction.

Principles of Treatment

1. Prompt recognition of any specific or treatable primary cause of cholestasis e.g. galactosemia, fructosemia etc and institution of appropriate therapy to prevent further hepato cellular injury.
2. Medical management of cholestasis.
3. Treatment of the specific cause.

Medical Management

A. *Nutritional support:*

a. In breast fed babies, continue breast feeding and supplement medium chain triglyceride (MCT) based diet (use of cocoanut oil) because they do not require the presence of intraluminal bile acids for absorption. In older infants, diet should be rich in calories (200 Kcal/kg/day), rich in MCT with protein (1-2 gms/kg) from vegetable source. At least 2-3% calories should come from essential fatty acids.

b. These infants are prone to develop deficiency of fat soluble vitamins viz A, D, E, K. They should be monitored and supplemented with water soluble preparations of vitamin A and D till cholestasis resolves. The vitamins A, D (water soluble preparations) is recommended in a dose 5 times the normal requirement. Vitamin E supplementation 50-200 mg/day orally. Vitamin K 5 mg/day IM for 3 days and then 5 mg weekly. Water soluble vitamins supplementation in twice the daily recommended doses.

B. *Management of associated problems:*

a. *Pruritus:* Pruritus can be reduced by giving Phenobarbitone (5 mg/kg/day) along with UDCA (10-20mg/kg/day). Other drugs which can be tried are Cholestyramine (4-8 mg/day), terfenedine (1-3 mg/kg/day).

b. *Portal hypertension:* Variceal bleeding should be controlled with endoscopic sclerotherapy.

c. *Ascites:* Bed rest, salt restriction (0.5-1 gm/ day of salt), diuretics (frusemide + spironolactone), and paracentesis in intractable ascites.

d. *Hepatic encephalopathy*: Should be treated in the usual line.

e. *Infection:* Infection should be suspected in the presence of ascites and end stage liver disease. A full work up for infection including ascitic fluid culture and sensitivity should be under taken. Cefotaxime should be used for peritonitis. If septicemia is suspected amikacin or gentamicin should be added which may be modified later as necessary.

Treatment of Specific Cause

1. Surgical treatment for biliary atresia.
2. *Galactosemia:* Elimination of lactose from diet. Supplementation with Soy protein based lactose free formula.
3. *Fructosemia:* Elimination of fructose and sucrose from diet.
4. *Infections:* Treatment of congenital syphilis, toxoplasmosis, sepsis etc.
5. *Choledochal cyst:* Surgery.
6. *EHBA with decompensated liver disease:* Liver transplantation.
7. *Idiopathic neonatal hepatitis:* Supportive treatment.

Prognosis

Prognosis depends on the primary cause of cholestasis. In idiopathic neonatal cholestasis, 60-70% will recover with no evidence of hepatic structural or functional impairment. Approximately 5-10% will have persistent fibrosis or inflammation and a smaller percentage will have more severe disease viz. cirrhosis.

Preventable metabolic causes and infections have a good prognosis with timely intervention. Choledochal cyst has good prognosis with timely intervention.

Patients with biliary atresia usually dies from liver failure before 2 years age when untreated. Even after operative treatment they have persistent inflammation of the intrahepatic biliary tree and in most cases a degree of hepatic dysfunction persist. Around 2/3 of the patients ultimately need liver transplantation.

In the familial variety of cholestasis, 20-30% will recover; 10-15% will acquire chronic liver disease with cirrhosis.

SUGGESTED READINGS

1. Ramesh Agarwal and A.K. Deorari. Unconjugated hyperbilirubinemia in newborns: Current perspective. Ind. Pediatr. 2002;39:30-41.
2. Bhutani VK, Johnson L, Sivieri EM. Predictive ability of a predischarge hour specific serum bilirubin for subsequent significant hyperbilirubinemia in healthy term and near term newborns. Pediatrics 1999;103:6-14.
3. Awasthi S, Rehman H. Early prediction of neonatal hyperbilirubinemia. Indian J Pediatr 1998;65:131-139.
4. Hinkes T Michael and Cloherty P John. Neonatal Hyperbilirubinemia. In Manual of Neonatal care 3rd edition 1991. Published by Little Brown and Company, USA.
5. American Academy of Pediatrics. Practice parameter: Management of hyperbilirubinemia in healthy term newborn. Pediatrics 1994;94:558-567.
6. Martin R. Camilia and Cloherty P. John. Neonatal hyperbilirubinemia in Manual of neonatal care, 5th edition, 2004 Published by Lippincott, Williams and Wilkins, Philadelphia, USA.
7. Consensus report on Neonatal cholestasis syndrome. Pediatric gastroenterology subspeciality chapter of Indian Academy of Pediatrics. Ind. Pediatr. 2000; 37:845-851.

21 Phototherapy

Abhinandan Das

Crammer and colleagues (1958) were the first to observe that exposure of preterm babies to sunlight and blue fluorescent light produced a fall in serum bilirubin concentration. Since then visible light in the form of phototherapy has been used extensively throughout the world as an important therapeutic armamentarium in the management of neonatal hyper bilirubinemia.

Effectiveness of Phototherapy

1. The maximum effect of phototherapy is seen during the first 24-48 hours of therapy after which its effect wanes.
2. It is more effective than exchange transfusion in achieving prolonged reduction of bilirubin levels in infants with non-hemolytic jaundice.
3. It modifies the course of hyperbilirubinemia in ABO and Rh hemolytic disease and reduces significantly the need for exchange transfusion.
4. It detoxifies bilirubin instantaneously and continuously regardless of the serum bilirubin levels.

Sunlight is Ineffective

Sun light is ineffective as a means of phototherapy because:

1. Its blue content is low.
2. It causes dehydration and hyperpyrexia.

3. Skin burns can occur due to prolonged exposure.

Hence sunlight cannot be recommended as a means for lowering serum bilirubin concentration. It must be remembered clearly that irrespective of the source of light from various phototherapy equipments, it is the blue content of light that is acting on the bilirubin molecule.

Factors Influencing Efficacy of Phototherapy

The bilirubin molecule can absorb only light of certain colors or wavelengths. As bilirubin is a yellow pigment, only light of certain colours or wavelengths like blue, green, violet can be absorbed. When infants are treated with a broad-spectrum white light, only a portion of the white light is acting on the bilirubin molecule. Bilirubin does not absorb different colours of light equally. Following factors influence the efficacy:

1. *Wavelength and irradiance:* Blue light at 450 nm is most readily absorbed while green is less well absorbed. Special blue lamp with a peak output at 425-475 nm is the most efficient for phototherapy. Irradiance should exceed 5 uW/cm^2/nm. To reach the bilirubin molecule, light must penetrate the skin. The depth upon which light penetrates the skin depends upon the wavelength of light. Longer the wavelength deeper is the penetration.
2. *Area of skin exposed:* Body surface area exposed to phototherapy determines the efficacy. Therefore babies exposed to double surface phototherapy are reported to have faster decline of bilirubin levels than those exposed to single surface phototherapy.
3. *Gestational age:* In premature babies, the light waves penetrate deeper due to thin skin. Extended posture in preterm babies leads to exposure of greater surface area resulting in greater efficacy.

4. *Intermittent vs continuous phototherapy:* Intermittent Phototherapy has been found to be more deleterious than continuous phototherapy to the genetic material of human cell in tissue culture.
5. *General condition of neonates:* Well or sick neonates does not affect the efficacy of phototherapy.
6. *Distance of light source from the baby:* Further the phototherapy unit from the patient lesser will be the irradiance delivered and lesser will be its effectivity.

Phototherapy Equipment

Various light sources are used in phototherapy units:

a. Fluorescent lamps.
b. Halogen lamps.
c. Fibreoptic lights.

A. **Fluorescent lamps:** Blue lamps with a peak output at 425- 475 nm are most efficient. Fluorescent white light with a peak at 550-560 nm (range 380-700 nm) is used and has been shown to be equally effective. Ideal phototherapy to be used is a bank of 4 special blue and 4 daylight lamps, which have been found to be most effective.

The fluorescent lights are covered with plexiglass to screen out ultraviolet light below 300 nm and infra-red energy over 650 nm and it prevents injury to infants in case of glass break.

B. **Halogen (halide spot) lamps:** It consists of a 150 W, 20 V halogen bulb fixed overhead. Light source recommendations are 425-475 nm. It produces intense light that is far brighter than light produced by ordinary fluorescent lamps. It also produces appreciable amount of heat. These lamps are costly and its efficacy is not superior to the renewable fluorescent lamps. Moreover, the field of irradiance of these halide lamps is extremely heterogeneous with high intensity in the center and gradually decreasing towards the periphery, which may impair the efficacy in relation to the energy output.

C. **Fibre optic lights:** Light source recommendations are 425-475 nm. Fibre-optic light systems have been developed that deliver light from a high intensity lamp to a fibre optic pad or blanket. The pad is cool and can be placed in direct contact with the baby. Two types of devices are available.

Mechanism of Action of Phototherapy

Phototherapy is a mechanism for detoxifying bilirubin. It does it by converting bilirubin to photoproducts that are less lipophilic than bilirubin. These products partially bypass the liver conjugating system and can be excreted out of the body without further metabolism. When bilirubin absorbs light, three chemical reactions occur:

1. Photoisomerisation.
2. Structural isomerisation.
3. Photo-oxidation.

Photoisomerisation (Configurational Isomerisation)

Here the natural isomer of unconjugated bilirubin (4Z, 15Z) is instantaneously converted to less toxic isomer (4Z, 15E) that diffuses into the blood and is excreted into bile without conjugation. However, excretion is slow and the photo isomer is converted back to unconjugated bilirubin, which is reabsorbed from the gut if the baby is not having stools. After about 12 hours of phototherapy, the photo isomers make up about 20% of total bilirubin. Photoisomerisation occurs at low dose phototherapy ($6uW/cm^2/nm$) with no significant benefit from doubling the irradiance.

Structural Isomerisation

In this reaction intramolecular cyclisation of bilirubin occurs to form lumibilirubin. Lumibilirubin makes up 2-6% of serum concentration of bilirubin during phototherapy and is rapidly excreted in the bile and urine with out conjugation. Unlike photoisomerisation, the conversion of bilirubin to lumibilirubin is irreversible and it cannot be reabsorbed. It is the most important pathway for the lowering of serum bilirubin levels and is strongly related to the dose of phototherapy used in the range of 6 to 12 uW/cm^2/nm.

Photo-oxidation

It converts bilirubin to small polar products that are excreted in the urine. It is the least important reaction for lowering bilirubin levels. It is a slow process and is probably a minor contributor to elimination of bilirubin during phototherapy.

Indication of Phototherapy

While deciding to go for phototherapy we should consider the following:
- Rate of rise of bilirubin.
- Baby's age.
- Contributing etiological factors.

Guidelines of starting phototherapy in the healthy term babies, preterm babies, ABO incompatibility and Rh incompatibility are given in the previous chapter.

Side Effects of Phototherapy

1. Insensible water loss has been demonstrated in infants undergoing phototherapy and specially infants under radiant warmer. Loss may be upto 40% in term babies and 80% to 90% in preterms. The loss can be minimized with the use of servo-controlled warmer.

2. Increase in skin temperature, heart rate and respiratory rate occurs. Servo control warmers prevent their rise.
3. There is an increase in the incidence of watery diarrhea. There is an increased incidence in fecal water loss and also loss of fecal sodium, potassium and nitrogen.
4. Tanning of skin of black infants occur. Increased skin and muscle blood flow is observed.
5. Retinal damage is observed in experimental animals so the eye should be shielded with eye patches. Care should be taken so that eye patches do not obstruct the nose and cause respiratory distress.
6. Increased risk of hypocalcaemia has been seen in preterm babies on phototherapy.
7. "Bronze baby syndrome" characterized by greyish brown discoloration of skin, urine, and serum is seen in babies with cholestatic jaundice undergoing phototherapy. This is due to lumibilirubin undergoing free radical reaction in the form of polymerization to bilifuscin.
8. DNA strand breaks, mutations, chromatid exchanges has been described in cell culture. Bilirubin acts as a photosensitivity agent for these reactions. Intermittent phototherapy appears to produce more DNA damage than continuous phototherapy. As it is likely that light penetrates the thin scrotal sac and perhaps even reaches the ovary, it has been suggested to shield the gonads with diapers during phototherapy.
9. Phototherapy upsets infant mother interaction.

Technique of Phototherapy

- Infant is placed naked underneath the light banks/ spot or fibre optic light source used. Irradiance of 6-9 uw/cm^2/nm at 425-475 nm is used.

- Eyes are shielded with eye patches and gonads are covered with diapers. Distance of the baby from the light source is adjusted as per the requirement but ideally should not exceed more than 30-45 cm.
- Brief interruption for breast-feeding is allowed.
- Extra fluids are given as per the needs.
- Phototherapy is stopped once the safe level of bilirubin for age and gestation is reached.

Monitoring

1. Position of the baby is to be changed every two hours or after each breast feed if under single surface phototherapy unit.
2. Temperature to be closely monitored.
3. Daily record of the baby's weight to be kept.
4. Hydration status to be checked.
5. Stool frequency and urine output to be recorded.
6. Serum bilirubin to be checked 12 hourly.

Single and Double Surface Phototherapy

Phototherapy efficiency depends upon the body surface area exposed to light. With the introduction of fibre optic light systems, along with banks/spots; it has become easier and more convenient to give double surface phototherapy. A significant fall of serum bilirubin is seen following the use of double surface phototherapy. Fibre optics light systems have proved very useful.

How to Achieve Intensive Phototherapy

- Maximum surface area is to be exposed.
- A requirement of 2 or more light sources is a must. (Any combination of overheads, spots or biliblankets).
- Distance of the overheads should be as close to the infant as possible without hyperthermia or burns.

Precautions

Phototherapy is associated with increased insensible water loss. Between 10-20% extra fluid should be given, over the usual requirement, to compensate for the increased insensible water loss.

When to Stop Phototherapy

A. When the serum bilirubin is low enough to eliminate the concern of its toxic effects.
B. Risk factors for toxic levels of serum bilirubin are gone.
C. Baby is old enough to handle increased levels of serum bilirubin.
   13.0 +/- 0.7mg/dl (term babies).
   10.7+/- 1.2 mg/dl (preterm babies).

Contraindication of Phototherapy

a. Direct hyperbilirubinemia.
b. Certain porphyrias.

Maintenance of Equipment

- Periodic checking is a must.
- The tubes are to be checked every 3 months or 1000 hours or as soon as effective output declines as shown by the fluxmeter.
- If the fluxmeter is lacking, a record of working hours is to be kept.
- If the fluxmeter shows the output to be less than 2/3rds of its required value, the tubes then need replacement.
- Lamps are to be kept cool.
- Darkening of the fluorescent lamps by rings of degraded phosphorus if seen needs immediate replacement.

CONCLUSION

Phototherapy is the most preferred method in the management of neonatal hyperbilirubinemia. It is a non-invasive method and relatively free from complications. It is convenient, easy to use and even it can be used in home situations. It is inexpensive in terms of personal, equipment and disposables.

SUGGESTED READINGS

1. Maisles M. Jeney. Neonatal Jaundice in Neonatology-Pathophysiology and management of newborn. 4th edition G B Avery. Lippincott Co.
2. Camilia R. Martin and Cloherty P. John. Neonatal Hyperbilirubinemia in Manual of neonatal care, 5th edition, 2004, Philadelphia, USA.
3. Deorari AK. Bilimeter for phototherapy units. Bulletin NNF Vol. 11:4:4748.
4. Saili A, Agarwal A. Phototherapy. Bulletin NNF Vol 12: 3:47-48.

22 Fluid and Electrolyte Balance in Newborn

Amritlal Saha

In the fetus, the ECF (extracellular fluid) volume is larger than the ICF (intracellular fluid) volume and decreases with age. After, parturition, there is a sudden efflux from the ICF to the ECF compartment. This increase in the ECF compartment floods the neonatal kidneys eventually resulting in a salt and water diuresis within 3-5 days. This results in a physiological weight loss in the first week of life. Since the ECF compartment is larger in more preterm neonates, the weight loss is greater in preterm neonates (10-15%) than term neonates (5-10%).

Fluid balance in the newborn infant is tenuous because of very high rates of insensible water losses (IWL) and immature renal function. Prior to 34 weeks of gestation the premature infant greatly has a reduced glomerular filtration rate (GFR). Although the GFR increases after 34 weeks of gestation, the rate of filtration is still below adult values, even in the full term infant. Sodium reabsorption is reduced in the full term infant and even more reduced in the preterm infants. Because of this, the fractional excretion of sodium is higher in the VLBW infant (upto 4%) than in the full term infant or older child (less than 2%). Thus, although the required sodium intake of term infant is 1-3 mEq/Kg/24hr, the VLBW infant may require 3-5 mEq/Kg/24hr to prevent sodium wasting and hypothermia. The newborn infant also has a limited ability to excrete diluted or concentrated urine.

Maximum urinary concentrating ability of newborn is 600-700 mOsm/L compared with 1200-1400mOsm/L in the adult. Urine osmolarity should be maintained between 50 and 300 mOsm/L, which corresponds to a urine specific gravity of 1.003-1.012. Over hydration is a risk when urine osmolality is below 20-30 mOsm/L. Additional signs of immaturity of renal function in the newborn include reduced Na HCO_3 reabsorption, diminished capacity to acidify urine and reduced excretion of drugs.

Table 22.1: Factors affecting IWL in neonates

Increased IWL	*Decreased IWL*
• Increased respiratory rate	• Use of incubators
• Conditions with skin injury	• Use of plexiglass heat shields
• High ambient temperature	• Plastic blankets
• Increased body temperature	• PVC film
• Decreased ambient humidity	• Intubations
• Use of radiant warmers, phototherapy	• Increased ambient humidity
• Surgical malformations (Gastrochisis, omphalocele, neural tube defects)	

Causes of Increased IWL in Preterm Babies

1. Large surface area with thin skin.
2. Rapid respiratory rates.
3. Greater use of radiant warmers.
4. Phototherapy.

Table 22.2: Fluid requirements according to weight (ml/Kg)

Days of life	*>1500 gms*	*1000-1500 gms*	*<1000 gms*
1	60	80	100
2	75	95	115
3	90	110	120
4	105	125	145
5	120	140	160
6	135	155	175
7th day onwards	150	170	190

Table 22.3: Extra fluid needed in certain conditions

Condition	*Gestational age and weight (Full term)*	*LBW (Less than 2500)*
Phototherapy	20cc/kg/day	30cc/kg/day
Radiant warmer	20cc/kg/day	30cc/kg/day
High ambient temperature	10-20 cc/kg/day	30cc/kg/day
Hyperthermia	10-20 cc/kg/day	5-10cc/kg/day

Assessment of Hydration

Hydration can be assessed by clinical monitoring and laboratory investigations. Daily weight measurement can be used as a guide to estimate the fluid deficit in newborns. Term neonates loose 1-2% of their birth weight daily with cumulative loss of 5-10% in the first week of life. Acute changes in TBW result in weight changes. Therefore body weight must be measured atleast daily.

Signs of dehydration include tachycardia, sudden weight loss (more than 3% per day in early neonatal period), depressed anterior fontanel, sunken eye-balls, feeble pulses, fall in BP, shock–delayed capillary filling.

Signs and symptoms of over hydration include weight gain without edema, puffiness of face, pedal edema, and hepatomegaly, bulging fontanel, convulsion, altered sensorium, oliguria. Laboratory investigations e.g. Blood urea nitrogen (BUN), Na^+, urine output and urine specific gravity reflect the hydration status.

Laboratory Investigations Include

1. Serum electrolytes and plasma osmolality.
2. Urine electrolytes and specific gravity.
3. Serum blood urea nitrogen, creatinine.
4. Fe-Na (fractional excretion of sodium) reflects balance between glomerular filtration and tubular reabsorption.
5. Blood gas analysis.

Table 22.4: Laboratory investigations and their interpretations

Investigation	*Dehydration*	*Overhydration*
Serum Na^+	Hyponatremia	Hyponatremia
BUN	Azotemia	Normal
Urine osmolality and urine specific gravity	Raised	Normal

Situations Requiring Intravenous Infusions

1. Birth weight of less than 1200 gms. Intravenous infusion is needed for the first 3-4 days.
2. Severe birth asphyxia.
3. Respiratory distress syndrome.
4. Apneic attack.
5. Hypoglycemia.
6. Seizure.
7. Intestinal obstruction.
8. Dehydration.

Fluid Management of Specific Conditions

Disorders of fluid and electrolytes are common in neonates, particularly in preterm and critically sick neonates.

The goals of fluid and electrolyte therapy are:

- To maintain appropriate ECF volume, and
- To maintain appropriate ICF and ECF osmolality.

The Premature Infant

In the premature infant body weight may decrease upto 5-15% over first 5-6 postnatal days. In the first two days 10% dextrose should be given. Babies weighing less than 1000 should be given 5% dextrose. Electrolytes are added from the 3rd day. Fluid should be adjusted to maintain a stable weight until an anabolic state is achieved and growth occurs. Fluid and electrolyte status should be reassessed frequently during the first 2 days of postnatal life in order to define requirements.

Asphyxia

In severe birth asphyxia if the baby is in shock.

1. *Immediate therapy:*
   - Normal saline/fresh plasma or albumin 10-20 cc/kg in 1-2 hours followed by 10% dextrose infusion.
   - Sodium bicarbonate to be used only after ventilation is established (1:1 dilution with distilled water, given I.V. slowly in the dose of 1 ml/kg).
2. *Post resuscitation:*
   - Restrict fluids to 2/3rds of normal requirements.
   - Na^+ and K^+ as per normal requirement of postnatal age.

Dehydration

Dehydration is defined as loss of fluid in excess of 3% of body weight. The normal postnatal loss is 1-2%/day and birth weight is regained by 10 days.

Etiology

1. Excessive vomiting, diarrhea.
2. Paralytic Ileus.
3. Hyperpyrexia, under radiant warmer.
4. Salt loosing congenital adrenal hyperplasia.

Diagnosis

Dehydration is manifested by:

- Weight loss (> 3%/day or cumulative loss of >20 %).
- Decreased urine output <1ml/kg/hr.
- Increased urine specific gravity (>1.020).
- Increased urine osmolality (>400mOsm/L).
- Increased serum sodium (Na > 145 mEq/liter).

Infants less than 32 weeks gestation may not demonstrate oliguria in response to hypovolemia. Poor skin turgor, tachycardia, hypotension, metabolic acidosis and increased BUN may co-exist.

Therapy

Sodium and water administration should be liberalized to correct the deficit and then adjusted to equal maintenance plus ongoing losses.

Volume of deficit (in liters) = weight in kg × estimated weight loss/100.

1. Only 2/3rds of the calculated fluid and sodium deficit is to be corrected in the first 24 hours.
2. Total fluid requirement include 2/3rd deficit, maintenance and ongoing losses.
3. Types of Fluid depends on whether dehydration is hyponatremic (serum sodium below 135 mEq/L), isonatremic (serum sodium in between 135-150 mEq/L or hypernatremic (serum sodium above 150 mEq /L).

Electrolyte Imbalance

1. *Hyponatremia due to ECF volume depletion:* Predisposing factors are diuretics, osmotic diuresis, VLBW with renal water and sodium wasting, adrenal or renal tubular salt loosing disorders, gastrointestinal losses (vomiting, diarrhoea) and third space losses of ECF (skin sloughing, early necrotizing enterocolitis). Decreased weight, poor skin turgor, tachycardia, rising BUN, and metabolic acidosis suggests the diagnosis. If the renal function is mature, decreased urine output, increased specific gravity co-exists.

   Treatment:

   If possible reduce ongoing losses. Liberalization of sodium and water intake will replete deficits and allow for maintenance plus ongoing losses.

2. **Hyponatremia with normal ECF volume:** Predisposing factors include excess I.V. fluid and the syndrome of inappropriate hormone secretion (SIADH). Factors that may cause SIADH include pain, opiate administration, intraventricular hemorrhage, asphyxia, pneumothorax and positive pressure ventilation. Weight gain without edema, hyponatremia, decreased urine output and increased urine osmolality suggests the diagnosis.

   Treatment
   Water restriction is the therapy for SIADH.
   If serum sodium concentration is less than approximately 120 mEq/L or neurologic features such as obtundation or seizure develop; furosemide 1mg/kg IV every 6 hours can be initiated while replacing urinary sodium excretion with hypertonic NaCl (3%). These strategies leads to loss of free water with no change in total body sodium. Fluid restriction alone can be utilised once serum sodium exceeds 120 mEq/L.
3. **Hyponatremia due to ECF volume excess:** Predisposing factors include sepsis with decreased cardiac output, late necrotizing enterocolitis, congestive heart failure and neuromuscular paralysis. Weight increase with edema is suggestive of diagnosis, decreasing urine output, rising urine specific gravity and BUN.

   Treatment: Should be directed towards ameliorating the underlying disorders. Water restriction, sodium restriction and efforts to improve cardiac output may be beneficial.
4. **Hypernatremia with normal or deficient ECF volume:** predisposing factors include VLBW infants with increased insensible water loss. (e.g. radiant warmers and phototherapy) and renal water loss (e.g. deficiency secondary to IVH). Weight loss, tachy-

cardia and metabolic acidosis can occur. Decreasing urine output and rising specific gravity may develop. Hypernatremia in a VLBW infant in first 24 hours of life is almost always due to free–water deficits.

Treatment: The development of Hypernatremia does not necessarily imply excess total body sodium. The rate of water administration should be increased. If signs of ECF depletion or excess develop, sodium intake also should be adjusted.

5. **Hypernatremia with ECF volume excess:** Predisposing factors include excessive administration of isotonic or hypertonic fluids. Hypernatremia and edema can be pronounced in infants predisposed to sodium retention because of reduced cardiac output. Weight increase with edema is suggestive of this diagnosis.

   Treatment: Reduce the rate of administration by reducing the sodium administration by reducing the sodium concentration of fluids, restricting the rate of fluid administration.
6. **Disorders of potassium balance:** Potassium is the fundamental intracellular cation. Of note is the fact that potassium concentration (3.5 to 5.5 mEq/L) does not reflect total body potassium stores, since the distribution of extracellular and intracellular potassium is also dependant on the pH of the body compartments. An increase of 0.1 pH units in serum pH results in approximately a 0.6-mEq/L fall in serum potassium concentration due to an intracellular shift of potassium ions. Total body potassium is regulated by the balance of potassium intake (1-2 mEq /Kg per day) and potassium excretion through the urine and G.I. tract.

Hypokalemia can lead to arrhythmias, ileus, renal concentrating defects and obtundation in the newborn. Predisposing factors include nasogastric or ileostomy drainage, chronic diuretic use or ileostomy drainage, chronic diuretic use, and renal tubular defects.

Diagnosis is made by determining serum electrolytes and pH and an ECG (prolonged QT interval and U wave).

Therapy should focus on reducing abnormal renal or gastrointestinal losses of potassium and gradually increasing oral or parenteral potassium salts as needed.

Hyperkalemia can result in malignant arrhythmias in the newborn, including ventricular fibrillation. Predisposing factors include medication errors, hemolytic anemia, congenital adrenal hyperplasia, renal failure/ oliguria and extreme prematurity.

Diagnosis is based on the determination of nonhemolysed serum and urine electrolytes as well as serum pH and Calcium concentration. An ECG can demonstrate signs of prolonged QRS, and eventually ventricular tachycardia/fibrillation.

Treatment

a. Stabilization of conducting tissue by calcium gluconate at 1-2 ml/kg I.V., and lidocaine or bretylinium for ventricular tachycardia.
b. Dilution and intracellular shifting of potassium by administration of $NaHCO_3$, 1-2 mEq/Kg IV, slowly.
c. Hyperventilation.
d. Insulin in glucose infusion.
e. Nebulization with salbutamol.
f. Enhanced K^+ excretion can be achieved by furosemide 1 mg/kg IV or peritoneal dialysis or double volume exchange transfusion.

Acid Base Disturbances

Metabolic Acidosis

It may occur due to hypoxia, diarrhea, vomiting and starvation or excessive protein intake. It is clinically characterized by deep and rapid breathing. Blood pH is less than 7.3 and plasma bicarbonate below 18 mEq/L. The requirement of sodium bicarbonate can be calculated from pH of blood and base deficit. Base deficit × weight in kgs × 0.3 = mEq or ml of 7.5% sodium bicarbonate needed. One half of the calculated dose is given immediately as 7.5% sodium bicarbonate solution, half diluted with distilled water or two volumes of 5% dextrose solution and the rest is administered in the next 4-8 hours. In general, total dose of sodium bicarbonate should not exceed 10 to 12 mEq/kg per 24 hours and watch should be kept on the serum sodium level. In management of acidosis, the correction of predisposing factors, such as hypoxia, shock and starvation are of fundamental importance.

SUGGESTED READINGS

1. Singh M. in Care of the newborn, 4th edition, 1991, Sagar Printers and Publishers, New Delhi.
2. Charles F. Simmons Jr. Fluid and electrolyte management of the newborn in Manual of neonatal care, 3rd edition, 1993. Edited by John P. Cloherty and Ann R. Stark. Little Brown and Company, USA.
3. Adelman D. Raymond Solhung J. Michael. Pathophysiology of body fluids and fluid therapy in Nelson Textbook of Pediatrics. 15th edition, edited by Behrman, Kliegman and Arvin. W B Saunders Company. Prism Books Pvt. Ltd., Bangalore., India.
4. Fernandez A in Manual of neonatal care. 1st edition, 1996. B.I. Churchill Livingstone.

23 Oxygen Therapy in the Newborn

Arati Deka

INTRODUCTION

Oxygen is the most commonly used intervention in the management of any critically ill child. Its ubiquitous nature tends to foster a casual attitude towards its application. The survival of term and preterm newborns has improved considerably through better neonatal care, which includes better understanding of oxygen use in treatment. It is still the mainstay of treatment of various respiratory problems. However, it must be realised that oxygen at enriched levels is a drug with well characterized toxic effects like any other drugs. Therefore, it must be used carefully like any other pharmacological agent. Proper understanding of this important agent is essential to minimize its toxicity.

Physiological Consideration

Oxygen enters the blood by diffusion across the pulmonary epithelium-vascular epithelium membrane according to the oxygen pressure difference between the alveolus (PAO_2) and plasma (PaO_2). Oxygen dissolves in plasma and binds to hemoglobin. The quantity of oxygen bound to hemoglobin is dependent on the partial pressure of oxygen. The dissociation curve of fetal hemoglobin being towards the left at any PaO_2 below 100 mm of Hg, fetal blood binds more oxygen than adult hemoglobin. This increased oxygen affinity of fetal hemoglobin though an advantage in fetal life, releases less oxygen at any partial pressure to tissues after birth, compared to adult hemoglobin. As a result these infants can look pink at very low PO_2 values. It also makes the clinical recognition of hypoxia more difficult since cyanosis is observed at oxygen tensions (32-42 mmHg) lower than the partial pressure (50 mmHg) at which tissue suffers hypoxia. Thus cyanosis loses its importance as an early sign of hypoxia during neonatal period. The flattening of oxygen dissociation curve at high PaO_2 level makes it almost impossible to estimate oxygen tension above 80 mm of Hg, while monitoring artificial oxygen tension. This should be kept in mind when using pulse oximetry in neonatal intensive care units.

Indication of Oxygen Therapy

The main indication of oxygen therapy is arterial hypoxia secondary to any cause. They are:

1. Birth asphyxia.
2. Cyanosis (excluding congenital heart disease without cardiac failure and methemoglobinemia).
3. Respiratory distress due cardiac failure, HMD, pneumonia, and congenital malformation.
4. Hypothermia.
5. Recurrent apneic attack.
6. Pneumothorax or pneumomediastinum-inhalation of 100% oxygen would facilitate earlier resorption of air.
7. Shock,·septicemia, anemia.

Signs and Symptoms of Hypoxemia

Hypoxemia affects practically every system of the body. As a result, the clinical manifestations are non-specific. In mild to moderate hypoxemia—there is tachycardia, tachypnea, nasal flaring intercostal retraction and grunting.

In severe hypoxemia there is bradycardia and apnea; decreased level of activity, muscle tone, alertness also indicates increasing hypoxemia. Cyanosis is a sign of hypoxemia. Healthy newborn infants commonly demonstrate poor peripheral perfusion, polycythemia as a result of which there is peripheral cyanosis; which is not because of hypoxemia. Therefore central cyanosis if present in well perfused warm areas of a neonate's body may indicate low oxygen content. For true cyanosis to be detected, the presence of 5gm/dl of reduced hemoglobin is required. This is equivalent to arterial saturation of 80% or PaO_2 of 50 mm Hg in adults. As fetal hemoglobin (HbF) has an increased affinity for oxygen, resulting in higher oxygen saturation at a given PaO_2, cyanosis therefore occurs late.

Source of Oxygen

The two main sources are oxygen cylinders and oxygen concentrators.

Oxygen Cylinders

These are reusable cylinders, which are filled from a bulk supply and then transported to the point of use. Their short life span; bulk and cost are major hurdles in the use of this form of oxygen.

Oxygen Concentrators

They have an electric pump to force compressed air through synthetic aluminum silicate, which reversibly binds oxygen; they deliver about 2-4 L/min of gas containing 90% oxygen. The initial costs of these concentrators are more than the oxygen cylinders but the running cost is lower. They should be used in places only where there is reliable electric supply and adequate servicing facilities.

Methods of Oxygen Administration

Several methods are available for use in neonates:

1. **Nasal cannula:** This is a small tube of hard plastic held beneath the nostrils by tape. It has two prongs placed at the anterior nares. Oxygen flows through the tubes and prongs into the nose. Administration of oxygen via nasal cannula has become a common practice in neonatal and pediatric respiratory cases, because of its ease of administration. Low flow flowmeters are recommended to allow more precise titration of oxygen. The advantages are that this is a more comfortable way of administration of oxygen than nasal catheter and the risk of gastric distention is also minimal. Thus the effectiveness is limited. Placement of nasal cannula on the face is important. Care should be taken to keep tubing away from the chin and neck to prevent airway obstruction. They should not be taped to the face because skin breaks down or blistering could occur.
2. **Nasal catheter:** This consists of a soft catheter inserted into the nostril to a length equal to the distance from the side of the nose to the tragus. The nasopharynx and oropharynx acts as a natural reservoir. This is probably the most effective way to oxygenate children with respiratory infection. It is cheap and requires low flow rates of oxygen. However, gastric distension can occur, if the catheter is prolonged too far. The gas must also be humidified. Some children will not tolerate the tubes and will gag. If this continues for a few minutes, then the tube must be pulled back by 1-2 cm. A flow rate of 2L/min can be achieved and FiO_2 of upto 70% in small infants. The nasal catheter must be cleared frequently so that nasal secretions do not block the holes in the tubes.

3. **Nasopharyngeal catheter:** Nasopharyngeal catheter consists of a soft catheter with several distal holes inserted into the nostril to a length equal to the distance from the side of the nose to the tragus. It is cheap and requires low flow meter of 2L/min to achieve a FiO_2 of 0.7. Humidification is needed. Frequent cleaning of the holes is required.
4. **Oxygen mask:** Various types of mask are available for use in pediatric population, which includes simple masks, partial rebreathing masks and venturi devices. The masks should be soft pliable and transparent. These are not very popular because of the increased risk of aspiration and potential airway obstruction. Flow rate adjustment is critical with the mask as rebreathing of CO_2 may occur if the flow rate is inadequate. Venturi masks have the advantage of providing precise amounts of FiO_2 needed. At present face mask are not recommended except for providing supplemental oxygen in the moderate range for a short period of time e.g. during procedures and for transport in emergency situation.
5. **Oxygen hoods:** An oxygen hood is a small box made of transparent plastic. Oxygen enters through an aperture at the top of the box. A continuous flow of gas ensures flushing out of exhaled gases and deliver controlled oxygen concentration to the head and face of neonates and small children. Oxygen concentration can be adjusted between 30-100%. They also offer an easy visibility to the baby. Some hoods also maintain temperature. Total flow of at least 3L /min must be ensured to prevent rebreathing of CO_2. The actual concentration fall each time the head box is opened to give access to the head. The concentration of oxygen in the box should be periodically checked with an oxygen analyzer.

6. **Closed Incubators:** Closed Incubators are very effective at providing a humidified neutral thermal environment, but are poor devices for providing oxygen. The baby's head should be enclosed in a oxygen hood and oxygen is allowed to flow inside the box rather than the incubator to achieve better ambient oxygen concentration around the face. In deeply cyanosed babies, 100% oxygen can be administered through a tightly fitting oronasal mask for a period of 10-15 minutes.
7. **Continuous positive airway pressure (CPAP):** This is a mode of delivery of oxygen in which O_2 is delivered at a positive pressure of 3-8 cm of water as a continuous humidified flow. It acts by preventing airway collapse especially towards end of expiration. It can be delivered through nasal prongs, naso-pharyngeal airway or endotracheal tube. The positive pressure can be generated by the help of ventilator or by commercial device. The most important use of CPAP has been in patients suffering from HMD and in weaning of patients from ventilators.

Essentials of Oxygen Therapy

1. Oxygen must be administered adequately humidified. Dry oxygen increases insensible water losses from the airway and also causes inspissation of secretion, increasing the work of breathing of the neonates.
2. Oxygen administration should be warm to prevent unnecessary cold stimulus to a sick neonate.
3. VLBW babies on ventilators can imbibe water from the humidified gas mixer being supplied. Therefore, strict control of fluid balance in such babies is critical.

Humidification

Humidification of gases is essential for proper oxygenation. Humidity represents the amount of water vapour in the gas. Normally inspired gases contain some degree of humidity. These are further humidified as they pass through the upper respiratory tract, so that gases reaching the lungs are at 100% relative humidity. Since delivery of oxygen sometimes involves the use of pathways which bypass the respiratory tract, humidification of gases does not occur leading to impairment of ciliary activity, retention and thickening of secretion, inflammation of ciliated pulmonary epithelium, atelectasis and pneumonia. A number of devices are, therefore devised to overcome this problem.

a. **Simple Humidification:** These have no mechanism to heat the delivered gas mixture to body temperature. They can thus achieve a relative humidity of 100% only at room temperature. The simplest is a pass over humidifier in which the gases are passed over the surface of water prior to administration. Bubble humidifiers are devices where the gas are bubbled through water. The level of humidification fall drastically if the water level in these humidifiers fall below a specific level. Undulated bubble humidifiers are commonly recommended for use with low flow oxygen device like nasal cannula and simple oxygen masks in tropical countries.
b. **Heated humidifiers:** It involves a heating element that heats the mixture of inspired gases besides humidifying them. These are more efficient but complex to operate. The degree of humidification of gases leaving the unit depends on a number of factors, including the temperature setting of the thermal unit, the flow rate and length of the circuit. Newborns should receive warmed O_2 to lower the risk of hypothermia and resultant increase in oxygen consumption.

Monitoring of Oxygen Therapy

The goal of oxygen therapy is to provide adequate tissue oxygen without risk of its toxicity. The infant should be assessed for clinical signs of hypoxemia while on oxygen therapy. Signs such as skin colour, peripheral perfusion, respiratory rate and pattern, use of accessory muscles of respiration should be monitored. In general, care should be taken to administer the lowest % of inspired oxygen to maintain a PaO_2 of 60-80 mm of Hg depending on the age of the patient. Oxygen concentration administered should be monitored atleast every 2 hourly. Both hypoxia and hyperoxia are potentially harmful. Objective tests are required to provide oxygen support that is sufficient yet minimally toxic. Oxygen therapy should not be stopped abruptly but discontinued slowly by decreasing FiO_2 by 0.1 at a time. Before stopping oxygen therapy the child should be given a trial period with out oxygen.

1. **Monitoring inspired oxygen concentration:** In spite of employing oxygen blender to deliver desired oxygen concentration, a small error in the setting and possibility of further dilution before reaching infants lungs should be assumed and therefore measurement of oxygen concentration is mandatory in infants airway. Three types of analyzers are available:
   a. Thermal conductivity analyzer.
   b. Paramagnetic susceptibility analyzer.
   c. Electrode sensor which is the most frequently used monitor. It detects oxygen by diffusion of oxygen molecule through a Teflon membrane in the electrode. The variation in oxygen concentration causes a change in sensor current that is proportional to partial pressure of oxygen. It permits continuous monitoring, rapid calibration and the use of an alarm to signal undesirable fluctuation. Oxygen monitor should be calibrated atleast once a day.
2. **Monitoring arterial oxygenation:** Monitoring partial pressure of oxygen in arterial blood is mandatory in

all infants undergoing oxygen therapy. This helps in adjusting the respiratory support accurately thereby minimizing oxygen toxicity. Arterial oxygenation can be evaluated in neonates by invasive and non-invasive methods.

a. *Invasive techniques:*
- Indwelling arterial catheter.
- Intermittent arterial puncture.
- Arterial capillary sampling.

Table 23.1: Comparison of invasive techniques for oxygen monitoring

Particulars	*Advantages*	*Disadvantages*
a. Indwelling catheter	• Steady state gases • Easy access • Allowing continuous monitoring	Potential for major complication
b. Intermittent punctures	Allows access to arterial blood	Patient may not be in a steady state
c. Capillary sampling	• Accurate, pH, CO_2 • Low complication rate • Ease of sampling	Not reliable for PaO_2

b. *Noninvasive techniques:*
- Transcutaneous oxygen monitor.
- Pulse oximetry.
- Infrared spectrometry.

A. **Transcutaneous oxygen monitor ($TcPO_2$):** It utilizes a skin electrode to measure tissue oxygenation. By measuring the diffusion of extra cellular oxygen through heated skin. Sensor sites should be chosen as centrally as possible like chest, abdomen to minimize errors. The site of the sensors should be changed every four hours to reduce skin injury.

Calibration is required at the beginning and after each site change. The skin should not be gelatinous and immature or the sensor will cause burn. These monitors are practically useful for measuring outside the range of accuracy of pulse oximetry. The combination of pulse oximetry provides additional information that can help identify the source of hypoxia.

B. **Pulse oximetry:** It utilizes spectroscopic principle to determine oxygen saturation with each arterial pulsation. It measures the ratio of oxygenated and reduced hemoglobin. The accuracy of pulse oximeter is perfusion dependant. The pulse oximeter is thus unusable in patients with shock. The pulse oximeter is extremely sensitive to identify hypoxia but hypoxia may be overlooked due to shift of oxygen diffusion curve to the left in newborn. On the other hand if the PaO_2 is > 100-mmHg oxygen saturation by pulse oximetry remains 100%, thus hyperoxia can be missed. So, it should be supplemented with intermittent blood gas analysis while monitoring a child on oxygen therapy. The sensor should be shielded from direct light (phototherapy or procedure light) by covering it effectively.

C. **Infrared spectrophotometry:** infrared light penetrates skin, bone and tissues and can be detected by electrodes placed on opposite side of infant's skull. It is used in neonate for assessment of cerebral tissue oxygenation and alteration of cerebral blood flow.

Besides these two methods, some other methods for measuring the sufficiency of oxygenation in mitochondrial respiratory chain, the final common pathway of hypoxia are being evaluated, which has not been possible with existing method.

Complications of Oxygen Therapy

Oxygen like any other drug has reported toxic effects. The goal of oxygen therapy should be "to relieve hypoxemia while minimizing its toxic effects".

Toxic effects of oxygen therapy in infants include retinopathy of prematurity and bronchopulmonary dysplasia. The degree of oxygen toxicity any patient experiences is a function of host tolerance, PaO_2 and duration of oxygen administration. Premature infants with immature lung growth develop toxic oxygen effects more quickly at a lower PaO_2 and FiO_2 levels than term infants.

Retinopathy of Prematurity

A 40 to 70% incidence of retinopathy of Prematurity has been reported in infants below 1000 grams, but oxygen therapy is not the only factor. Infants in room air have also been diagnosed with retinopathy of prematurity.

The immature retinal vasculature constricts in response to elevated oxygen tension. If constriction is prolonged it may become irreversible. The vasculature then proliferates in an attempt to oxygenate the retina. This may lead to retinal detachment and even blindness. The risk of retinopathy of prematurity is low if the PaO_2 is maintained in the 60-80 mmHg range or saturation in the 87-92% range.

The attempts at early diagnosis of retinopathy of prematurity have been unrewarding due to vitreous haziness in preterm babies. It is recommended that a baby should be evaluated by an experienced ophthalmologist at discharge or at 8 weeks and again at 3 months to monitor eye toxicity.

Bronchopulmonary Dysplasia

It is a chronic neonatal lung disease that develops as a result of prolonged mechanical ventilation and increased FiO_2. Clinically patients demonstrate a need for increased oxygen concentration and ventilatory support beyond the normal recovery period for respiratory distress syndrome. Excess mucus secretion, air trapping and lobar atelectasis occur. Ventilation/perfusion ratios are altered and hypercarbia develops. In the final stages, there is interstitial edema, left to right shunting through a patent ductus and pulmonary hypertension.

Various studies have evaluated number of antioxidant for prevention of oxygen toxicity. The only one that appears promising is superoxide bismutase to prevent pulmonary damage.

SUGGESTED READINGS

1. Kumar H, Antony TJ, Sharma D. Oxygen therapy in pediatric practice. Indian Pediatr 1993;30:62-63.
2. Saili A. Oxygen therapy in Challenges in neonatology editor A. Saili 1st edition, Jaypee Brothers Medical Publishers (P) Ltd., Daryaganj, New Delhi.
3. Singh M. Organization of a special care neonatal unit in Care of normal newborn, 5th edition, 1999. Sagar Publications, New Delhi.
4. Bulletin, NNF, vol. 4, 1990.

24 Neonatal Hypoglycemia

J.N. Sharma

The normally grown, healthy, term infant is born with a blood glucose concentration of 60-70% of the maternal level and it falls during the first 24 hours, the lowest value is seen at the age of three hours. This is followed by a transient rise in blood glucose level during next 24 hours which again falls at around the age of 72 hours before stability is achieved. After delivery, relatively high blood lactate concentrations help to fuel the neonatal brain. Subsequently, ketone concentrations rise, providing further alternative fuels and thus minimizing the baby's glucose requirement while maternal lactation is established. Because of this ability to utilize alternative substrates, the term baby is probably not at risk of hypoglycemia associated neuronal injury over the first few days, whereas preterm and SFD babies do not produce ketones and are at risk.

Incidence of hypoglycemia is reported to occur in 8.1% of full term large for gestation (LGA) infants, 14.4% of term small for gestation (SGA) infants, 47% of infants of diabetic mothers, 67% and 38% of preterm SGA and preterm LGA infants respectively.

Definition

The normal range of blood glucose is different for each newborn and depends upon a number of factors including birth weight, gestational age, body stores, feeding status as well as presence or absence of disease.

There is no agreed definition of hypoglycemia in the newborn. A recent consensus has been to evolve an 'operational threshold' which defines neonatal hypoglycemia as that concentration of plasma or whole blood glucose at which clinicians should consider intervention. This threshold is currently believed to be a blood glucose value of less than 40 mg/dl (plasma glucose level less that 45 mg/dl) irrespective of the gestational age and age after birth.

Classification and Causes

It is useful to classify neonatal hypoglycemia as transient and persistent.

Causes of Transient Neonatal Hypoglycemia

1. Small for gestational age (SGA) infants.
2. Prematurity.
3. Birth asphyxia.
4. Hypothermia.
5. Septicemia.
6. Congenital heart disease.
7. Polycythemia.
8. Starvation.
9. Hyperinsulinism e.g. Infants of diabetic mothers, erythroblastosis fetalis, maternal drugs, maternal glucose infusion, Beck-with Wiedman syndrome.

Causes of Persistent Neonatal Hypoglycemia

1. *Hyperinsulinism:* Insulinoma, nesidioblastosis.
2. *Inborn errors of metabolism:* Glycogen storage disease (type-I, III, IV), galactosemia, maple syrup urine disease, methyl malonic aciduria, hepatic gluco-

neogenetic deficiencies (fructose 1, 6 diphosphatase, pyruvate carboxylase), mitochondrial fatty acid oxidation defects.

3. *Hormonal deficiencies:* Congenital hypopituitarism, cortisol deficiency states, congenital adrenal hyperplasia, glucagon deficiency.

Screening for Hypoglycemia

Blood glucose should be routinely estimated in the following at risk situations:

1. Very low birth weight babies (< 1500 gms).
2. Small for gestational age (SGA) babies (weight < 10th percentile for gestation).
3. Large for gestational age infants (wt > 90th percentile for gestation).
4. Preterm infants (gestation < 35 weeks).
5. Infant of diabetic mother (insulin dependent and gestational diabetes).
6. Rh- hemolytic disease of newborn.
7. History of maternal therapy with terbutaline, propranolol, oral hypoglycemic agents.
8. Neonatal conditions: Perinatal asphyxia, polycythemia, sepsis, shock, hypothermia.

Time Schedule for Screening

Hypoglycemia after the first 2-3 hours is a biochemical symptom and usually means that the baby has failed to make adequate perinatal metabolic adaptation. Hence babies at risk of such metabolic maladaptation should be identified early and managed prospectively. Blood glucose monitoring should be done as follows:

1. For neonates apparently well but belonging to at risk group at 3, 6, 12, 24, 72 hours.
2. For infants of diabetic mothers and gestational diabetes at 1, 2, 3, 6, 12, 24, 36, 48, 72 hours.

3. After exchange transfusion with CPD blood at 2 hours following exchange.

Point to be Noted

All the readings of blood sugar should be taken prior to feeding as far as practicable.

Screening Should be Stopped When

1. At the end of 72 hours, an at risk infant has not developed hypoglycemia.
2. An infant on total oral feeds having 2 (two) consecutive blood glucose values >50 mg/dl.

Methods of Glucose Estimation

1. **Reagent strips (Glucose-oxidase):** Though popular and widely used, estimation of blood glucose by reagent strips is not accurate especially at blood glucose levels less than 40 mg/dl. Low values should be always confirmed by laboratory estimation before diagnosis of hypoglycemia is made.
2. **Laboratory estimation:** This is the most accurate method. Blood samples should be quickly estimated to avoid erroneously low levels because the glucose level in a blood sample can fall @ 18 mg/dl/hour in a sample that waits analysis.

Diagnosis

Asymptomatic hypoglycemia: This diagnosis is made when the blood glucose level is below the operational threshold (to be confirmed by laboratory estimation) in the absence of clinical signs.

Symptomatic hypoglycemia: A diagnosis of symptomatic hypoglycemia is made on the basis of the Whipple's triad viz.

1. Presence of signs attributable to hypoglycemia:
   - Lethargy, limpness, stupor, coma.
   - Apnea, cyanosis.
   - Weak or high pitch cry.
   - Poor feeding, vomiting.
   - Seizure, tremor, jitteriness, irritability.
2. Low blood glucose documented by accurate, sensitive and precise method.
3. Resolution of clinical signs within minutes to hours once the blood glucose level is normalized. If the clinical signs are not alleviated by IV glucose, then other diagnostic possibilities should be considered.

It is worth mentioning that cerebral fuel deficiency in term babies may be manifested as a reduction in the level of consciousness and/or seizures. Jitteriness is not a useful discriminating symptom in such babies. As the level of consciousness drops, the cry changes, movements decrease, feeding becomes poor, and there are long respiratory pauses or apnea. Infants of diabetic mothers (IDM), are usually quiet and lethargic rather that jittery. Further, the hypoglycemia of most IDM's usually respond to treatment and resolve by 24 hours.

Management

Asymptomatic Hypoglycemia

If blood sugar level < 20 mg/dl, Glucose infusion should be started @ 6-8 mg/kg/minute.

If blood glucose level is between 20-40 mg/dl:

Oral feeds have to be started and blood glucose level repeated after 1 hour.

If repeat blood glucose is < 40 mg/dl: Glucose infusion should be started @ 6-8 mg/kg/hour.

If repeat blood glucose > 40 mg/dl, 2 hourly oral feeds should be continued. Blood glucose has to be monitored

6 hourly for 48 hours.

No IV glucose bolus is required in asymptomatic infants.

What Oral Feed to be Given?

Breast milk is the best, either direct or expressed (if baby is unable to suck). If breast milk is not available formula feeds in term and SFD babies and IV infusion with 10% dextrose in preterms as per daily fluid requirement can be given.

Milk contains nearly twice the energy of 10% glucose; promotes ketone body production; enteral feeding, especially with breast milk, promotes metabolic adaptation. Oral feeding with milk should not be discontinued if the baby becomes hypoglycemic while on weaning.

Symptomatic Hypoglycemia

Treatment consist of a bolus dose followed by continuous infusion.

Bolus Dose

200 mg (2 ml) / kg of 10 % glucose IV over one minute to be followed by continuous infusion. Besides symptomatic hypoglycemia, a bolus dose may be necessary in the following situations:

1. Intolerance to oral feeding.
2. Oral feedings not able to maintain normal blood glucose levels.
3. Blood glucose level less than 25 mg%.

Continuous Infusion

- Immediately after the bolus dose, a glucose infusion at an initial rate of 6-8 mg/kg/minute (4 ml/kg/hr) should be started.

- Blood glucose should be checked after 1 hour.
  1. If blood glucose is > 50 mg/dl infusion should be continued for 24 hours. Blood glucose to be monitored every 6 hours. If two consecutive blood glucose levels are above 50 mg/dl, start weaning.
  2. If blood glucose level is between 40 and 50 mg/dl infusion is to be continued. Blood glucose to be checked after 1 hour.

After 1 hour: If blood glucose is > 50 mg/dl, proceed as (1).

If blood glucose is < 40mg/dl, increase glucose infusion rate.

@ 2 mg/kg/minute till a maximum of 12mg/kg/min.

Monitor blood glucose 1 hourly till euglycemia then 6 hourly.

When to Start Weaning?

If two consecutive blood glucose values are > 50 mg/kg/minute in or after 24 hours of infusion, the infusion can be tapered @ 2 mg/kg/minute every 6 hours with glucose monitoring after every 30 minutes of every change in infusion rate. Tapering has to be accompanied by concomitant increase in oral feeds.

When to Stop Infusion?

i. When an infusion rate of 4mg/kg/min is achieved.
ii. Oral intake is adequate.
iii. Two consecutive blood sugar levels at 6 hours interval are above 50 mg/dl.

Recurrent /Resistant Hypoglycemia

Definition

This condition has to be considered when there is a failure to maintain a normal blood glucose level despite a glucose infusion rate of 12mg/kg/minute or when stabilization of blood glucose level is not achieved by 5-7 days of life.

In this situation, besides increasing the rate of infusion, investigations have to be considered on the basis of clinical suspicion and drugs may have to be tried in the treatment. One should avoid using dextrose infusion of > 12.5% through a peripheral vein due to the risk of thrombophlebitis.

Investigations to be Considered

1. *Serum Insulin level.
2. Serum Cortisol level.
3. Growth hormone level.
4. Blood ammonia.
5. Blood lactate level.
6. *Urine Ketones and reducing substances, ketone bodies in blood.
7. Urine and serum amino-acidogram.
8. *USG upper abdomen, CT scan abdomen (to exclude insulinoma of pancreas).

* Initial minimum investigations to be ordered

Treatment

Most neonatal hypoglycemia will resolve in 2-3 days. A requirement of more than 8 mg of glucose/kg/minute suggests increase utilization due to hyperinsulinism. This is usually transient as in infants of diabetic mothers. If it lasts for more than 7 days, endocrine evaluation may be necessary to rule out excess insulin secretion. Blood samples for insulin estimation should be drawn in presence of hypoglycemia. If the insulin level is high in presence of low blood glucose it will indicate inappropriate secretion of insulin. If the insulin level is normal for the blood glucose level, other causes of persistent hypoglycemia viz. a metabolic disorder (carbohydrate and protein metabolism) and endocrine causes should be considered.

a. *Drugs:*

1. **Inj Hydrocortisone:** 10 mg/kg/day in 2 divided doses IV. Hydrocortisone reduces peripheral glucose utilization, increases neoglucogenesis and increases the effects of glucagons. Before administration of hydrocortisone, blood samples for estimation of glucose, insulin and cortisol levels should be obtained. Hydrocortisone can be rapidly tapered in a few days after a stable and adequate blood glucose level is achieved. Administration of Hydrocortisone usually results in stable and adequate level of glucose.
2. **Diazoxide oral:** 2-5 mg/kg/dose 8 hourly per oral. It inhibits insulin release by acting as a specific adenosine triphosphate (ATP)—sensitive potassium channel agonist in normal pancreatic Beta cells and decrease insulin release. It may be given in infants who have persistent hyperinsulinemia. A positive response is usually seen in 48-72 hours.
3. **Inj. Glucagon:** 0.025-0.3 mg/kg (max. 1.0 mg) IM. For infants of diabetic mothers, the dose is 0.3 mg/kg (max 1.0 mg). Glucagon is given as an emergency measure until an intravenous access is obtained for glucose administration. It acts by mobilizing glucose and hence should be used in hypoglycemic infants with good glycogen storage. The effect is temporary and glucose level falls by 2-3 hours as the effect of glucagon wanes off.
4. Epinephrine and growth hormone are used rarely.
5. Mother's milk or formula can be started and advanced unless there is a suspicion of a metabolic disorder. As the feedings are increased the intravenous infusion is tapered with monitoring of blood glucose levels.

b. *Surgery:* A subtotal pancreatectomy may be necessary for insulin secreting tumours.

Prevention of Neonatal Hypoglycemia

1. *Antenatal care of diabetic mother:*
   a. All pregnant women with a family history of diabetes should have a glucose tolerance test done routinely during pregnancy.
   b. No oral antidiabetic agents should be used to control diabetes during pregnancy or gestational diabetes.
   c. All diabetic pregnant women should maintain a fasting glucose level of less than 105 mg/dl and post prandial level of 120 mg/dl (especially during the 3rd trimester).
   d. Large doses of glucose infusion should not be given to mothers before or at delivery.
2. Drugs such as sabutamol, terbutaline, isoxpurine, and chlorothiazide should be avoided.
3. All small for date babies are particularly at high risk of hypoglycemia and should be carefully monitored.
4. Feeding started early and given frequently (atleast 8 feeds/day). The aim should be for a total of 90 ml/kg/day on day 1. Continuous nasogastric feeds may be considered if the baby is intolerant of volume.
5. During intensive care clinical detection of hypoglycemia is not possible in sick or preterm babies or babies prone to seizure for some reason other than hypoglycemia. In these conditions routine measurement of blood glucose is the only option. When clinically stable, glucose should be measured once daily but more frequently in the sick or unstable child.

SUGGESTED READINGS

1. Narayan S, Aggarwal R, Deorari AK, Paul VK. Hypoglycemia in the newborn. Indian J Pediatrics, 2001; 68: 963-965.

2. Hypoglycemia of the newborn: A review of literature. WHO/CHD 1997;97(1):1-55.
3. Bear A, Cornblath M, Gentz J, Kellum M *et al*. Neonatal hypoglycemia: A discussion. J. Pediatr, 1971;79:314.
4. Richard E Wilker. Hypoglycemia and hyperglycemia in Manual of neonatal care, 5th edition 2004. Edited by John P. Cloherty, Eric C Eichenwald, and Ann R. Stark. Published by Lippincott Williams Wilkins, Philadelphia, USA.

25 Management of Infant of Diabetic Mother

Saumendu Bhattacharjee

INTRODUCTION

Diabetes mellitus is the most common endocrinal disorder during pregnancy. The risk of complications is minimal in gestational diabetes, although macrosomia and neonatal hypoglycemia are sometimes seen. Most difficult maternal, fetal and neonatal problems occur in women with renal, cardiac or retinal disease. Diabetic women with vascular disease have an increased risk of intrauterine growth retardation.

The duration and severity of maternal diabetes mellitus and quality of its control during pregnancy determine the outcome of the offspring.

Management During Pregnancy

All pregnant women with a family history of diabetes mellitus should have a glucose tolerance test (GTT) done routinely during pregnancy. Oral hypoglycemics are contraindicated during pregnancy due to risk of teratogenesis and intractable hypoglycemia in newborn. Patients having gestational diabetes are managed by dietary therapy. They should be evaluated weekly, as 15% eventually will require insulin.

All diabetic pregnant women should maintain a fasting blood glucose level less than 105 mg/dl and postprandial levels less than 120 mg/dl. Maternal HbA1c should be measured at 12th week and 3 monthly thereafter. HbA1c should be maintained below 7.1%. Ultrasonography should be done at 18 weeks to rule out congenital anomalies. Ultrasonography is repeated at 26 to 28 weeks of pregnancy. Mothers should be monitored for glycemic control, polyhydramnios, pre-eclampsia, premature labour. Amniocentesis may be performed at 38 weeks to assess pulmonary maturity unless there is enough reason to deliver earlier. A Lecithin/Sphingomyelin (L/S) ratio of over 3.5 and SPC (saturated phosphatidylcholine) level greater than 1000ug/dl is considered safe mature indices in case of diabetic mother.

Delivery Management

Insulin requiring pregnancies should continue to 38 to 39 weeks unless there is evidence of fetal compromise. In case of emergency delivery, because of difficulty in controlling maternal diabetes, while waiting for an effect, steroids are avoided unless L/S ratio is less than 2:1 and SPC level is less than 500 ug/dl. Intrapartum maternal blood glucose should be maintained around 120 mg/dl.

Evaluation of the Neonate Following Delivery

Soon after the baby is born, assessment is made to determine the need for any resuscitative efforts. A glucose level and pH may be determined on cord blood. A thorough physical examination is done to rule out any major congenital anomalies and placenta examined.

In the nursery, supportive care should be given while a continuous evaluation of the infant is made. Infants of diabetic mothers, have a significant risk of hypoglycemia, hypocalcemia, hyperbilirubinemia and polycythemia. Therefore, following laboratory studies should be performed:

1. Blood glucose levels are checked at 1,2, 3, 6,12, 24, 36, 48, and 72 hours.
2. Hematocrit levels are checked at 1 and 24 hours.
3. Calcium levels are checked if the baby appears jittery or is sick.
4. Bilirubin levels are checked if the baby appears jaundiced.

Specific Problems Frequently Observed in Infants of Diabetic Mothers

Pregnancy in insulin dependent diabetic mothers is commonly complicated by one or more of a wide variety of problems in the fetus and newborn. These include:

- Sudden fetal death late in the 3rd trimester.
- Premature birth by induction to avoid 3rd trimester fetal death.
- Macrosomia.
- Birth trauma caused by macrosomia.
- Intrapartum asphyxia.
- Caesarean section to avoid birth trauma and intra-partum asphyxia.
- Neonatal respiratory distress from several causes.
- Hypoglycemia.
- Hypocalcemia.
- Hyperbilirubinemia.
- Polycythemia and hyper viscosity.
- Persistent pulmonary hypertension syndrome.
- Cardiomyopathy.
- Congenital anomalies .

Respiratory Distress

The infant of diabetic mothers is at risk for several forms of neonatal respiratory distress. The most important of these is hyaline membrane disease.

Pathophysiology: In Infants of diabetic mothers, surfactant production and incorporation of choline with lecithin to form saturated phosphatidylcholine (SPC) is delayed due to hyperinsulinemia. Hyperinsulinemia may also block the cortisol induced lung maturity predisposing them to HMD. Other causes of respiratory distress besides HMD are transient tachypnea of newborn (TTN), hypertrophic obstructive cardiomyopathy, birth asphyxia, trauma, polycythemia, pneumonia, cardiac and pulmonary anomalies.

Following studies should be done in infants with respiratory distress: (i) Chest X-ray, (ii) Blood gases, (iii) ECG, BP measurements, (iv) Blood cultures.

Management of RDS should be done in the usual lines.

Hypoglycemia

About 50% of IDMs and 1/5th of IGDMs suffer from hypoglycemia in the first 12 hours.

Pathophysiology of hypoglycemia: Maternal hyperglycemia is reflected in fetal circulation and leads to islet cell hyperplasia of fetal pancreas and a hyperinsulinemic state. Few other hypotheses include decreased response to counter-regulatory hormones, decreased secretion of counter-regulatory hormones, and inadequate substrate mobilization (decreased hepatic glucose production, decreased oxygenation of fatty acids). Hypoglycemia in SFD infants born to mothers with vascular disease may be due to inadequate glycogen stores.

The onset of symptoms in IDMs is frequently within 1 to 2 hours of age and is most common in macrosomic babies. IDMs are usually quiet and lethargic rather than jittery. Other symptoms such as apnea, tachypnea, respiratory distress, hypotonia, shock, cyanosis and seizures may occur.

Management of hypoglycemia is in the usual lines.

Hypocalcaemia and Hypomagnesemia

Early hypocalcaemia (S.Calcium <7mg/dl or ionic calcium <4 mg/dl) occurs in 50% of all IDMs in the first 3 days.

Patho physiology of hypocalcemia: It is secondary to temporary parathormone deficiency. Physiological hypercalcemia of pregnancy is exaggerated in diabetic mothers leading to excessive fetal parathormone suppression. It is also due to Vit. D antagonism at the intestinal level from elevated cortisol and hyperphosphatemia due to tissue catabolism. Prematurity and birth-asphyxia are other contributory factors.

Pathophysiology of hypomagnesemia: Hypomagnesemia (<1.5 mg/dl) in the baby is a reflection of hypomagnesemia in mother due to urinary magnesium losses from diabetes-induced polyurea.

Management: Both hypocalcaemia and hypomagnesemia usually resolves spontaneously. But if symptomatic (apnea, cyanosis, seizure) 2 m/l/kg of 10% Ca-gluconate should be given to control seizures followed by oral or I.V. calcium therapy. If there is associated magnesium deficiency, it is treated by inj. MgSo4 solution 0.1-0.2 ml/kg I.M. daily for 3 days. Oral supplementation may follow.

Polycythemia, Hyperviscosity, Thrombocytopenia, Coagulopathies

Central hematocrit >65% or Hb>21gm/dl causes hyperviscosity, intravascular sludging, ischemia, hypoxia. Typical ruddy appearance is seen in 20-40% of cases.

Pathophysiology: In IDMs, polycythemia may be secondary to elevated HbA1 in both maternal and fetal serum, which may lead to reduced oxygen delivery and increased erythropoetin. In SGA infants' polycythemia may be related to placental insufficiency, causing fetal hypoxia and increased erythropoetin.

Thombocytopenia is thought to be due to impaired thrombopoiesis from marrow crowding by excess of erythroid precursors.

Thrombotic episodes like renal vein thrombosis occurs due to sludging, and inhibitors of fibrinolysis.

Management: Asymptomatic infants with a peripheral venous hematocrit between 60-70% can usually be managed by increasing fluid intake and repeating hematocrit after 4 to 6 hours.

Symptomatic infants should have a partial exchange transfusion with 5% albumin or normal saline, if the peripheral venous hematocrit is more than 65%. The total volume exchanged is usually 15 to 20 ml/kg of body-weight.

Renal vein thrombosis postnatally may present with hematuria, flank mass, hypertension, or embolic phenomena. Most renal vein thrombosis can be managed conservatively.

Hyperbilirubinemia: Hyperbilirubinemia is quite common in IDMs.

Pathophysiology: Several causes leads to increased frequency of hyperbilirubinemia in IDMs:

1. Insulin causes increased erythropoetin and thereby polycythemia.
2. Decreased erythrocyte lifespan because of less deformable cell membrane related to glycosylation of RBC membrane.
3. Immature liver function, birth trauma, asphyxia, prematurity, increased enterohepatic circulation of bilirubin due to poor feeding etc. are other contributory factors.

Management: Hyperbilirubinemia in IDMs is diagnosed and treated as in any other infant and is discussed in details in a separate chapter.

Congenital anomalies: Major congenital anomalies are seen in 5-9% of IDMs and this account for 30-50% of perinatal death.

Pathophysiology: Hyperglycemia per se is teratogenic. A relationship exits between elevated HbA1 in the first trimester and major anomalies in IDMs. Secondary effects of hyperglycemia, which leads to increased congenital anomalies are thought to be due to (a) reduced arachidonic acid and myoinositol levels, (b) increased free oxygen radical, hyperperoxides, sorbitol etc. Euglycemic control should start before conception to prevent congenital anomalies. The types of congenital anomalies seen in IDMs involve:

1. CNS (anencephaly, meningocoele syndrome, holoprosencephaly).
2. Cardiac (VSD, ASD, situs inversus, cardiomyopathy).
3. Vertebral, Skeletal and Caudal regression syndrome (sacral agenesis).
4. Renal (agenesis, hydronephrosis).
5. GIT (Duodenal atresia, lazy colon). The incidence of Down's syndrome may also be increased.

Preterm labour and still births: Spontaneous Preterm labour occurs in about 17% cases and is mostly due to UTI and polyhydramnios (due to fetal macrosomia, placentomegaly).

Unexplained death occurs in last 2 weeks of pregnancy and is related to pre-eclampsia (25%), impaired uterine blood flow and increased fetal oxygen demand.

Macrosomia: Birth weight over ninetieth percentile, chubby, cushinoid babies with hairy pinna are typical of IDMs especially seen in mothers with elevated blood sugar in their 3rd trimester. Incidence of macrosomia is 15-45% depending on diabetic control. All organs except brain and kidney are enlarged in macrosomic infants.

Pathophysiology of macrosomia: Insulin is an anabolic hormone; thus, the hyperinsulinemic state of the fetus plays a major role in the development of macrosomia. This augmented insulin production by the fetus, plus excessive maternal glucose and amino-acids, stimulates, protein, lipid and glycogen synthesis to cause macrosomia. Macrosomia increases the risk of preterm delivery, shoulder dystocia, brachial plexus injury, birth trauma and asphyxia, and increased incidence of cesarean section.

Poor feeding: Poor feeding in IDMs may be due to immature behavior of the babies themselves. Several complicating problems like RDS, CCF, hypoglycemia etc. may also contribute to it.

Myocardial dysfunction: Cardiomegaly is common and CCF is seen in 5-15% of babies. Transient hypertrophic sub-aortic stenosis resulting from ventricular septal hypertrophy in IDMs is seen. Fetal heart is particularly rich in insulin receptors and hyperinsulinemia may lead to hyperplasia and hypertrophy of myocardial cells. Most symptoms resolve by 2 weeks of age and septal hypertrophy resolves by 4 months.

Small left colon syndrome: It may present as generalized abdominal distension because of inability to pass meconium. After well hydration of the baby is ensured, a gastrograffin enema often will make the diagnosis and will result in evacuation of the colon as well.

Persistent pulmonary hypertension: IDMs are at increased risk of persistent pulmonary hypertension, and several factors may contribute. One factor is increased smooth muscle thickness in the pulmonary arteries in IDM. These babies are also often asphyxiated, one of the predisposing conditions for this syndrome. They may be polycythemic and hyperviscous, which causes a greater, rise in pulmonary than in systemic vascular resistance.

Long term outcome: Poor diabetic control, birth asphyxia, birth trauma, prolonged hypoglycemia, RDS, are found to be associated with developmental delay, mental retardation, cerebral palsy etc. Macrosomic babies (IDM) have a greater chance of becoming obese after 5 years of age. The fact that obesity in childhood correlates with amniotic fluid insulin concentration suggests that altered fetal β cell secretion of insulin is related to long-term postnatal growth.

Poor maternal control during 2nd and 3rd trimester particularly alterations in ketone metabolism, can be directly correlated with abnormal neonatal behavior and with poor indices of infant development at age 2 years and of intelligence at age 4 years. Offsprings of women with diabetes have a 1 to 9% incidence of developing diabetes during later life; this is significantly greater than the general population. The mechanism responsible for this is complex and is beyond the scope of this write up.

SUGGESTED READINGS

1. Aviva Lee—Parritz and Cloherty, J.P. Maternal condition that affect the fetus—Diabetes in Manual of Neonatal Care, 5th edition, edited by Jon P Cloherty, Eric C. Eichenwald and Ann R. Stark. Lippincott Williams and Wilkins, Philadelphia, USA.
2. Reece, E.A., *et al*. Infant of the diabetic mother. Semin Perinotol 1994;18:459.
3. Fee B, Weil W: Body composition of infants of diabetic mothers by direct analysis, Ann N Y Acad Sci 1963;110-869.
4. Grabbe SG, Mestman JH, Freeman RK, *et al.*: Management and outcome of pregnancy in diabetes mellitus, classes B to R. Am J Obstet Gynecol 1977;129;723-732.
5. Haworth JC, McRae KN, Dilling LA: Prognosis of infants of diabetic mothers in relation to neonatal hypo-

glycemia. Dev. Med Child Neurol 1976;18:471-479.

6. Widness JA, Susa JB, Garcia JF, *et al.*: Increased erythropoeisis and elevated erythropoetin in infants born to diabetic mothers and in hyperinsulinemic rhesus fetus. J Clin Invest 1981;67:637-642.
7. Rizzo TA, Ogata ES, Dooley SL, Metzger BE, Cho NH: Perinatal complications and cognitive development in 2 to 5 years old children of diabetic mothers. Am J Obstet Gynecol 1994;171:706-713.
8. Pedersen J: The pregnant diabetic and her newborn. Problems and management. Baltimore, Williams and Wilkins 1967.
9. Naeye R: Infants of diabetic mothers: A quantitative morphologic study. Pediatrics 1965;28:980.
10. Petersen MB, Pedersen SA, Greisen G, Pedersen JF, Molsted—Pedersen L: Early growth delay in diabetic pregnancy: Relation to psychomotor development at age 4.Br Med J Clin Res Ed 1988;296:598-600.
11. Buchnan TA, Kitzmiller JL: Metabolic interactions of diabetes an pregnancy. Ann Rev Med 1994;45:245.

26 Parent to Child Transmission of HIV

J.N. Sharma and Palash Ranjan Gogoi

The HIV infected adult male can transmit the infection to women and thus HIV infection becomes a serious threat to children of such parents. In India, sexual route is the most common route of transmission of HIV. After implementation of effective blood safety programme, parent to child transmission (PTCT) has emerged as the second important cause of infection. It is the most important cause of HIV infection in children and this resulted in majority of the 700,000 new infections in children globally in 2003.

In India, it is estimated that about 28 million deliveries occur annually, of which 1.4 lakh occur amongst HIV infected mothers. Presuming an approximate rate of 30% transmission to the child, about 40,000 babies get HIV infection via vertical transmission.

Perinatal transmission accounts for 2.14% of the total cases of HIV infection in India. In the developing countries like India, most of the mothers are getting infection from their husbands through the sexual route i.e., fathers are equally responsible for the transmission of HIV to their children. Hence, in order to ensure that mothers alone should not be blamed for mother to child transmission (MTCT), MTCT has been renamed as PTCT (Parent to child transmission) in India.

Incidence

There are very scanty reports on PTCT in India. The first Indian seropositive infant was reported in 1987. In India, the PTCT rate has been reported in the range of 13 to 60% in different studies. A PTCT rate of 48% has been reported by Kumar *et al.*, and 36% has been reported by Dongaoker *et al.*

Timing of Vertical Transmission

Vertical transmission can occur during pregnancy, labour and delivery as well as breast feeding. The incidence of the different routes is as follows:

1. Intra-uterine: 30 to 40%
2. Intra-partum: 60 to 70%
3. Post-partum: 29%, when mothers acquire HIV infection post-nataly and 14%, when mothers have chronic HIV infection.

Postulated Mechanisms of PTCT

Parent to child transmission of HIV virus can occur by the following mechanisms:

1. Transplacental micro-transfusion, especially during late pregnancy.
2. Exposure of the baby's muco-cutaneous surface to maternal blood and cervical secretions of the mother during delivery.
3. Virus transmission through breast milk.

Prevention of PTCT

India has launched a PPTCT (Prevention of parent to child transmission) programme to monitor and to take measures to prevent perinatal transmission. PTCT blockage involves 4 strategies:

- Primary prevention of HIV infection among the child bearing age parents and prevention of unwanted pregnancy among HIV positive females.

- Measures to decrease viral load in HIV infected mothers by administration of anti retroviral therapy (ART) to mothers.
- Measures to decrease exposure of baby to maternal fluids by promotion of delivery by elective LSCS and avoidance of breast feeding.
- Measures to decrease chances of HIV in exposed baby by administration of ART to the baby.

Interventions to Prevent PTCT

Different interventions undertaken to prevent vertical transmission include:

1. Antiretroviral therapy
2. Infant feeding issues
3. Elective LSCS
4. Cleaning of birth canal during delivery
5. Vitamin A prophylaxis
6. Immunotherapy.

Antiretroviral Therapy

The most successful intervention decreasing vertical transmission is the use of anti-retroviral (ARV) drugs during pregnancy, labor and postnatally to mother and baby. Most extensively and successfully used drug is Zidovudine, used as monotherapy since 1994. Nevirapine has also been used successfully as monotherapy since 1999. Of late combination of two drugs or more has been used successfully bringing down the vertical transmission to < 2%.

Mechanisms of Actions of ARV Drugs

The antiretroviral drugs act by the following mechanisms:

- Reduces the viral load in the mother so that a lesser quantity of virus goes into the infant.
- Prevent the virus from “fixating” itself in the child (post-exposure prophylaxis). ARV drugs reduce transmission not only when started before and during delivery but also within 48 hours after delivery.

Some important trials of anti retroviral therapy are shown in a tabular form below:

Table 26.1: Showing important t

Trial	*Ante partum*	*Intrapartu*
PACTG 076 (1994) protocol	From 14-34 weeks, oral ZDV* 100 mg 5 times/day	IV ZDV 2 r over 1hr, f by 1mg/kg
Thai-CDC protocol (1998, short course	From 36 weeks, oral ZDV 300 mg	Oral ZDV every 3 hr

THE MERITS AND DEMERITS OF THE DIFFERENT PROTOCOLS

PACTG 076 Protocol:

Though 076 protocol is ideal, it has many practical problems for India.

1. It is a lengthy protocol both for mother and baby.
2. It leads to increased cost, decreased compliance and failure in majority.
3. It needs early registration (14 weeks) and HIV testing of all mothers, which is difficult.
4. IV AZT/ZDV is not available in India.
5. It needs elective LSCS, which is not available and not safe all over the country.
6. It recommends only top feeding in babies, which may not be desirable, safe, affordable and acceptable to mothers.

Hence there is need for a shorter, less complicated protocol for developing countries.

Thai-CDC Protocol (Short Course ZDV Protocol):

This protocol was tried in Bangkok, Thailand in 1998 in collaboration with CDC keeping in mind the need for simple, short term ZDV/AZT protocol for developing countries. The merits and demerits of this protocol are:

1. It is a short protocol, only for mother and for just 1 month.
2. This is affordable, acceptable by many, leading to better compliance.
3. Mother can be enrolled even if they register as late as 35 weeks.
4. LSCS is not mandatory.
5. No need of intravenous ZDV.
6. Only oral ZDV is used that too only for mother.
7. The only drawback is avoidance of breast feeding,

yet this protocol is ideally suited for developing countries.

Nevirapine Protocol (HIV NET 012):

Nevirapine as monotherapy was used in this protocol in Uganda in 1999. The merits of this protocol are:

1. It involves only a single dose (400 mg) to mother at onset of labor, and single dose (2 mg/kg/dose) to baby soon after birth.
2. This protocol is very cost effective, acceptable with good compliance.
3. It can also be given to mothers who register at last moment or even to unregistered cases.
4. Elective LSCS is not mandatory.
5. Breast feeding is allowed.

All these make this protocol acceptable by many in developing countries. Both Thai-CDC and HIV NET 012 were adapted in India, tried in 11 medical colleges with efficacy of 66% in each. The National AIDS Control Organization (NACO) recommends the Nevirapine protocol for use in India for prevention of parent to child transmission in the PPTCT programme in India.

Infant Feeding Issues

The advantages of breast feeding are well known. It is a complete food till 6 months of age. It prevents G.I. and respiratory infections. Some immunoglobulin components of milk and colostrum might provide some protection against HIV-1 in the breast milk. Human milk contains a lot of protective factors like mucins, lysozyme, lactoferrins, cytotoxic T cells, protease inhibitors, high carotenes, epidermal growth factors (EGF) and IgA. The IgA carpets the GIT mucosa and EGF enhances the maturity and integrity of intestinal epithelium and prevents the entry of HIV. Others decrease the binding of HIV to the epithelial cells of G.I.T. and thus reduce the risk of transmission.

Replacement feeding with formula or animal milk prevents transmission of HIV, but the child is exposed to other serious infections.

Mixed feeding with breast milk and animal milk/ formula has been shown to be definitely associated with a higher HIV transmission as the integrity of G.I. epithelium is disrupted due to G.I. infections with top feeding. Mixed feeding can injure the gut epithelium by infection and allergy and thereby increase the gut permeability for HIV transmission.

A study done in Durban, South Africa in 1999 compared HIV transmission among exclusively breast fed babies, exclusively top fed babies and babies given mixed feeding (i.e., breast feeding with animal/formula milk).

Table 26.1: Showing feeding pattern and risk of transmission

Feeding pattern	*Risk of transmission at 3 months*	*Risk of transmission at 15 months*
Exclusively breast fed	14.6%	24.7%
Exclusively top fed	18.8%	19.4%
Mixed feeding	24.1%	35.0%

At 3 months, it appeared that the transmission was less in exclusively breast fed babies than in exclusively top fed babies and both were significantly better than mixed feeding. Long-term follow-up results at 15 months showed that the advantage of exclusive breast feeding seems to be negated as compared to exclusive top feeding. However both were significantly better than mixed feeding.

Hence, HIV infected mothers should not give mixed feeding. If she decides to breast feed, it should be exclusive breast feeding and if she decides to give replacement feeding, it should be exclusive artificial milk feeds.

Policy of Breast Feeding

To minimize the risk of HIV transmission to infants, while at the same time not increasing their risk of other causes of morbidity and mortality, United Nations (WHO/ UNICEF/UNAIDS) recommendations states that "When replacement feeding is acceptable, feasible, affordable, sustainable and safe, avoidance of breast feeding by HIV positive mothers is recommended. Otherwise, exclusive breast feeding is recommended during the first months of life" and should then be discontinued as soon as feasible. The recommendations further states that "When HIV infected mothers choose not to breast feed from birth or stop breast feeding later, they should be provided with specific guidance and support for at least the first two years of the child's life to ensure adequate replacement feeding".

Hence it may be concluded that it will be optimal to exclusively breast feed the baby till 6 months and then abruptly wean off completely in next 10 to 15 days.

However, it should be an informed choice by the mother. The role of counselor and pediatrician should be to give correct information on various options and they should not be biased or judgmental towards any option. The informed choice taken by mother should be respected even if it appears incongruent socio-economically. In the west, mothers prefer not to breast feed. In India, the choice should be left to mother. But whatever is the choice, it should be either exclusive breast feeding or exclusive replacement feeding and not mixed feeding.

Safe Delivery Practices

Elective lower section CS: Many studies have shown that elective LSCS, done at 38 weeks, before rupture of membrane or onset of labor reduces the risk of HIV transmission by 20-50%. Elective cesarean section reduces HIV transmission in the following ways:

1. Reduces transplacental hemorrhage occurring during labor.
2. Reduces the length of exposure of baby to vagino-cervical secretions or maternal blood.
3. Reduces the quantum of infective material.
4. Reduces swallowing of infected material by baby; and
5. Reduces chances of ascending infection to baby.

Table 26.3: Showing interventions and risk of PTCT

Interventions	*Risk of PTCT*
NO intervention	20%
With ZDV alone (076 protocol)	17%
With elective LSCS alone	8%
Combined LSCS and ZDV	0%

However, elective LSCS in all HIV infected mother is an enormous task. It may increase maternal mortality as it may not be safe in some parts of our country. It will also increase the cost of therapy. Hence, decision has to be individualized depending upon the set-up and stage of HIV in mother.

Vaginal delivery: Vaginal delivery leads to more chances of HIV infection. Studies have shown that the risk of transmission of HIV was 8% with LSCS and 20% with vaginal delivery. The chances increased to 29-31% if interventions are done during vaginal delivery like traumatic delivery or episiotomy. Hence episiotomy and other procedures should be avoided during vaginal delivery in HIV infected mothers.

Cleaning of birth canal at delivery: Vaginal and cervical secretions are the most important sources of HIV infection to the baby during delivery. Cleaning of birth canal with virucidal/antiseptic agent at the time of delivery has been proposed as a means to decrease vertical transmission. Such an ideal agent that is effective, safe and inexpensive is still not available. Studies have been done in Africa using chlorhexidine for this purpose and were found to decrease vertical transmission. Other studies have failed to get the desired results. Hence search for the ideal agent still continues. Interestingly all these studies showed decrease in mortality in babies due to decreased incidence of neonatal sepsis. Hence cleaning of birth canal is beneficial both ways.

Vitamin A and nutritional support: Vitamin A deficiency is known to lead to high maternal HIV viral load as well as increased viral titers in breast milk, both of which lead to increased rate of vertical transmission. HIV itself leads to Vitamin A deficiency leading to a vicious cycle. Earlier studies have shown beneficial role of Vitamin A supplementation. However, a recent study from Malawi in South Africa has shown no benefit of Vitamin A supplementation in HIV infected mothers on vertical transmission. Improving nutrition also helps to decrease symptomatology of mothers and decrease the rate of vertical transmission. Simple advice of improving diet from available local home food can lead to better nutrition and better outcome of pregnancy.

Immunotherapy: Maternal anti-HIV antibodies help to decrease vertical transmission. Some HIV exposed individuals do not get infected due to presence of HIV specific CD_8 + cytotoxic T cells. Such manipulation of cell mediated immunity can be exploited to decrease vertical transmission. Vaccination of pregnant women who are HIV positive using purified gp 120 and gp 40 has been tried so as to boost up the antibody titers in mother, which will decrease vertical transmission. Such studies are in trial in the USA.

Care of HIV Exposed Infant

The actual HIV status of the newborn cannot be obtained upto 18 months of delivery, as maternal antibody are present in the neonate till 10-18 months (average 13 months)of age. If the mother is infected with HIV-1 then HIV-1 DNA PCR test is the preferred diagnostic test. Current recommendation is to test the newborn at birth, at 1-2 months of age and then at 4-6 months of age. A neonatal blood sample should be taken for the first test. A cord blood sample should not be taken because it gives a high false positive result. If the baby is not breast fed, HIV infection can be reasonably excluded if the all 3 tests are negative. However, follow-up serologic testing should be performed until disappearance of passively transferred maternal antibodies.

An exposed infant is considered uninfected when there are no physical findings suggestive of HIV-1 infection, virologic tests are negative, immunologic tests results (CD_4 count and percentage) are normal, and after the infant is 12 months of age or older, two or more

HIV antibody test results are negative. If mother is infected with HIV-2 which is much less common, then HIV-2 PCR test should be asked for in the infant.

All babies born to HIV positive mothers should be given bath immediately after birth. They can be advised exclusive breast feeding upto 6 months and then abruptly stopped within 10-15 days. However the decision on feeding shall be taken by the parents after proper counseling. According to the present recommendation of NACO, one dose of Nevirapine (2 mg/kg/dose) should be given at birth.

Ideally all exposed infants should be advised Pneumocystis Carinii pneumonia (PCP) prophylaxis till perinatal HIV infection is excluded. In addition, it is worth considering additional 6-9 months chemoprophylaxis against tuberculosis, to be started as two drug INH and RMP regimen at birth, in view of the high prevalence of tuberculosis and its coexistence with HIV infection, especially in developing countries.

Asymptomatic babies can be vaccinated according to the schedule. In symptomatic babies oral polio and BCG vaccines are contraindicated.

The PPTCT (Prevention of Parent to Child Transmission) Programme

The Government of India has launched the programme of PPTCT (Prevention of parent to child transmission) with an aim to control PTCT (parent to child transmission). Implementation of this comprehensive programme in our country needs to be given top priority in prevention of AIDS in children as PTCT is the major route of acquisition of HIV in children.

All the components of the PPTCT programme must be adequately emphasized for achieving the primary goal of reducing overall maternal and infant morbidity and mortality. Any specific intervention package to reduce

PTCT of HIV should be fully integrated in the overall antenatal, obstetrical and pediatric care. The components of the PPTCT programme include:

- Information, education, counseling.
- Condom promotion.
- VCTC (Voluntary counseling and testing centre) for HIV/AIDS.
- Treatment of STDs in mother.
- Good antenatal care.
- Prevention of transmission with antiretroviral therapy (ART).
- Safe delivery practices.
- Counseling and support for safe infant feeding practices.
- Community action in order to make the programme successful and safeguard future generation.

SUGGESTED READINGS

1. Holla RG, Nair MNG, Trends in the Prevention of Neonatal HIV; Journal of Neonatology; Oct to Dec'2004, Vol 18, Issue no.4, 5-11.
2. Jain Shikhar, Jaiswal SP, Parent to Child Transmission of HIV-Indian Scenario Journal of Neonatology; Oct to Dec 2004, Vol 18, Issue no.4, 12-17.
3. Bagga Rashmi, The Mother with HIV; Journal of Neonatology; Oct to Dec 2004, Vol 18, Issue no.4, 18-21.
4. Gupta G, Singh D, Management of Neonates with HIV infection; Journal of Neonatology; Oct to Dec 2004, Vol 18, Issue no.4, 26-37.
5. Dadhich JP; Guidelines on infant feeding and HIV; Journal of Neonatology; Oct to Dec 2004, Vol 18, Issue no.4, 38-41.
6. Manual for management of HIV/AIDS in children, 2005, NACO/IAP/UNICEF/WHO, 13-30.
7. Women and HIV infection including Mother to Child Transmission; Specialist's Training and Reference Module, NACO 2004, 164-176.

27 Birth Trauma: Congenital Brachial Palsy and Intracranial Hemorrhage

J.N. Sharma

Birth trauma is physical injury to an infant during birth process. Injuries may occur antenatally, intrapartum, or during resuscitation. The following factors contribute to an increased risk of birth injury:

1. Primipara.
2. Small maternal stature.
3. Maternal pelvis abnormality.
4. Prolonged or unusually rapid delivery.
5. Oligohydramnios.
6. Malpresentation of the fetus.
7. Use of mid forceps or vacuum extraction.
8. Versions and extraction.
9. Very low birth weight/extreme prematurity.
10. Fetal macrosomnia or large fetal head.
11. Fetal anomalies.

Evaluation at birth: Every neonate at risk should be thoroughly examined at birth to exclude birth trauma. Birth trauma may be minor or major. Minor traumas are asymptomatic and recover spontaneously. Major traumas may require urgent intervention medical or surgical.

The present write-up includes two birth injuries which are potentially disabling conditions with long-term effects if not managed properly at diagnosis.

CONGENITAL BRACHIAL PALSY

Congenital brachial palsy can be defined as a flaccid paralysis of an arm, rarely both arms, presenting at birth when on examination, the range of passive motion is greater than the active arm.

Classification

A useful classification has been described by Narakas based on the clinical findings in the first week of life.

Group I: Paralysis of shoulder and biceps (C5 and C6).

Group II: Paralysis of shoulder, biceps and forearm extensors (C5, C6 & C7).

Groups I and II constitute Erb's palsy with the difference of involvement of wrist extensors in Group II.

Group III: Complete paralysis of the limb (flail arm) (C5 to T1).

Group IV: As in three with ipsilateral Horner's syndrome due to sympathetic involvement.

Injury to C8 and T1 roots alone, described in association with breech delivery, which is clinically manifested as a claw hand (Klumpke's paralysis) is reported to be rare.

Pathogenesis

Although it is established that congenital brachial palsy is the result of injury to the brachial plexus or a part of it, controversy as to whether injury occurs before or at delivery, exists. However, three important risk factors have been identified viz. a heavy baby, shoulder dystocia and breech delivery. It is thought to be due to excessive traction on the head, neck, and the arm during birth.

The injury usually involves the nerve root; especially where the nerve roots come together to form the nerve trunks of the plexus. It varies in extent and severity. In general, the more extensive the injury, the more severe it is. Four types of injuries can occur:

1. Neuropraxia where only the myelin sheath is damaged producing conduction block and is reversible.
2. Axonotmesis where there is disruption of some or all of the axons but there is preservation of the sheath which allows recovery.
3. Neurotmesis (post ganglionic) where there is post ganglionic rupture of the nerve.
4. Neurotmesis (preganglionic) where there is avulsion and the spinal nerve is torn from the spinal cord.

Assessment and Diagnosis

The injury to the shoulder, clavicle, humerous and the lower cervical spine may mimic a brachial plexus injury. In these conditions passive movements are restricted because of muscle spasm and pain. One should exclude these conditions before carrying out a detailed neurological examination of all the four limbs.

The newborn infant usually presents with lack of movements of an arm but with presence of full passive movements of the shoulder, elbow and wrist joints. In groups I and II, the deltoid, infraspinatus, biceps, supinator and the brachioradialis and the extensors of the wrist and fingers may be weak or paralyzed. The functions of the small muscles of the hand are preserved. The infant adopts the typical "waiter's tip" with the arm adducted and internally rotated at the shoulder, extension and pronation at the elbow and flexion of the wrist and fingers. The Moro, bisceps, supinator reflexes are absent on the affected side. The grasp reflex is intact. Sensation is variably affected and diaphragm is affected in around 5% cases.

In group III with total brachial plexus injury, the entire arm is flaccid. All reflexes including the grasp reflex and sensation are absent. Injury to the sympathetic fibres at T1 results in ipsilateral Horner's syndrome (group IV). There may be autonomic changes in the skin of the affected limb viz. coolness, dryness to touch and a marble like appearance.

In the rare form of injury to C8 and T1 alone, the lower arm paralysis affects the intrinsic muscles of the hand and the long flexors of the wrist and fingers. The biceps and supinator reflexes are present, the grasp reflex is absent. There is sensory impairment on the ulnar side of the forearm and hand and ipsilateral Horner's syndrome.

Role of Investigations

1. A chest radiograph should be ordered if there is respiratory difficulty to exclude diaphragm paralysis.
2. Radiographs of the shoulder and upper arm may be necessary to rule out bony injury.
3. A CT myelography may be necessary to identify the presence of pseudomeningoceles associated with root avulsion. An MRI is useful to demonstrate neuromas associated with root rupture.
4. Electromyography and nerve conduction velocities are seen as an adjunct to clinical examination. It helps to distinguish an avulsion from stretch injury in those with slow recovery.

Course and Prognosis

The outcome of congenital brachial palsy depends on the extent and severity of the lesion. In general the outcome is better in the upper plexus than in the lower or total plexus injury. Notable clinical improvement in the first two weeks after birth indicates that normal or near normal function will return. If significant recovery is to occur, the rate of progression is relatively rapid in the first 3 months and then slows down. Studies of nerve injury and regeneration have shown that in neuropraxia complete recovery can be expected in 3-4 months whilst in axonotmesis it may take many months. After rupture or avulsion, the chances of significant spontaneous recovery are poor in the former and nill in the latter.

Management

The management aims at achievement of maximal nerve injury recovery, maintenance of optimal passive ranges of movements of the affected joints and strengthening the affected muscles thereby minimize long term disability. This requires the input of a multidisciplinary team of experts viz. orthopedic surgeon (brachial plexus expert), physiotherapist, occupational therapist, orthotist and a pediatric anesthetist. The pediatricians play the pivotal role. The services of a social worker and a clinical psychologist may also be required.

The initial management is conservative and is the responsibility of the pediatrician and the physiotherapist. The duties of the pediatrician include counselling the parents, assessment of severity and extent of lesion. The role of the physiotherapist is to teach, support, monitor and record progress. The best therapists are the parents.

In the first week, the arm should be rested and protected from excessive movement. Physiotherapy should be started after the second week when the post injury neuritis has resolved. The “statue of liberty” splinting, practised earlier, should be avoided because it may lead to contractures in the shoulder girdle.

The parents are instructed to treat the child atleast three times a day in the following manner:

a. Passive abduction and external rotation of the shoulder, placing the hands above the head.

b. External rotation of the shoulder with elbow flexed and kept at the infant's side placing the back of the hand on the bed.
c. These exercises should be done with both arms simultaneously to stabilize the trunk and scapula.
d. To stretch the posterior scapulohumeral angle, the arm is stretched across the chest towards the opposite shoulder. The hand should be placed behind the back and behind the head. The elbow, wrist and fingers should be put through all the movements to prevent contractures.

Surgical Treatment

The selection of infants who will benefit from surgery and when to intervene is still a dilemma. The emerging consensus is that the infants with a total flail arm with incomplete recovery at 1 month, and infants with less extensive lesion with incomplete recovery at 3 months, should be referred for specialist assessment.

INTRACRANIAL HEMORRHAGE

The human brain, during the perinatal period is vulnerable to a variety of insults which may produce life long consequences in the survivors. The ELBW infant is more vulnerable with a high incidence of neurological sequelae.

Development of the Cerebral Circulation

The arterial system supplying the brain is established externally by about 7 weeks of gestation. Internal vascularization and penetration of the cerebrum starts from 7 weeks with the development of superficial capillary network and later deep branches to the subependymal bed at 12 weeks of age. The subependymal layer or the germinal matrix consists of a mass of glioblastic cells supplied by a vascular network. It is the source of 80% of intraventricular hemorrhage. The vascular structure of the germinal matrix consists of arteries connecting with veins through capillary network. The source of hemorrhage appears to be from the venous side of the network. The capillary network in the germinal matrix supplies the superficial and deep parts leaving the centre relatively avascular. At 24 weeks, the developing cortex is supplied by spiral perforating medullary arteries. The germinal matrix thins out after 30 weeks of gestation and become vestigial in the more mature brain.

The cerebral venous system develops from a number of venous plexuses which extensively communicate and are remodeled greatly during fetal development. Eventually the thin walled dural sinuses and the deep or Galenic system remain. The cortex is drained by regularly branching veins which develop in parallel to the cortical arteries but are fewer in number.

Classification of Intracranial Hemorrhage

1. Subdural which may be (a) supratentorial and (b) infratentorial.
2. Subarachnoid.
3. Intraventricular and Periventricular hemorrhage.
4. Cerebellar and brain stem rarely detected in life.

How to Suspect Intracranial Hemorrhage?

Intracranial hemorrhage should be suspected after a traumatic delivery or in asphyxiated newborn infants. Subarachnoid hemorrhage and small periventricular hemorrhages are often asymptomatic. The clinical presentations include cerebral depression, seizures, apnoea, circulatory collapse, poor temperature control and a rapid fall in hematocrit.

Choice of Investigation

1. *Cranial ultrasound:* The first choice for supratentorial subdural hematoma.
2. *CT scan:* Useful for posterior fossa and subdural collections.
3. *MR scan:* Less useful for hemorrhagic lesion.
4. *Coagulation screen:* In infants > 34 weeks gestation.

Subdural Hemorrhage

Subdural bleeds can result from tentorial tear in the anterior end of the insertion of the falx cerebri into the tentorium cerebelli where the great cerebral vein and the inferior sagittal sinus combine to form the straight sinus. This area is easily damaged during a difficult delivery of the fetal head. Subdural bleeds can also result from tearing of the bridging veins over the vault.

The signs of subdural hemorrhage usually include those of severe asphyxia, of raised intra cranial pressure, or blood loss. The anterior fontanel is often bulged primarily as a result of cerebral edema. The diagnosis can be confirmed by ultrasonography. If not well visualized (e.g. in infratentorial bleeds) CT or MRI may be required.

Treatment includes treatment of coexistent asphyxia. A large subdural hematoma will need drainage by a subdural tap. A formal neurosurgical intervention may be considered after assessment of the prognosis of the accompanying HIE. Small bleeds do not require any intervention.

Supra tentorial bleeds are rarely directly fatal but infratentorial types are usually fatal.

Subarachnoid Hemorrhage

Subarachnoid hemorrhage occurs as a result of damage to the veins traversing the subarachnoid space. It is much more common than is generally realized. Small amounts of venous or capillary bleeding occur during mildly traumatic or asphyxial deliveries. The condition is usually asymptomatic but may present with seizures, jitteriness or irritability during the first few days.

Diagnosis is confirmed by obtaining a uniformly blood stained CSF on lumber puncture. A cranial USG may be done to exclude other types of intra cranial hemorrhage. A subarachnoid hemorrhage however cannot be detected with USG.

Symptomatic treatment of seizures and coexistent asphyxia is all that is required. There is no need for repeat lumber puncture to drain CSF. The condition usually resolves spontaneously. Prognosis is good.

Intraventricular Hemorrhage

Intraventricular hemorrhage (IVH) is a common injury in the preterm brain. The incidence and severity of IVH increase with decreasing gestation with the highest incidence in the ELBW infants. The ELBW infants not only have a higher incidence but also suffer severe grades of bleeding.

Intraventricular hemorrhage can be broadly divided into early and late onset. Early bleeds (within 12 hours of birth) occur more often in infants with lower gestational age and birth weight. It appears to be closely related to evidence of fetal distress, acidosis and mode of delivery. Premature rupture of membrane and maternal pregnancy induced hypertension appear to protect against early hemorrhage. Late onset type is seen in rather more mature preterm infants and is seen to be related to post natal events such as respiratory distress syndrome, derangement of blood gases, pneumothorax, endotracheal tube suctioning, hypothermia and excessive use of heparin. Intraventricular hemorrhage is rarely seen as an initial event 4 or 5 days after birth.

The reason remains unclear. Immediately after birth, the cerebral vasculature is relatively dilated and unreactive. Changes in vascular permeability occurs as a result of lowering of the prostacyclin levels 2-3 days after birth from the existing high levels, even in sick infants.

Pathogenesis

Intraventricular hemorrhage originates in the germinal matrix in infants at 26-32 weeks of gestation. The germinal matrix is a structure which is abundant over the head of the caudate nucleus and can also be found in the periventricular zone. The germinal matrix involutes early in the third trimester making germinal matrix intraventricular hemorrhage (GMH-IVH) rare in infants over 32 weeks gestation and 1.5 kg birth weight. In the preterm infant GMH-IVH originates from the fragile involuting vessels of the subependymal germinal matrix. The hemorrhage may be confined to the subependymal layers, rupture into the ventricle or pass into the subarachnoid space, and may be associated with separate hemorrhagic lesions in the periventricular parenchyma. It may be followed by complete resolution or post hemorrhagic hydrocephalous and may be associated with periventricular leucomalacia.

The pathogenesis of GMH-IVH has been shown to be related to various risk factors which may be divided into intravascular, vascular and extravascular. The intravascular factors are probably the most important and are also the factors most amenable to preventive efforts.

The intravascular factors include ischemia/reperfusion (rapid infusion in hypovolemic states), increases in cerebral blood flow (as a result of pneumothorax, seizures, hypercarbia, anemia, and hypoglycemia), fluctuating cerebral blood flow (while breathing out of synchrony with ventilator, presence of a large PDA) or increases in cerebral venous pressure (in preterm with high CPAP, tracheal suctioning, fetal head compression during labour, pneumothorax). In addition, impaired coagulation and platelet dysfunction are also intravascular factors that can contribute to the pathogenesis of GMH-IVH.

The vascular factors include the fragile nature of the vessels of the germinal matrix. These vessels have no muscularis mucosa and little adventitia. The vessels are of relatively large diameter and thin walled. All these factors make the vessels particularly susceptible to rupture.

The extravascular risk factors include deficient extravascular support and likely excessive fibrinolytic activity.

Intraventricular hemorrhage may rarely occur in term infants when it is usually from the choroid plexus with a history of the baby being delivered by forceps or ventouse. It may occur in association with deep venous sinus thrombosis, thalamic infarction and from the small remnants of subependymal germinal matrix. The other causes of IVH include vitamin K deficiency or a coagulopathy associated with hypoxic ischemic encephalopathy.

Complications of GMH-IVH

The two major complications include periventricular hemorrhagic infarction (PVHI) and post hemorrhagic hydrocephalous (PHH).

The PVHI represents a hemorrhagic venous infarction which results from obstruction of flow in the terminal vein by a large IVH. It is usually seen on the side of the larger IVH. A Doppler USG show markedly decreased or absent flow in the terminal vein on the affected side. Neuropathological studies demonstrate a fan shaped hemorrhagic infarction in the distribution of the medullary veins that drain into the terminal vein.

PHH may develop over days to weeks following IVH. There is progressive dilatation of the ventricles which relates to obliterative arachnoiditis that prevents CSF resorption, and obstruction of the aqueduct or the foramina of Luschka or Magendie by particulate clot. Brain injury which results is largely due to regional hypoxia-ischemia and mechanical distension of the periventricular white matter. In addition, injury to the immature oligodendrocytes in the white matter can be caused by reactive oxygen species generated by non protein bound iron present in CSF of infants with PHH. Post hemorrhagic hydrocephalous may present with increasing head growth, bulging fontanelle, separated sutures, decreased level of consciousness, sun setting sign, apnea, feeding difficulties and respiratory difficulty on one hand and may be asymptomatic on the other hand in preterm newborns. Serial cranial USG are necessary for diagnosis in the preterm newborn. 40% of these infants have spontaneous resolution. The rest 60% require medical or surgical treatment of which 15% die during the neonatal period.

Clinical Features

Uncomplicated germinal matrix hemorrhage is usually asymptomatic. With a larger hemorrhage, infants often become limp and unresponsive, may develop short tonic fits with decerebrate posturing and divergent squint.

If the infant was breathing spontaneously, it becomes apnoeic. They are difficult to resuscitate because they have become hypotensive and acidemic. These changes are due to blood loss as well as due to reflex changes in the pulmonary vasculature following an abrupt rise in intracranial pressure.

Characteristically, the PCV will drop by 5-10% after a few hours, and they often look pale with peripheral vasoconstriction. If the GMH—IVH is very large, the neonate develops a tense anterior fontanelle or an acute increase in head circumference.

The term newborn with IVH presents with seizures, apnoea, irritability or lethargy and a full fontanelle. It is rarely catastrophic unless there is associated subdural hemorrhage or parenchymal hemorrhage.

Diagnosis

In the preterm infant, GMH-IVH can be readily diagnosed with cerebral ultrasound examination. A GMH can be recognized as an echogenic area between the caudate nucleus and the ventricle (Fig. 27.2). An IVH can be recognized as an echogenic clot within the normally echolucent ventricle (Fig. 27.3). If an intraparenchymal lesion accompanies a GMH-IVH, it is usually globular and is seen on the same side. It evolves over a period of weeks into a porencephalic cyst (Fig. 27.4).

A routine cranial ultrasound should be performed in all infants born at < 32 weeks gestational age, in older infants born > 32 weeks of gestational age who have risk factors viz. perinatal asphyxia or pneumothorax and in those infants who present with abnormal neurological signs. The first cranial ultrasound examination should be done on day 3. However, in very sick, VLBW neonates it may be done within 24 hours of birth. An ideal schedule for USG examination may be day 3, 7, 30 and 60 for infants born < 32 weeks gestation (or birth weight < 1.5 kg).

Prevention

Traumatic intracranial hemorrhage can be reduced by judicious planning for management of cephalo pelvic disproportion (CPD) and operative delivery viz. forceps, ventouse and CS.

Prevention of preterm birth is the most effective method of prevention of IVH. In the event of preterm labour the following are advisable:

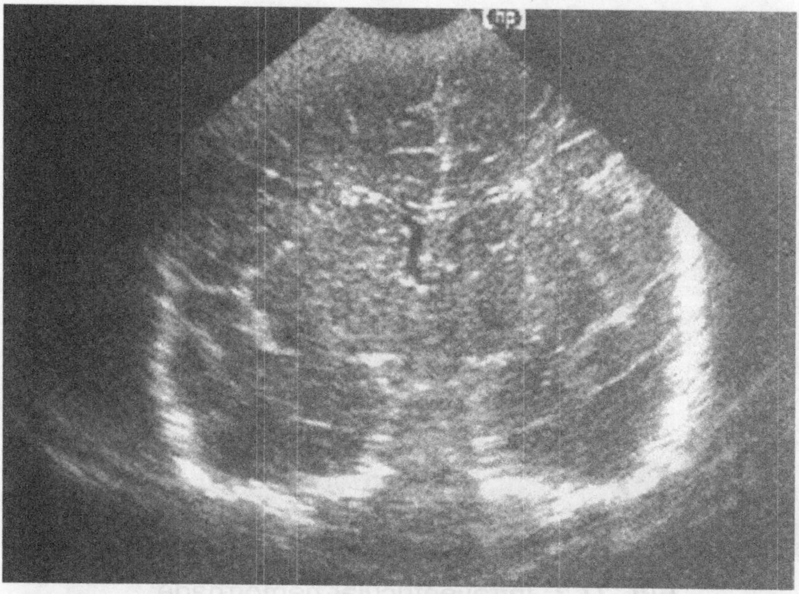

Fig. 27.1: Normal ventricles

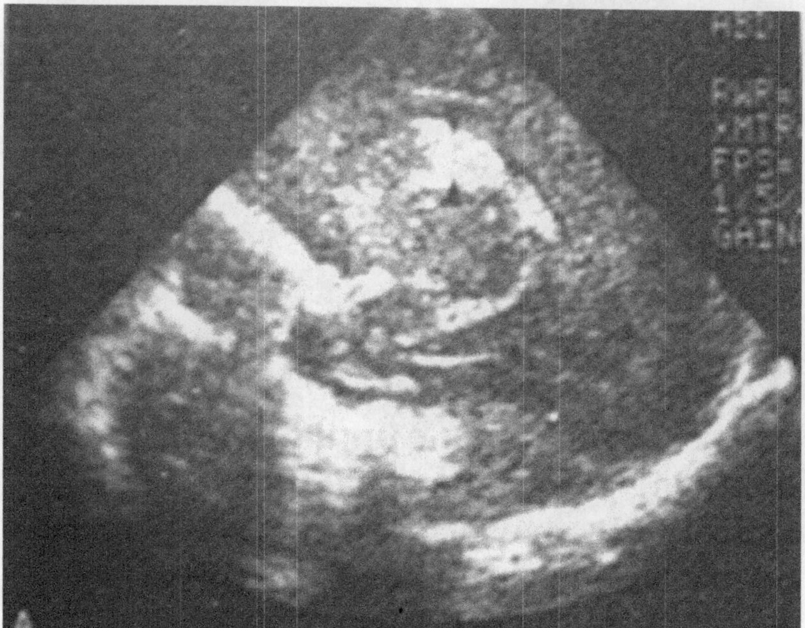

Fig. 27.2: Germinal matrix hemorrhage

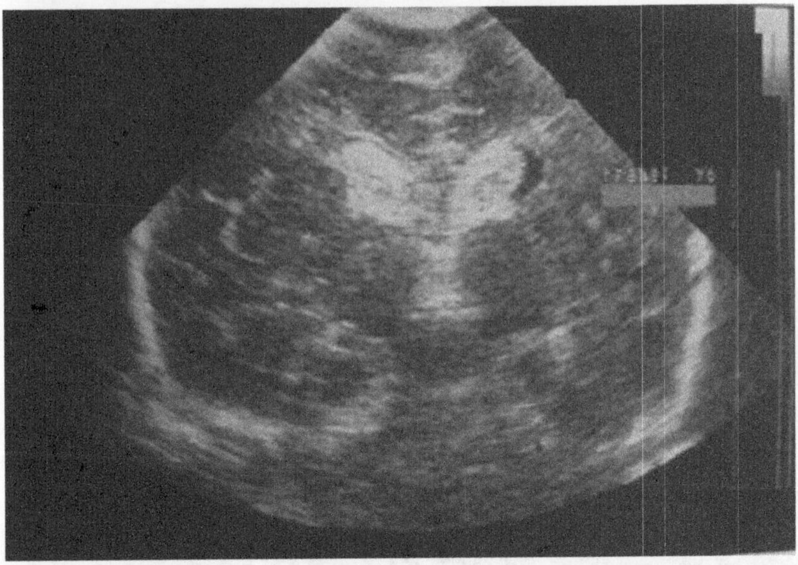

Fig. 27.3: Intraventricular hemorrhage

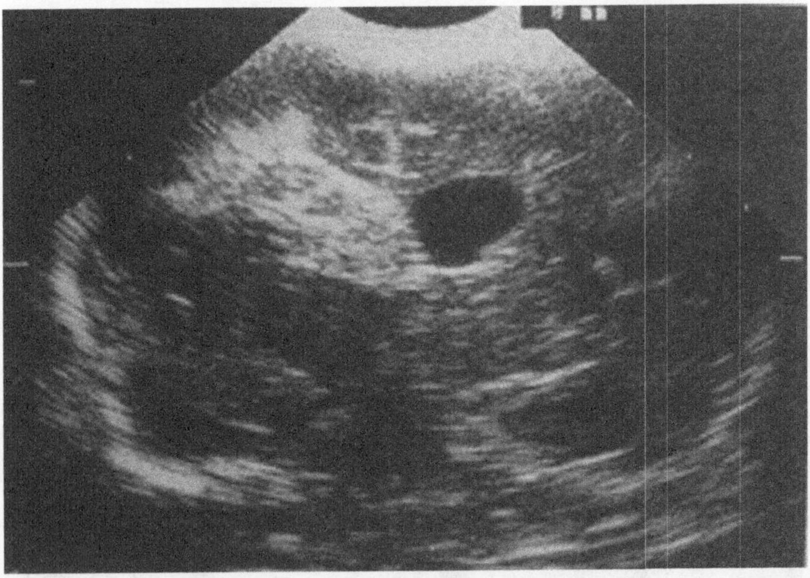

Fig. 27.4: IPL with porencephalic cyst

1. The birth of the infant should be planned in a hospital equipped for high risk deliveries. The risk of IVH is more in infants transported after birth.
2. Care should be taken for appropriate resuscitation, with vigilance in avoiding hyperventilation, hypoxia or low PCO_2, maintaining mean arterial pressure (MAP) and avoiding excessive handling and tracheal suctioning to prevent elevations in cerebral blood flow.
3. Designing ventilator techniques for elimination of cerebral blood flow (CBF) fluctuation related to mechanical ventilation which reduces the incidence of pneumothorax.
4. Avoidance of rapid infusion of sodium bicarbonate and volume expanders. In particular, infusion of colloid and hyperosmolar solutions should be given slowly.

Pharmacotherapy in Prevention

Several clinical trials have studied the effects of different pharmacotherapy to reduce the incidence of IVH in low birth weight infants. Among the various medications used, antenatal administration of glucocorticoids has clearly shown a decrease in the incidence of GMH-IVH. Other drugs viz. antenatal phenobarbitone, vitamin K, magnesium sulphate, indomethacin, vitamin E, ethamsylate has not shown conclusive evidence to prevent GMH-IVH.

Management

No specific treatment is available. Treatment is essentially supportive. Anemia—shock requires packed cell transfusion. Acidosis may require judicious and slow administration of sodium bicarbonate. Seizures should be aggressively treated with anticonvulsant. Coagulation abnormalities if present should be corrected.

Management of PHH consists of careful monitoring of ventricle size by serial cranial USG and appropriate intervention to reduce CSF accumulation.

Enlargement of the ventricles can be imaged with US long before clinical symptoms or excessive head growth. In many newborn post-hemorrhagic ventricular dilatation (PHVD) is mild, transient and asymptomatic. Progressive hydrocephalous is very likely if the CSF pressure is more than 15 cm H_2O. Hence a lumber puncture has to be performed once a PVHD is detected on USG. A CSF analysis will also help to exclude a low grade infection as a cause of ventricular enlargement and measure the CSF protein concentration to decide regarding the need of a shunt.

Once a PHVD has been recognized, serial measurements of ventricular size and head circumference are mandatory. Neurosurgical placement of an external ventriculostomy catheter may be needed in the early stage of uncontrolled, symptomatic PHH. When a VLBW is large enough, a permanent ventricular peritoneal shunt is placed. Serial lumbar punctures, repeated ventricular taps, diuretics (Frusemide, glycerol) + Acetazolamide therapy have been suggested but have shown to have no role in the management of PHH. Symptomatic large subdural hemorrhage in term babies should be treated by removal of the fluid by a subdural tap.

SUGGESTED READINGS

1. L. Gareth Evans–Jones, Rolfe Birch. Congenital brachial palsy in Recent Advances in Pediatrics (22) 2005 edited by T.J. David. Published by the Royal Society of Medicine Press Ltd., London W1 G 0 AE, UK.
2. J.M. Rennie and N.R.C. Roberton. Intracranial hemorrhage in A manual of neonatal intensive care. 4 the edition, 2004. Published by Arnold, 338 Euston Road, London NW1 3 BH.

3. Ashima Madan, Shannon E.G. Hamrick and Dona M. Ferriero. Central nervous system injury and neuroprotection. In Avery's Diseases of the newborn, 8th edition, 2005. Edited by H.William Taeusch, Roberta A. Ballard and Christine A. Gleason, Saunders.
4. Jannet S. Soul. Intracranial hemorrhage in Manual of neonatal care, 5th edition 2004, edited by John P. Cloherty, Eric C. Eichenwald and Ann R. Stark Lippincott, Williams and Wilkins, Philadelphia, USA.

28

Neonatal Transport

Pradipta Sanker Guha

All pediatricians from time to time have to make a decision of when, how and whom to refer a critically ill newborn. Neonatal transport should be considered when the care required by a sick neonate exceeds the capabilities of the referring hospital. Physicians should always be knowledgeable about the levels of services that are provided by the nearby government and private setups.

Which Newborns to Refer?

Maternal-fetal transport should always be preferred in the event of a high-risk pregnancy. The following neonatal conditions are guidelines to be used when considering the possibility of neonatal transport.

1. Prematurity and/or birth weight <1500 g.
2. Gestational age <32 weeks.
3. Respiratory distress requiring ventilatory support (CPAP, ventilation).
4. Seizures.
5. Congenital anomalies and/or inborn errors of metabolism.
6. Congenital heart disease or cardiac arrhythmias requiring cardiac services.
7. Severe hypoxemic-ischaemic injury.
8. Other conditions requiring neonatology consultation and consideration for transfer:

- Severe hyperbilirubinemia possibly requiring exchange transfusion.
- Infant of diabetic mothers.
- Severe intrauterine growth restriction.
- Birth weight between 1500 and 2000 g and gestational age between 32 and 36 weeks.
- For procedures unavailable at the referring hospital.

Responsibilities of the Referring Hospital

Stabilization

Unless there is a surgical emergency it is preferable to stabilize the child and keep the patient in the referring hospital awaiting the arrival of a trained pediatric transport team. While awaiting the transport staff the referring team should:

1. Maintain airway, oxygenation, and thermal stability.
2. Normalize circulatory deficits.
3. Maintain adequate blood glucose concentration.
4. Maintain umbilical venous/artery access if appropriate.
5. Insert a nasogastric tube and decompress the stomach.
6. Do appropriate studies (sepsis screen, cultures, X-ray) and initiate antibiotics.
7. Documentation:
   - Obtain initial transport consent from parents.
   - Complete transfer record. Note down all procedures and drugs given to the infant.
   - Ensure that the receiving hospital has the necessary facilities (i.e. surfactant, nitric oxide, surgery, ECMO etc.).

Stabilization Checklist

1. **Thermoregulation:**
   - Provide neutral thermal environment.

- Place under preheated radiant warmer with servo control or in a preheated incubator, or
- Place under a 200 watt bulb with infant well covered from head to foot.

2. **Respiration:** Prevent hypoxia and prevent hyperoxia in premature infants:
   - Maintain airway by positioning and suctioning as needed.
   - Give oxygen when necessary. If supplemental oxygen is required, it should be warm, moist and blended.
   - Give stimulation, if there is apnoea.
   - Have bag and mask, oxygen, oxygen blender and pressure manometer at bedside. Bag and mask ventilation and cardiac massage if resuscitation is required. Intubate if needed for positive pressure ventilation.
3. Place on a **pulse oximeter** with alarms: Set heart rate (HR) at 100-200, saturation percent as recommended by receiving facility. If not available the respiration, heart rate and temperature monitored. Observe for cyanosis.
4. If available, obtain arterial blood gas if requiring supplemental oxygen or having respiratory distress.
5. **Circulation:** Maintain blood pressure and perfusion.
   - Use volume expanders (normal saline, Ringers lactate) 10 ml /kg if hypovolemic.
   - Provide hydration with intravenous 10% dextrose solution.
6. **Metabolism:** Prevent hypoglycemia and acidosis.
   - Assess glucose by reagent strip according to institutional protocol. If no facilities available infuse 10% glucose 2 ml/kg/dose. Maintain glucose over 40 mg/dl.
   - **Correct acidosis** by treating underlying cause.
     a. *Respiratory acidosis:* May require mechanical ventilation.

b. *Metabolic acidosis:* May require sodium bicarbonate.

THE TRANSPORT

Members of the Transport Team

It is necessary that members of the transport team have the cognitive and technical skills necessary for treating newborn patients. A pediatrician having expertise in either neonatal special care or pediatric emergency medicine should ideally train them. Basic necessities of a transport team should include ability to:

1. Manage the airway.
2. Provide respiratory support.
3. Obtain vascular access.
4. Basic knowledge of pediatric drug dosing.
5. Knowledge of the basic pathology of pediatric diseases and the transport environment.

A team member's experience and skill in caring for a critically ill neonate is more important than ones educational degree. An experienced non-physician team member via phone contact can manage many situations.

Equipments with the Transport Team

1. Resuscitation equipments.
2. Medications.
3. Monitors.
4. Suction equipment.
5. Infusion pumps.
6. Oxygen cylinder.

Mode of Transport

Any pediatrician should always be aware of the vehicles/ambulances that are at his disposal in addition to their phone numbers.

Factors to consider in selecting a vehicle, ground or air, are:

1. Severity of illness.
2. The distance to the tertiary/specialized care center.
3. Transit time required.
4. Weather conditions.
5. Vehicle availability.
6. Equipment needs.
7. Expense.

All Vehicles must be Able to Provide:

1. On board oxygen.
2. Electrical power and suction.
3. Adequate space for supplies and equipment including oxygen tank, pharmacy pack, respiratory therapy devices, infusion pumps.
4. Stretchers.
5. Monitors.

Experience or Speed

The level of expertise and experience should always be given precedence over the speed of transport.

En Route to the Specialized Care Center

Once the child is stabilized continuous direct observation of the infant is one of the most important forms of monitoring during transport. The benefit of handling the child and taking vital signs should be weighed against the possibility of an accidental extubation or thermal loss. All medications should be at hand and cell phones should be used to maintain direct contact with the referral center to deal with any unexpected event. After arrival at the receiving center the transport team should ring up the referring center and the parents that the child has reached safely.

Points of Importance During the Transport Process

- To prevent injury during the transport process due to incidents of sudden unexpected acceleration/ deceleration, the neonate and equipments should be properly secured/restrained.
- The neonate should be restrained in such a way as to permit visual access at all times.
- In the event of inclement weather, the need for transport shall not outweigh safety considerations of the transport personnel and neonate.
- The patient care environment should be adequately lighted.
- Equipment should be kept operational through regularly scheduled inspection.

COMMUNICATION

Communication with the Receiving Staff

It is essential that the referring staff provide the receiving physician with accurate clinical information regarding the neonate and the mother. If the clinical status of the neonate changes prior to the arrival of the transport team, the referring hospital should contact the receiving hospital regarding additional recommendations for care.

The following information should be available from the transport team:

- Neonatal history and assessment.
- Reason(s) for transport.
- Gestational age.
- Birth weight.
- Perinatal history:
    1. Duration of rupture of membranes.
    2. Treatment of mother with antibiotics, when she received the first dose.

3. Antenatal steroid administration.
4. Hepatitis B surface antigen status.
5. Syphilis status.
6. Results of Human Immunodeficiency Virus (HIV) testing.
7. Blood type and coombs.
8. Presence of thick or thin meconium.

- Temperature, respiratory rate, heart rate, blood pressure, color.
- Investigation reports. Oxygen requirement and blood gas results.
- Therapy administered, including drugs and dosages.
- Signed consent forms, as required by the receiving hospital.

Communication with the Parents

1. The referring physician should discuss transport plans with the parents. Consent for transfer and appropriate procedures should be obtained.
2. An opportunity should be provided to the parents to see and touch their neonate.

Information to be Provided to the Parents Includes:

1 A picture of the neonate.
2. Printed materials including the names and telephone numbers of the neonatologist(s), neonatal nurse, directions to the hospital, and breastfeeding information.
3. The parents should be notified of the neonate's status after arrival at the receiving center. The parents are encouraged to visit the neonate as soon as they are able to do so.

Referred neonates who have received the maximal benefits of specialized care, but are not yet ready for discharge, may be transported back to the hospital from which they originated, if appropriate.

Management of Special Situations

1. **Congenital diaphragmatic hernia:** Immediate intubation and mechanical ventilation. Decompress the stomach.
2. **Cyanotic congenital heart disease:** PGE_1 infusion should be ideally transfused at the referring hospital through a central venous line. Observe for the side effects apnea, hypothermia and hypotension. Endotracheal intubation may be warranted.
3. **Anemia:** Infants in urgent need of a transfusion can be given non cross matched type O-negative packed cells until matched blood is available.
4. **Abdominal wall defects:** Both gastroschisis and omphalocele are treated by placing a nasogastric tube and immediately wrapping exposed abdominal contents with warm, sterile, saline soaked (non-cling) gauge.
5. **Neural tube defects:** Should be wrapped in warm sterile saline soaked (non-cling) gauge.
6. **RDS** may require surfactant administration before transport. Wait for at least 30 minutes before transport to provide time for direct observation and monitoring for any ventilatory changes.
7. **Air transport:** Barometric pressure decreases as altitude changes leading to decrease in oxygen tension. Oxygen saturation should be monitored and FiO_2 should be increased to result in an adequate PaO_2. With decrease of barometric pressure gases trapped in closed spaces expand leading to deterioration of the child. Gas expansion should be drained or vented regularly.
8. **Nitric Oxide** may reduce the need for ECMO in critically ill term or near term infants with pulmonary hypertension and hypoxemic respiratory failure. Anticipating prolonged transport times it may be

appropriate to begin inhaled nitric oxide on transport under the supervision of an experienced physician.

TRANSPORT OF SICK NEONATE FROM A PRIMARY HEALTH CENTRE (PHC)

A very sick newborn infant attending the primary health centre has to be transported to the district hospital for adequate care. At the PHC, only immediate care can be provided.

Immediate Care

Immediate care in the PHC level consist of:

1. *Provision of warmth:* The neonate should be kept under a radiant warmer in a warm room. If a radiant warmer is not available, a lamp with a conical shade and a 200 watt bulb can be used. The lamp should be kept at a distance of 45 cm over the surface of the well covered infant. The room should be kept warm with adequate numbers of room heater.
2. *Stabilization:*
   a. Maintenance of airway, breathing and circulation: The neonate should be kept in the supine position with the neck slight extension and suction of airways should be done if necessary. In case of apnea, the child may need physical stimulation, mouth to mouth breathing or bag and mask ventilation (if available), chest compression and medications. If the capillary refill time is prolonged (> 3 seconds), normal saline 10 ml/kg/dose I.V. should be given.
   b. If possible, the blood sugar should be checked and maintained > 40 mg/dl. If facilities are not available, all sick neonates should be given one bolus dose of Inj 10% dextrose, 2 ml/kg I.V.
   c. *Feeds and fluids:* The neonate can be given

expressed breast milk with a cup if unable to feed on the breast. Gavage feeding may be tried but should not be insisted upon. If the infant is very sick, it is advisable to stop enteral feeding, start IV infusion and quick transport emphasized.

d. *Specific therapy:* All very sick neonates should be given 1 mg Vitamin K IM and the first dose of an antibiotic (Ampicillin 50 mg/kg + gentamycin 2.5 mg/kg IM stat) to cover both gram positive and gram negative organism. Oxygen administered if necessary.

3. *Communication:* The condition of the infant should be explained to the parents and reassured. The need for referral should be explained. Care to be taken during transport should be explained to the persons accompanying the sick infant.
4. *Organization of transport:*
   a. The mother should be encouraged to accompany the baby. In case she cannot accompany immediately, she should be encouraged to reach the facility at the earliest. A doctor/nurse/dai/health worker should accompany to provide care en route.
   b. A precise note providing details of the condition of the baby need for referral and treatment given should always accompany.
   c. The referral hospital should be informed before hand.
   d. Care during transport: The accompanying person should be explained to ensure that:
      i. The infant's neck should be in slight extension to keep the airway open.
      ii. The trunk as well as the soles and palms should feel warm to touch.
      iii. The nose and the mouth should not be covered. Secretions if present should be suctioned with a Dee Lee's mucus trap.

iv. That the baby is breathing normally. If apneic to give stimulation, positive pressure ventilation.
v. If intravenous fluid is running, the attendant should make sure that the number of drops/ minute is correctly maintained and if necessary regulated.

5. The sick infant should be transported to the nearest referral facility by the shortest route and by using the fastest possible mode of transport.

SUGGESTED READINGS

1. Contemporary neonatal transport: Problems and solutions, L Cornette Arch Dis Child Fetal Neonatal Ed 2004; 89:F212–F214.Doi: 10.1136/adc.2003. 046201.
2. Agostino R, Antsaklis, Bre´art G, *et al.* (EUROPET Expert group). New decision rules: Regionalization in perinatal care and indications For perinatal transfer. Prenat Neonatal Med 1999;4:104-07.
3. Barry PW, Ralston C. Adverse events occurring during interhospital transfer of the critically ill. Arch Dis Child 1994; 71:8-11.
4. Agostino R, Fenton AC, Kolle´e LAA, *et al.* Organization of neonatal transport in Europe. Prenat Neonatal Med 1999;4:20-34.
5. Shenai JP. Neonatal transport. Outreach educational program. Pediatric Clinic N Am 1993;40:275-85.
6. King BR, Foster RL, Woodward GA, *et al.* Procedures performed by pediatric transport Nurses: How "advanced" is the practice? Pediatric Emergency Care 2001;17:410-13.
7. Watts C. The role of the ANNP: Nurse-led Neonatal transports. J Neonatal Nurse 2001;7:196-200.
8. Rashid A, Bhuta T, Berry A. A regionalized transport service, the way ahead? Arch Dis Child 1999; 80:488-92.
9. Woodward GA, Insoft RM, Pearson-Shaver AL, *et al.* The states of pediatric inter-facility transport: Con-

sensus of the second national pediatric and neonatal interfacility transport medicine leadership conference. Pediatr Emerg Care 2002;18:38-43.

10. Guidelines for air and ground transport of neonatal and pediatric patients, 1993, American Academy of Pediatrics.
11. Edge WE, Kanter RK and Walsh RF, Reduction of morbidity in Interhospital transport by specialized pediatric staff, Critical Care Medicine 1994;22:1186-91.
12. Newborn care training and operationalisation at Primary health centres. Resource book - P III. Training of PHC Medical officers. WHO collaborating centre for training and research in newborn care. All India Institute of Medical Sciences, New Delhi.

29 Care of the Surgical Neonate

H.K. Borah

By definition, critically ill neonates present life threatening problems that must be solved quickly with little margin for error. Although critical care is inherently a multi-speciality discipline, the physician who assumes primary responsibility must be familiar with the pathophysiology of a wide range of problems and possess a working knowledge of specialized techniques of diagnosis and life support.

Monitoring is vital in critical care medicine. As such, the concern clinician should be well versed in the parameters of hemodynamic and respiratory monitoring. Moreover, one should also be familiar with endotracheal intubation and mechanical ventilation, acid base disorders, fluid and electrolyte balance, nutrition and alimentation, medication administration, maintenance of thermo neutral environment, acute renal failure and a host of other aspects of critical care.

Neonatal surgical problems are usually caused by congenital malformations and majority of these malformations are severe which makes the baby critically ill. The malformation generally involve a particular organ/ system, very often, they occur in association involving different organs/systems.

It is common knowledge that in the developing countries, the rates of morbidity and mortality are very high in neonatal surgical conditions, although over the years, there has been a considerable improvement in the outcome expectancy in the developed countries. To attain good results in the practice of neonatology and neonatal surgery in a developing country, very close collaboration and team work is essential between the obstetrician, pediatrician, public health medical worker, community physician, nursing personal along with the cooperation of the members of the family. The role of the pediatrician is very significant because after the birth of the baby, they are primarily responsible for the assessment of the baby and detection of any medical or surgical problem and prompt referral to a specialist center after taking adequate emergency care before and during transportation. The care of the surgical neonate after successful surgery again becomes the responsibility of the pediatrician.

Since over 85% babies are born in the rural parts of India, the role of medical/paramedical personnel in the initial management of the neonate is very important, because pediatricians are not yet accessible to many people in the remote areas. In fact much depends on this initial management for the ultimate outcome. Although critical care is essentially delivered in the neonatal intensive care unit (NICU), the emergency treatment provided to the neonate at the periphery and the precautions taken during its transportation to a referral center also form an essential component of the critical care management.

Causes of High Morbidity and Mortality

The causes of high morbidity and mortality in the surgical neonate can be summerised as follows:

a. Failure or delay in diagnosis, inadequate or faulty preoperative management, delay in transfer, all these result in many of the babies being moribund on admission to hospital.

b. Failure to concentrate these babies in one hospital. It is obvious that wide dispersal of these relatively rare cases does not allow individuals working in isolation to gain sufficient experience in the complicated management.
c. Failure to concentrate these babies in one ward of the hospital, hence the babies cannot get the necessary special nursing care which they need or conversely, they get all the nurses attention to the detriment of the other patients in the ward. Ideally these babies are best managed in a NICU.

Presentation of the Surgical Neonate

The surgical neonate can present with bilious vomiting, with respiratory difficulty, with significant skin defect, with large swellings or with urinary obstruction.

Bilious Vomiting

It is said that green vomit by a neonate should always be considered to be due to intestinal obstruction unless proven otherwise. The conditions seen under this group are:

1. ***Imperforate anus***: The condition should be obvious at birth if a thorough physical examination of the neonate is made. Unfortunately, it is detected much later when baby starts vomiting and develops abdominal distension following feeding. The baby with imperforate anus who presents with gross abdominal distension is usually a male and it has a high type of anomaly i.e. the blind rectal pouch has ended at a level higher than the levator diaphragm and frequently, there is an associated fistulous communication with the urethra.

   An invertogram taken in the lateral position is the most important radiological investigation which is required to confirm the diagnosis. These babies need a transverse/pelvic colostomy as an emergency palliative measure which has to be followed by an anorectal reconstruction (PSARP procedure) at around one year of age. The low type of anomalies (viz. anal stenosis, anal membrane) can be tackled through a perineal approach without a covering colostomy. In the female babies, the usual mode of presentation is passage of stool per vagina. As there is not much vomiting or abdominal distension associated with this condition during the neonatal period, there is no need of any emergency surgical intervention in these conditions. A well planned reconstructive surgery is preferred which is done at a much later time during infancy.

2. ***Intrinsic lesions of the bowel:*** Atresia and membrane obstruction may occur at any level of the alimentary tract. These babies may have a maternal history of hydramnios. An erect X-ray of abdomen may show a single bubble (*pyloric stenosis*), a double bubble (*duodenal atresia*) a triple bubble (*jejunal atresia*) and multiple air fluid levels (*ileal obstruction*). The lower is the site of obstruction, the greater abdominal distension and later is the onset of vomiting. These babies may not pass meconium. *Hirschsprung's disease* sometimes presents very early. The condition is more common in males. There is history of failure or delayed passage of meconium, abdominal distension and vomiting. Rectal examination causes a forceful expulsion of flatus and meconium/feces on withdrawal of the examining finger. Erect X-ray of abdomen shows grossly dilated bowel loops with fluid levels. Barium enema study is helpful in diagnosis, which should be confirmed by a rectal biopsy. If the condition is not relieved by repeated rectal irrigations with glycerine in warm normal saline, an emergency

colostomy is indicated to be followed by a definitive surgery later. Enterocolitis is a common complication of this disease during the neonatal period.

3. ***Intraluminal obstruction***: Meconium ileus and meconium plug syndrome are two conditions causing intra luminal obstruction. *Meconium ileus* is associated with cystic fibrosis of the pancreas. The lumen of the distal small bowel is obstructed by thick blackish green bitumen like meconium. An erect X-ray shows multiple fluid levels and soap bubble appearance caused by air trapped in the inspissated meconium. The condition needs immediate surgery. In *Meconium plug syndrome* there is an inspissated plug of meconium at the head of the column of meconium in the rectum or lower colon. A rectal examination may be diagnostic as well as curative; the plug is passed followed by meconium and gas.
4. ***Extrinsic obstruction:*** Intestinal malrotation and midgut volvulus, Ladd's bands are conditions under this group. Erect x ray suggests intestinal obstruction and confirmatory diagnosis is made at laparotomy.

Management

In babies with bilious vomiting, the following measures are to be taken even before the case is referred to a pediatric surgeon. The initial supportive measures play an important role in the outcome and consist of the following:

1. Feeding is to be stopped immediately and the stomach is to be kept empty by repeated nasogastric aspiration through an infant feeding tube. The outside end of the tube should be kept open at all times for continuous decompression.
2. An erect posture plain X-ray of the abdomen should be done in all cases as it helps to make a working diagnosis.

3. If any delay is anticipated in transfer of the baby or the baby is dehydrated an I.V. infusion is to be started. The amount of fluid to be given should be calculated on the basis of need. Number 24 G I.V. canula and burette iv drip sets are preferred for use in neonate for infusing measured volumes of fluid accurately. It is always important to keep in mind that "it is safer to err on the dry side".
4. Special attention should be paid to maintain body temperature of the baby during physical examination and during transport.
5. The baby should be referred or transported to a speciality center as early as possible after stabilization.

With Respiratory Difficulty

The two common conditions under this group are as follows:

1. ***Esophageal atresia with tracheo esophageal fistula:*** The common type of this anomaly is where there is a blind upper pouch and a fistula to the trachea from the lower pouch. Suspicion should arise when a neonate, particularly one having a history of maternal hydramnios, continues to drool frothy saliva and developing rattling respiration despite repeated suctioning with a mucus sucker. In such a baby, the patency of the esophagus should be tested by passing down a well lubricated firm red catheter. If the catheter gets arrested at about 8-10 cms from the lips, the diagnosis is confirmed. There is good reason to perform this simple test in every newborn just after birth. Cases of TEF then would be detected soon after birth and before the baby is fed, because feeding causes aspiration into the lungs which deteriorates the prognosis. An erect infantogram is to be done in

these babies. Presence of gas in the stomach and intestine indicates that there is a fistula and absence indicates a pure atresia without a fistula. The upper blind pouch in TEF should be kept empty by repeated suctioning until surgical intervention is done.

2. ***Congenital diaphragmatic hernia:*** It is one of the most acute surgical emergencies in the neonates. It occurs as a result of failure of closure of the pleuro peritoneal cannal on the left chest (foramen of Bochdalek). It leads to the displacement of the abdominal contents into the chest and there is an association of the different degrees of hypoplasia of the left lung. The baby usually presents with respiratory distress and cyanosis immediately after birth. There is diminished movement of the chest on the left side, apex is displaced to the right side and the bowel sounds are heard in the chest. The abdomen is scaphoid. X-ray of the chest confirms the diagnosis. After birth, if the diagnosis of congenital diaphragmatic hernia is suspected, an infant feeding tube is passed into the stomach to keep it empty. This prevents further distention of the gut trapped inside the chest. If the baby requires assisted ventilation, an endotracheal tube is passed and bag and tube ventilation started. No attempt should be made to give positive pressure ventilation by a bag and mask because it will further distend the stomach and increase the respiratory distress. The baby should be nursed on a left lateral position keeping the head slightly elevated. It helps in better excursion of the unaffected right lung. The baby need emergency surgical intervention and should be referred to a pediatric surgeon or transferred to a better facility for further management after preliminary life saving measures looked after.

3. ***Other conditions:*** The other conditions of respiratory distress like congenital lobar emphysema, congenital cystic disease of lungs, and hypoplasia of the lung can be diagnosed by an X-ray chest. The former two requires urgent surgical treatment while the latter requires intensive care. Bilateral choanal atresia and Pierre Robin syndrome are two other rare surgical causes of respiratory distress in newborn.

With Significant Skin Defect

1. ***Exomphalus major:*** It is the most common condition under this group, in which there is a herniation of the abdominal viscera through a huge defect at the site of the umbilicus. The protrusion is covered by a membrane consisting of three layers—peritoneum inside and amnion outside separated by wharton jelly. Although the membrane is shiny and intact at birth, it soon becomes opaque, malodorous and necrotic because of the lack of blood supply. If untreated, it ruptures leading to the evisceration of the contents. In case of defects of less than 5 centimeters in diameter, it is usually possible to do an immediate surgical repair. In cases with larger defect, conservative management may be done by repeated application of 2% aqueous mercurochrome and keeping the area open without dressing. This may be resorted to when immediate surgery is not possible. By this treatment, a tough dry eschar is formed over the swelling. This eschar is gradually replaced by skin from the surrounding areas during a period of 8-10 weeks; the ventral hernia thus formed is treated much later.
2. ***Ruptured exomphalos and gastroschisis:*** There is an antenatal evisceration of the gut in this condition. The exposed viscera should be kept moist and warm by covering them with warm saline packs. During

transport to the hospital or within the hospital, it is convenient to enclose the exposed viscera in a transport polyethylene bag to prevent hypothermia and dryness. The conditions obviously require urgent surgery.

3. ***Extrophy of bladder:*** These cases are also managed by primary repair during the neonatal period, although the results are not uniformly satisfactory.

With Large Swellings

1. ***Sacrococcygeal and cervical teratomas:*** Should be excised during the neonatal period because of the risk of malignant transformation in them increases beyond that period.
2. ***Meningoceles and meningomyeloceles:*** Particularly those which have already ruptured or are proceeding towards impending rupture, should be repaired as early as possible, during the neonatal period. In the case of intact ones with a glistening covering, repeated application of 2% aqueous mercurochrome encourages the ingress of the surrounding skin, the lesion can then be managed electively sometime during later infancy.

With Urinary Obstruction

1. ***Posterior urethral valve*** is the commonest cause of urinary obstruction in the newborn. After adequate stabilization of the acid base and fluid electrolyte balance in the baby, and under proper antibiotic cover, early fulguration of the valves is the best form of treatment. In the absence of proper equipment for this procedure, a proximal diversion in the form of a cutaneous vesicostomy/ureterostomy is performed which is to be followed by ablation of the valves at a later time during the infancy.

2. ***A pin hole meatus*** is commonly diagnosed erroneously as phimosis subjecting the neonate to unnecessary circumcision. Gentle dilatation of the prepuce and a short time application of an ointment containing steroid usually solve the problem.

Noncritical Surgical Conditions

There are many other surgical conditions in the neonate where the baby is not critically ill but the parents are worried and seek advice of the physician for urgent solution. The conditions which do not require any urgent surgical intervention are cleft lip and palate, umbilical hernia, hypospadias, epispadias, undescended testis, cystic hygroma, cephalhematoma, hemangioma, umbilical granuloma. However, parents of babies with cleft palate need counseling on feeding problems.

Congenital vaginal hydrocele does not require any surgery during the neonatal period as majority of the cases regress spontaneously later during infancy following late obliteration of the patent processus vaginalis. Congenital inguinal hernias, on the other hand, require urgent repair because of high incidence of obstructive symptoms.

In cases of congenital talepes equino varus, plaster of paris immobilization following reduction should be started as early as possible during the neonatal period. It results in a better prognosis than in the cases where the treatment is started after the neonatal period, operative surgical reduction can thus be avoided in many cases. Cases of ambiguous genitalia need to be evaluated urgently because the assignment of gender to the neonate is a social emergency. Cases of congenital adrenal hyperplasia present in a critical state due to rapid loss of salts which need to be urgently replaced in addition to corticisteroids.

SUGGESTED READINGS

1. Annals of the National Academy of Medical Sciences (India), 1979.
2. Potts W.J. the Surgeon and the child. Published by W.B. Saunders., Philadelphia, USA.
3. Marini JJ, Wheeler AP. Critical care medicine—the essentials. Published by Williams and Wilkins, Baltimore, 1989.
4. Yadav KA. Care of surgical neonates in developing countries in textbook of neonatal surgery published by Vikas Publishing House Pvt. Limited, New Delhi, 1983.

30 Common Neonatal Procedures

J.N. Sharma

Hand Washing

Effective and thorough hand washing is regarded as the single most useful measure for prevention of nosocomial infection. The nails should be trimmed and no nail polish should be used. Rings, wrist watch, bangles etc. should be removed before entering the nursery. The hands should be washed for 2 minutes before entering the nursery and for 10 seconds in between touching two babies. The hands and arms should be washed upto the elbow with liquid soap in running water.

Indications

A thorough hand washing is mandatory before entering the nursery, before performing an invasive procedure, and after providing care to an infected infant.

Steps

1. The hand should be lathered covering all areas including nails, webs, and sides of the fingers which are known to harbour organisms.
2. The six steps of cleaning should be followed:
   - Palmer surface of the hands: 20 seconds.
   - Each dorsal surface: 10 seconds.
   - Knuckles: 10 seconds each.
   - Thumbs: 10 seconds each.

- Tip of the fingers: 10 seconds each.
- Wrist: 10 seconds each.

3. The hands should be washed with water upto the elbows and dried with autoclaved napkins, disposable sterile paper napkins or allowed to dry spontaneously.

How to Insert An Orogastric Tube?

Equipments

1. 8 F feeding tube (a larger tube may make it difficult to obtain a seal. Secretions can easily occlude a smaller tube).
2. 20 ml syringe.

Steps

1. Measure the length of the tube. The length should be equal to the distance from the bridge of the nose to the ear lobe and from the ear lobe to the xiphoid process.
2. Insert the tube through the mouth. The nose should be kept open for ventilation.
3. After the tube is inserted for the desired length, the stomach contents should be gently aspirated with a 20 cc syringe.
4. Then remove the syringe and leave the end of the tube open.

Tape the tube to the baby's cheek to ensure that the tip remains in the stomach.

Endotracheal Intubation

Indications

1. Prolonged positive pressure ventilation (beyond a few minutes).
2. Bag and mask ventilation is not resulting in good chest rise.
3. When chest compression is necessary.

4. Medication e.g. epinephrine, naloxone.
5. Meconium stain liquor and depressed baby.
6. Surfactant therapy.
7. Suspected congenital diaphragmatic hernia.
8. Extreme prematurity.

Equipments

1. Infant laryngoscope with an extra set of batteries and extra bulbs.
2. Blades: No. 1 (term newborn), No. 0 (preterm newborn) No. 00 (optional for extremely preterm newborn. Straight blades are preferred.
3. Sterile disposable endotracheal tubes with inside diameters of 2.5, 3.0, 3.5 and 4.0 mm.
4. Stylet (optional).
5. Carbon dioxide monitor (optional).
6. Suction setup with 10F or larger suction catheter, plus sizes 5F or 6F and 8F for suctioning the endotracheal tube.
7. Roll tape, ½ or ¾ inch, scissors.
8. Oral airway.
9. Self-inflating resuscitation bag and mask with oxygen reservoir.
10. Stethoscope.

Preparation of the Endotracheal Tube

1. Select the appropriate size tube.
2. *Cut the tube at 13-15 cm length:* Remove connector and cut the tube diagonally. Replace the connector.

Selection of appropriate tube size on the basis of weight/ gestation

Tube size (mm)	*Weight (gm)*	*Gestational age (wks)*
2.5	Below 1,000	Below 28
3.0	1,000-2000	28-34
3.5	2,000-3000	34-38
3.5-4.0	Above 3000	Above 38

Anatomical Landmarks

The following anatomical landmarks are important to understand the procedure of intubation:

1. *Vallecula:* A pouch formed by the base of the tongue and the epiglottis.
2. *Epiglottis:* A lid like structure over hanging the entrance to the trachea.
3. *Glottis:* The opening to the trachea; contains the vocal cords.
4. *Vocal cords:* Folds of mucous membrane on both sides of the trachea, just within the glottis.
5. *Esophagus:* The food passage situated just posterior to the tracheal opening.

Steps of Intubation

1. Position the baby with neck in slight extension.
2. Turn on the laryngoscope light and hold the laryngoscope in the left hand between the thumb and first two or three fingers with the blade pointing away from you. The laryngoscope is designed to be held in the left hand by both right and left-handed persons. If held in the right hand, the curved part of the blade will block the view of the glottis, as well as make insertion of the endotracheal tube impossible.
3. Visualisation of glottis and insertion of the tube: During actual resuscitation the following steps will need to be completed within approximately 20 seconds. Free flow oxygen should be delivered through out the procedure.
   a. *Stabilize the baby's head* with your right hand. A second person may be called to hold the head in the proper position.
   b. *Slide the laryngoscope blade from the left angle of the mouth*, over the right side of the tongue, pushing the tongue to the left side of the mouth,

and advance the blade until the tip lies in the Vallecula, just beyond the base of the tongue. You may need to use your right index finger to open the mouth to make it easier to insert the laryngoscope.

c. *Lift the blade by raising the entire blade* by pulling up in the direction the handle is pointing, to expose the pharyngeal area.

d. *Look for the landmarks*: If the tip of the laryngoscope is correctly positioned in the Vallecula, you should see the epiglottis at the top, with the glottic opening below. You also should see the vocal cords appearing as vertical stripes on each side of the glottis or as an inverted letter "V". If these structures are not immediately visible, you should quickly adjust the blade until the structures come into view. Applying downward pressure to the cricoid may help bring the glottis into view. The pressure may be applied with your own little finger or by an assistant. Suctioning of the secretions also may be helpful to improve your view.

e. *Insertion of tube*: Holding the tube in your right hand, introduce it into the right side of the baby's mouth. This will prevent the tube from blocking your view of the glottis. Keep the glottis in view and when the vocal cords are apart, insert the tip of the endotracheal tube until the vocal cord guide is at the level of the cords. This will position the tube in the trachea approximately halfway between the vocal cords and the carina.

f. *If the cords are together,* wait for them to open. Do not touch the closed cords with the tip of the tube. It may cause spasm of the cords. If the cords do not open within 20 seconds, stop and ventilate with bag and mask. After the heart rate and color have improved, you can then try again.

g. *Stabilize the tube* with one hand and remove the laryngoscope with the other. With the right hand held against the face, hold the tube firmly at the lips and/or use a finger to hold the tube against the baby's hard palate. Use your left hand to carefully remove the laryngoscope without displacing the tube. If the stylet was used, remove it from the endotracheal tube.

h. *Check to be sure that the tube is in the trachea:* If the tube is positioned correctly, one should observe:
   - A rise in the chest with each breath.
   - Breath sounds over both lung fields but decreased or absent over the stomach. Use a small stethoscope and place it laterally and high on the chest wall (in the axilla). A large stethoscope or a stethoscope placed too central or too low may transmit sounds from the esophagus or stomach.
   - No gastric distension with ventilation.
   - Vapour condensing on the inside of the tube during exhalation.
   - You can use the tip to lip measurement to estimate if the tube has been inserted the correct distance. Adding 6 to the baby's weight in kilograms will give a rough estimate to the correct distance from the tube tip to the vermilion border of the upper lip. Babies weighing less than 750 gms may require only 6 cm insertion.
   - Detection of presence of CO_2 in the endotracheal tube can serve as confirmatory evidence that the tube is in the trachea by using a CO_2 detector viz. capnograph or a colorometric device connected to the endotracheal tube. However, ELBW babies or babies with very poor cardiac output may exhale insufficient CO_2 to be detected reliably by CO_2 detectors.

Complications, possible causes and corrective action of endotracheal intubation

Complication	Possible causes	Corrective action
1. Hypoxia	Taking too long to intubate	Pre-oxygenation, free flow O_2 during procedure, halt intubation after 20 secs
	Incorrect placement of tube	Reposition tube
2. Bradycardia/ Apnea	Hypoxia	Pre- oxygenation with bag and mask
	Vagal response from	Free flow O_2 during procedure
	Laryngoscope/ suction catheter	Oxygenate after intubation with bag and tube
3. Pneumothorax	Over ventilation of one lung due to tube in right main bronchus	Place tube correctly Use appropriate ventilating pressure
4. Contusions or Lacerations of tongue, gums	Rough handling of laryngoscope or tube	Obtain additional practice/skill
	Inappropriate rocking rather than lifting of laryngoscope	
Or airway	Laryngoscope blade too long or too short	Select appropriate equipment
5. Perforation of esophagus	Too vigorous insertion of tube	Handle gently
	Stylet protrudes beyond end of tube	Place stylet properly
6. Obstructed endotracheal tube	Kink in the tube or tube obstructed with secretions	Try to suction tube with catheter. If unsuccessful consider replacing tube
7. Infection	Introduction of organism via hands or equipment	Pay careful attention to clean/ sterile technique

Lumbar Puncture

Indications

1. For evaluation of neonates who have symptoms and signs of meningitis, hemorrhage, metabolic and degenerative disorders.
2. As a part of sepsis screen.

Contraindications

1. Clinical signs of significantly increased intracranial pressure or midline shift.
2. Hemodynamic and pulmonary instability.
3. Soft tissue infection over the lumber puncture area.
4. Unresponsive coagulopathy or severe thrombocytopenia.

Complications

1. Acute respiratory or neurologic deterioration.
2. Epidural, subdural or sub arachnoid hemorrhage.
3. Cerebral herniation.
4. Temporary paralysis.

Technique and Steps

Lumbar puncture can be performed either in the lateral recumbent or sitting position. The sitting position is beneficial in newborn and in babies with pulmonary disorders because it may prevent hyper flexion of the neck that can precipitate respiratory distress with the recumbent technique. A neonatal lumbar puncture needle or a scalp vein needle can be used for the procedure. The scalp vein set has the additional advantage that the CSF pressure can be measured by holding the polythene tubing upright.

Steps

1. The neonate should be placed in the sitting position with the dorsal and lumbar spine flexed as much as possible or in the lateral position with the spine flexed. The neck should not be flexed.
2. The back should be sterilized with spirit—betadine —spirit.
3. The spine of the 4th lumbar vertebra should be identified by drawing a line joining the two iliac crests.

The needle should be inserted at the mid point between L4 and L5 spines and advanced anteriorly with the beveled end of the needle facing upwards. The space between L3 and L4 can be tried if no fluid is obtained. Higher taps can cause spinal cord injury because the spinal cord in newborn comes down to the L3 level.

4. The subarachnoid space in the newborn is usually reached within a depth of 1 cm but the sensation of penetrating the ligamentum flavum is often absent.

Subdural Tap

A subdural tap should be attempted to drain a subdural collection of fluid or blood confirmed by an ultrasound or CT examination. A short and wide bored needle with a stylet should be used instead of a lumbar puncture needle.

Steps

1. The anterior half of the scalp should be shaved and thoroughly washed with soap and water.
2. The baby should be completely wrapped. The head should be placed near the edge of the table.
3. The site of tap is in the coronal suture just lateral to the lateral angles of the anterior fontanel. If one side is dry, tap should be done on the other side.
4. After puncture, one should wait for about half a minute or so because subdural fluid is often thick and viscid. If no fluid comes out, the needle can be advanced further to a maximum depth of 1.0 to 1.5 cm. Suction with a syringe should not be applied.

Ventricular Tap

The indications of ventricular tap include: (i) diagnosis of intraventricular hemorrhage (ii) administration of antibiotics in treatment of ventriculitis and (iii) for relief of intracranial pressure in an infant with hydrocephalous waiting a shunt operation. A long lumbar puncture needle with a stylet should be used for a ventricular tap.

Steps

1. The preparation of the scalp is same as for subdural tap.
2. The site of puncture is also the same.
3. The needle should be pushed forwards and inwards directing it towards the nasion. The ventricle is generally reached at the depth of 2.5 cm. Suction with a syringe should be never attempted.
4. After removal of the needle the baby should be kept in the sitting posture and local pressure is applied to stop oozing CSF.

Umbilical Vessel Catheterization

Indications

1. Umbilical vein catherization:
   a. Exchange transfusion.
   b. Monitoring of central venous pressure.
   c. Infusion of fluids, blood or medication.
2. Umbilical arterial catheterization:
   a. For frequent monitoring of arterial blood gases.
   b. As a route for infusion of parenteral fluids.
   c. For continuous monitoring of arterial blood pressure.

Complications

1. Clot formation and release of micro emboli.
2. Liver necrosis following infusions of medications or parenteral nutrition.
3. Spontaneous perforation of vessel wall.
4. Portal hypertension.
5. Necrotising enterocolitis.

Technique

1. *Umbilical vein catheterization:*
   a. The infant is restrained by using a padded crucifix splint for fixing all four limbs.
   b. The umbilicus is prepared aseptically with spirit and iodine.
   c. The umbilical vein is identified by its 12 O' clock position, bigger and collapsed vessel with thin vessel wall, bleeding on removal of the clot.
   d. The length to be introduced is measured as 20% of the crown heel length and marked. The catheter is prepared by filling it with heparinised saline (prepared as 1 unit/500 ml of saline).
   e. The catheter is then gently pushed forward in a rotary movement till free flow of blood is obtained. The catheter should be never left open to the atmosphere because negative intra thoracic pressure could cause air embolism.
   f. The catheter should be fixed with a purse string suture as tightly as to stop bleeding and not to obliterate the catheter.
   g. The position of the catheter tip should be verified by X-ray. Only when it is in the inferior vena cava hypertonic solutions may be infused.
2. *Umbilical artery catherization:*
   1. Restrain and asepsis as in umbilical vein catheterization.
   2. The length of the catheter to be introduced should be measured 60% of the shoulder umbilical length. The catheter is prepared in the same way as in umbilical vein catheterization.
   3. The catheter is then introduced into one of the arteries identified by its 5 O' clock or 7 O' clock position, smaller and thick walled, no clot and absence of bleeding.
   4. The catheter is then introduced gently towards the caudal direction. The catheter tip may be

positioned at a high or low site. In highly positioned state the catheter lies between ductus arteriosus and origin of celiac axis (between T_4 and T_{11} vertebrae). In the lower location, the tip is positioned in the abdominal aorta between inferior mesenteric artery and aortic bifurcation (opposite L_4 vertebra). The lower location is associated with risk of cyanosis and gangrene of buttocks and legs. The feet and buttocks should be examined during this procedure.

5. The catheter should be removed slowly over a period of 30-60 seconds, allowing the umbilical artery to go into spasm at its proximal end, thus avoiding profuse bleeding.

Peripheral Vascular Access

Indications

1. Replacement of fluid.
2. Administration of blood and blood products.
3. Correction of electrolyte abnormalities.
4. Administration of medications.
5. Parenteral nutrition.

Equipment

Butterfly needles (23, 24, 25 G), IV canula (23, 24 G).

Selection of Site: The most commonly used IV sites are the superficial veins of the scalp, hand, arm, leg and foot. During emergency, the largest and most accessible veins, distant from the resuscitative efforts should be selected.

Technique

1. The vein should be visualized properly. It can be done by pressure by application of a rubber band tourniquet or hand pressure proximal to the vein.

2. An indirect puncture of the vein is better than the direct puncture to avoid double puncture. In indirect puncture, the skin is punctured and needle is carried along the wall of the vein for a distance and then the venous wall is punctured. In the direct puncture method, the skin and the venous wall is punctured in the same site, In both the methods the beveled end of the needle should face downward.

Complications

1. Phlebitis.
2. Extravasation, I.V. infiltration.
3. Air embolism.
4. Hematoma formation.
5. Infection: Risk diminishes if the canula are removed every 48-72 hours. And every 24 hours in case of cut downs.

Radial Artery Puncture

The radial artery puncture is done for collection of blood for ABG estimation. However if repeated arterial blood samples are required, it is best to cannulate the umbilical artery because it is easy and convenient. The radial artery lies in the centre of the lateral third of the flexor aspect of the wrist, just lateral to the tendon of flexor carpi radialis. It is difficult to palpate in the newborn.

Steps

1. The artery should be located.
2. Needle size 23-26 G should be used to minimize trauma to the vessel. The 1 ml syringe should be rinsed with 0.5 ml heparin.
3. With the bevel end of the needle facing upwards, the needle should be inserted just proximal to the proximal skin crease of the wrist at an angle of 25-45°.

4. The needle is withdrawn while maintaining gentle suction till blood flows into the syringe.
5. After collection of sample, pressure should be applied to the site of puncture for atleast 5 minutes.

Bladder Tap

Bladder taps are the best method to collect urine samples in newborn for culture. A sterile technique should be followed. Careful cleaning with iodine and alcohol solution over the prepubic region is essential.

Equipment

The bladder tap is done with a 5-10 ml syringe attached to a 22 or 23 gauge needle or to a 23 gauge butterfly needle. Before the tap it should be determined that the baby has not passed urine recently.

Steps

1. The pubic bone is located by touch.
2. The needle is placed in the midline, just above the pubic bone.
3. The needle is slid in, the direction of the infant's coccyx.
4. The urine is collected in a sterile container.
5. If the needle goes in more than 3 cm and no urine is obtained, it should be assumed that the bladder is empty.

Percutaneous Central Venous Catherization

Percutaneous central venous catheterization is useful for long-term venous access for intra venous fluids, particularly parenteral nutrition. Two veins are generally used. The subclavian vein in case of babies weighing more than 1200 gms and external jugular vein in case of babies weighing less than 1500 gms.

Subclavian Vein Catheterization

Equipment

The equipment required includes a 3.0 F catheter with an introducer needle and guide wire. Double lumen 4.0 F catheters may be used in larger babies (> 2.5 Kg).

Steps

1. The infant is sedated and placed in a supine position with a roll between the scapulae. The head turned away from the side of insertion. The shoulders should drop posteriorly.
2. The skin is prepared with an iodine containing solution and infiltrated with a local anesthetic.
3. The introducer needle is inserted through the skin immediately beneath the clavicle at the junction of one third and two third of the distance between shoulder and the midline. The needle should be almost parallel to the chest wall and aimed at the sternal notch.
4. When the blood flow is established, the guide wire is passed and the catheter is placed over the wire. The catheter tip should lie at the junction of the superior vena cava and right atrium. Catheter position should be determined radiographically.

Complications

Complications include pneumothorax, hemothorax, and inadvertent subclavian artery puncture. In view of the seriousness of the complications, subclavian venous catherization should be attempted by those who are thoroughly familiar with the technique.

External Jugular Vein Catheterization

Equipment: The equipment required includes a 1.9 F

to 2.1 F silicone catheter cut to the appropriate length, a splittable introducer needle and an iris forceps.

Steps

1. The site is prepared with an antiseptic solution.
2. The introducer needle is inserted into the vein until blood flows freely.
3. The silicone catheter is then inserted through the needle with the forceps and is slowly advanced the predetermined distance for central venous positioning.
4. The introducer needle is removed. The extra catheter length is coiled on the skin near the insertion site. The site is covered with transparent surgical covering.
5. The catheter tip is positioned at the junction of the superior vena cava and the right atrium to be confirmed by radiography.

Complications

Complications are rare. May include infection, thrombosis and thrombophlebitis.

Exchange Transfusion

The indications of exchange transfusion are as follow:
1. When phototherapy fails to prevent rise in the serum bilirubin level to toxic level.
2. To remove antibody and sensitized red cells and thereby stop hemolysis and bilirubin production.
3. To correct anemia and improve heart failure in hydropic infants with hemolytic disease.

Blood used in Exchange Transfusion

- Blood should be whole blood, collected in citrate phosphate dextrose (CPD).
- It should be as fresh as possible (<24 hrs old for hydropic or sick infants and< 72 hrs for all others).

- In Rh hemolytic disease, if blood is collected before delivery, it should be O Rh negative crossed matched against the mother. If collected after delivery, it also may be cross matched against the infant.
- In ABO HDN, the blood should be O Rh negative or Rh compatible with mother and infant cross matched against the mother and infant and have a low titre of naturally occurring anti A and anti B antibodies.
- For non-immune hyperbilirubinemia, blood is typed and cross-matched against the plasma and RBC of the infant.

Steps

1. Exchange transfusion can be done in the operation theatre or the nursery under strict asepsis.
2. The infant should be placed under a radiant warmer with cardiac and blood pressure monitors in place. The infant is restrained by using a padded crucifix splint for fixing all four limbs.
3. An assistant should be engazed to record the volumes of blood, observe the infant and vital signs.
4. The blood for exchange should be warmed to 37°C. The abdomen is sterilized with spirit—betadine—spirit.
5. The umbilical vein is catheterized. If it is not possible to insert the catheter into the umbilical vein, exchange transfusion can be performed through a central venous pressure line placed through the antecubital fossa or the femoral vein via the saphenous vein.
6. Normally, exchanges are done by the push-pull technique through the umbilical vein. The catheter should be inserted only as far as required to permit free blood exchange. In the push-pull method, blood is exchanged in aliquots of 5 ml in infants < 1500 g, 10 ml for infants 1500-2500 g, 15 ml for infants 2500-3500g, and 20 ml for infants > 3500g. The recommended time for exchange transfusion is 1 hour.

7. The blood should be gently mixed after every deciliter of exchange to prevent settling of RBC and exchange of anemic blood at the end.
8. A silk purse string suture should be applied around the vein after the exchange is completed. The tail of the suture should be left. This will facilitate localization of the vein for the next exchange. The cord tie should be kept tightened for an hour after the catheter is removed. It should be loosened after 1 hour to prevent necrosis of the skin.

Abdominal Paracentasis

Abdominal paracentesis is done to remove ascitic fluid. The therapeutic indications include respiratory distress in infants with hydrops fetalis and urinary ascites. Diagnostic indications include diagnosis of peritonitis.

Steps

1. The equipments required are an 18 to 22 G intravenous catheter, a three way stopcock, and a 50 ml syringe.
2. The lower abdomen is prepared with providone iodine solution and the area is drapped.
3. The bladder should be evacuated by manual pressure or by a urinary catheter.
4. 1% Xylocaine is infiltrated into the subcutaneous tissue when possible.
5. The catheter is inserted just lateral to the rectus sheath one third of the distance between the umbilicus and the symphysis pubis. Alternatively, the catheter can be inserted in the midline. The catheter should be advanced approximately 1 cm until the resistance of passing through the abdominal wall diminishes or fluid come out.
6. Five to 10 ml of fluid is obtained for diagnostic purpose.

For therapeutic effects 10-20 ml/kg should be removed.

7. The catheter is then removed and the site bandaged.

Complications

1. Tachycardia, hypotension and decreased cardiac output may result following removal of large amounts of ascitic fluid. Slow and calculated amount can prevent such complications.
2. Bladder or intestinal injury and aspiration may occur in presence of distended bladder or intestinal loops. These puncture sites usually heal spontaneously.

Thoracocentesis

In newborn infants with severe hemodynamic compromise, thoracocentesis may be a life saving procedure. Thoracocentesis can be done by needle aspiration with a butterfly needle/intravenous catheter with an inner needle or by chest tube drainage.

Needle Aspiration

1. A 23 or 25 gauge butterfly needle or a 22 or 24 gauge intravenous catheter is attached to a 10-20 ml syringe fitted with a three way stopcock.
2. The second or third intercostal space is identified and overlying skin is prepared with an antibacterial solution over the midclavicular line.
3. The needle is passed into the intercostal muscles just above the top of the third rib. As the needle is inserted, continuous suction should be applied with the syringe. A rapid flow of air will occur into the syringe when the needle enters the pleural cavity. When the pleural space is entered the needle should not be advanced further.
4. The needle can be withdrawn after the airflow has seized.

Chest Tube Drainage

Chest tube drainage is generally required for continuous drainage of the plural cavity.

Insertion of the Tube

1. A chest tube of appropriate size is taken i.e. no. 10 (smaller) and no 12 (larger) French catheters are adequate for most newborn infants. Use of a plain forceps is better than a trochar because it prevents injury to the lungs.
2. The 4th and 6th ribs are identified at the mid axillary line. The area is prepared with an antibacterial solution. The subcutaneous tissue is infiltrated with 1% zylocaine. A dose of narcotic may be administered to the infant for pain management.
3. A small incision (1.0-1.5 cm) is made through the skin, in the sixth space in the mid axillary line, parallel to the rib. The subcutaneous tissue overlying the rib is dissected and a subcutaneous track is made into the 4th intercostal space. The pleural sac is entered in the 4th ICS at the intersection of the nipple line just anterior to the mid clavicular line.
4. The forcep is pushed through the intercostal muscles and parietal pleura. Pleural penetration will be indicated by a rush of air. The opening is widened by spreading the tips and the forcep is kept in place.
5. The end of the chest tube is grasped with the tips of mosquito forceps. The chest tube and the forcep should be in a parallel orientation. The chest tube is then directed through the skin incision into the pleural opening between the open tips. After the pleural space has been entered, the chest tube should be directed anteriorly and cephalad by rotating the curved ends of the mosquito forceps. The forceps is released and the tube is advanced for a few centimeters.

6. The chest should be palpated around the entry site to confirm that the chest tube is not in the subcutaneous tissues.
7. The chest tube is attached to an under water drainage system.
8. The skin incision is closed by 3-0 or 4-0 silk with a purse string suture or a single interrupted suture on either side of the tube. The insertion site should be covered by a small dressing.
9. An AP and lateral chest X-ray should be obtained to confirm tube position and ascertain drainage of pleural air.

Removal of Tube

Suction has to be discontinued when the tube has not drained for 24-48 hours but tube should be kept under water seal. The chest should be removed if radiographic examination does not show reaccumulation in the next 12-24 hours.

The chest tube should be removed during expiration in spontaneously breathing infants and during inspiration in mechanical ventilated infants.

Mechanical Ventilation

Mechanical ventilation is an invasive life support procedure with a goal to optimize both gas exchange and clinical status at minimum FiO_2 and ventilator pressure/ tidal volume. The types of ventilatory support most frequently used in newborn include:

1. Continuous positive airway pressure (CPAP), and
2. Pressure limited, time cycled, continuous flow ventilators. Synchronized and patient triggered ventilators are adaptations of conventional pressure limited ventilators used for newborns. Volume cycled ventilators are rarely used. The high frequency ventilator

is an important adjunct to conventional mechanical ventilators in the newborn.

Continuous Positive Airway Pressure (CPAP)

Continuous positive airway pressure is a continuously applied distending pressure (CDP) used for maintenance of an increased transpulmonary pressure during expiratory phase of respiration in a spontaneously breathing sick infant. It differs from intermittent positive pressure ventilation (IPPV) or intermittent mandatory ventilation in which breathing is taken over by the machine completely and the increase in pulmonary pressure occurs during both inspiratory as well as expiratory phases.

CPAP can be administered by nasal prongs, either single or double, by endotracheal tube and face mask. The most commonly used method is delivery of CPAP by nasal prongs. These are useful and effective as neonates are obligatory nasal breathers. The prongs can be sterilized and reused making them cost effective. Endotracheal CPAP is not preferred because of its invasiveness and the risk of infection. Moreover, it increases the work of breathing by increasing the dead space. It imposes a higher resistance because the lumen of the endotracheal tube is narrower than the trachea and its length is considerably longer than the nasal prong.

A newer system, the bubble CPAP deliver continuous positive airway pressure with an under water seal. This has been shown to cause vibrations of the chest due to gas flow under water, which is transmitted to the infant's airway. These vibrations simulate wave forms produced by high frequency ventilation. Bubble CPAP has also been shown to reduce the need for intubation and mechanical ventilation and decrease chronic lung disease.

CPAP is less invasive than mechanical ventilation and causes less barotrauma. On the other hand it does not improve ventilation and may worsen it. It provides inadequate respiratory support in the face of severe changes in pulmonary compliance and resistance.

Indications

1. In Preterm infants with RDS:
   a. Early treatment in preterm infants with minimal respiratory distress and minimal need for supplemental oxygen to prevent atelectasis.
   b. Respiratory distress and FiO_2 requirement above 0.30 by hood.
   c. FiO_2 above 0.40 by hood.
   d. Clinically significant retractions and/or distress after extubation. Infants with RDS who require FiO_2 above 0.35 to 0.40 on CPAP should be intubated and given surfactant replacement therapy and put on mechanical ventilation.
2. Apneic spells.
3. Weaning chronically ventilator dependent infants.

Steps of Application of Nasal CPAP

1. Positioning the infant in supine position with the head elevated about 30 degrees with the neck in slight extension. Keep gas flow at 5-8 litres/minute. Start with FiO_2 0.50, and CPAP 5-6 cm H_2O.
2. Insert a 6 FG orogastric tube to reduce gastric distension. Leave the end open and aspirate 2 hourly.
3. Measure arterial blood gas within 30 minutes of starting CPAP and 4-6 hourly thereafter.
4. If oxygenation is inadequate, CPAP should be increased by 1 cm of H_2O upto a maximum of 8-9 cm of H_2O and FiO_2 gradually upto 0.80.

5. When the infant's condition improves, the FiO_2 should be gradually reduced by decrements of 5-10% and the CPAP by 1-2 cm of H_2O. The treatment should be stopped when CPAP is 3 cm H_2O and FiO_2 is 0.30.
6. If PaO_2 falls below 45 mm Hg on these settings or the $PaCO_2$ rises above 60 mm Hg, then the baby should be intubated and ventilated.
7. Tension pneumothorax is a common complication which should be always suspected if the baby's condition deteriorates on CPAP.

Indicators of Adequate CPAP

An adequate CPAP is indicated by the following:
1. A comfortable infant. Absence of retraction/grunt, cyanosis.
2. CRT < 3 seconds.
3. Oxygen saturation 90-95%.
4. PaO_2 60-80 torr, $PaCO_2$ 40-50 torr, pH 7.3-7.4.

Pressure-Limited, Time Cycled, Continuous Flow Ventilators

Principle

Continuous flow of heated and humidified gas is circulated past the infant's airway with a selected maximum inspiratory pressure (Pi), positive end expiratory pressure (PEEP) and respiratory timing (rate and duration of inspiration and expiration). The gas is a selected mixture of air with oxygen.

These ventilators are useful in any type of lung disease.

Indications

1. Prolonged apnoea.
2. PaO_2 below 50 mmHg or FiO_2 above 0.80 (not in cases with cyanotic congenital heart disease).

3. $PaCO_2$ above 60 mmHg with persistent acidemia.
4. Frequent intermittent apnoea unresponsive to drug therapy.
5. Administration of surfactant therapy in infants with RDS.

Ventilator Strategy in Specific Disease States

The ventilator strategy in four common disease states is described below. It needs mention that before initiating ventilatory support, one should exclude mechanical causes of respiratory distress viz. pneumothorax or airway obstruction.

1. **Hyaline membrane disease (HMD)/Respiratory distress syndrome**
   a. In mildly affected infants who do not require intubation and surfactant therapy are started on CPAP early in the course of the disease to prevent further atelectasis. CPAP is initiated at 5-6 cm H_2O and increased to a maximum of 7-8 cm H_2O by titrating on the basis of clinical assessment of retractions and respiratory rate and observation of O_2 saturation.
   b. In moderately severe HMD, intubation, surfactant therapy and a short period of mechanical ventilation followed by CPAP may be considered.
   c. Mechanical ventilation is indicated when ventilation perfusion scan (V/Q) mismatching is so severe that increased FiO_2 and CPAP are inadequate or in infants who tire from increased work of breathing. A preferred approach is to maintain the appropriate mean airway pressure (MAP) with a Ti (inspiratory time) initially set at 0.3 second and a rate of approximately 20-40 breaths per minute. The oxygen flow rate of 7 to 12 L/minute is needed. The inspiratory pressure (Pi) is initially estimated by good chest excursion and is usually 20-25 cm

H_2O. The PEEP is set at 4-5 cm H_2O; may go upto 6 cm H_2O. A higher PEEP should be avoided in HMD because it may interfere with cardiac output.

d. When the patient become stable, FiO_2 and Pi are weaned first, alternating with rate in response to assessment of chest excursion, oxygen saturation, and blood gas results. Extubation is usually successful when ventilator rates are about 15 breaths per minute.

2. **Meconium aspiration syndrome**
   a. Because of the obstructive ball valve effects of meconium aspiration, application of positive pressure may result in pneumothorax. So initiating mechanical ventilation requires careful consideration of the risks and benefits.
   b. Low levels of PEEP (4-5 cm H_2O) are helpful in splinting open the partially obstructed airways and equalizing V/Q matching.
   c. If pneumonitis is more prominent, more rapid rates can be used.
   d. Sedation or muscle relaxants can minimize the risk of air leak in severe MAS.
   e. Weaning may be rapid if the illness is primarily related to airway obstruction or prolonged if complicated by baro trauma and severe inflammation.
   f. Surfactant therapy should be considered in severe MAS. It may improve lung compliance and oxygenation.
3. **Apnoea**
   a. Infants with prolonged apnoea, completely dependent on the ventilator, require physiologic ventilation using moderate PEEP (3-4 cm H_2O), low gas flow and normal rates (30-40 breaths/minute) with Pi 10-18 cm H_2O adjusted to prevent hyperventilation.

b. For infants with intermittent but prolonged apnoea low rates (12-15 breaths/minute) may be sufficient.

4. **Air leak:** The two most common air leak syndromes are interstitial emphysema and pneumothorax. The primary aim is to reduce MAP through any of its components viz. Pi, Ti, PEEP and to rely on increased FiO_2 to provide oxygenation. Sometimes very rapid rates (upto 60/minute) may be required to ventilate the alveoli.

Adjuncts to Mechanical Ventilation

1. If agitation or distress in the infant is associated with excessive lability of oxygenation and hypoxemia sedation can be used. Lorazepam (0.05 to 0.1 mg/kg/dose given every 4-6 hours) can be used in mature infants. Morphine (0.05-0.1 mg/kg) may be used but may cause neurologic depression. In preterm infants, nonpharmacologic methods, viz. limiting environmental light and noise and providing behavioral supports, may help decrease agitation and limit the need of sedation.
2. Muscle relaxants viz. pancuronium bromide (0.1 mg/kg/dose, repeated as needed) is rarely necessary to be used. It may be indicated in (a) infants who continue to breathe out of phase with the ventilator after attempts at finding appropriate settings and sedation has failed, (b) Requirement of FiO_2 is over 0.75 or peak inspiratory pressure is over 30 cm H_2O. Prolonged use of muscle relaxants leads to fluid retention and deterioration in compliance. Sedation should be routinely administered to infants receiving muscle relaxants.
3. All infants on mechanical ventilation require continuous monitoring of oxygen saturation and intermittent ABG measurements.

Surfactant Administration

Indications

1. Prophylactic administration to infants at high risk of RDS i.e. babies with birth weight less than 1250 grams and larger infants with evidence of pulmonary immaturity.
2. Rescue therapy in infants with moderate to severe RDS (requirement of mechanical ventilation and FiO_2 higher than 40%).
3. Treatment of term infants with respiratory failure due to meconium aspiration syndrome, pneumonia and persistent pulmonary hypertension.

Timing of Administration

1. Prophylactic therapy as soon as possible after birth preferably within 2 hours.
2. Rescue therapy should be given immediately following the diagnosis of RDS.

Steps of Administration

1. The infant should be on mechanical ventilation.
2. The endotracheal tube should be suctioned to ensure patency. The correct anatomic location of the tube should be confirmed.
3. Surfactant is administered by instillation into a 5 French, end hole catheter inserted into the infant's endotracheal tube with the tip of the catheter protruding just beyond the end of the endotracheal tube and above the infant's carina.
4. The oxygen saturation and heart rate should be continuously monitored during administration of the doses. After administration of each dose, the ABG has to be monitored to detect and correct post dose abnormalities of ventilation and oxygenation.

Adverse Reactions During Administration Process

The adverse reaction during the administration process includes transient bradycardia, hypoxemia, pallor, vasoconstriction, hypotension, endotracheal tube blockage, hypercapnia, apnoea and hypertension.

SUGGESTED READINGS

1. Steven A. Ringer. Common Procedures in Manual of neonatal care. Editors John P. Cloherty, Eric C. Eichenwald, Ann R. Stark, 5th edition, 2004. Lippincott Williams and Wilkins, Philadelphia, USA.
2. Rakesh Sahni and Jen Tien Wung. CPAP—A gentler, noninvasive approach for managing neonatal RDS. Journal of Neonatology 2002;16:24-36.
3. Upadhyay Amit and Deorari A K. Continuous positive airway pressure—A gentler approach to ventilation. Indian Pediatrics 2004;41:459-472.
4. A Neonatal Vade—Mecum edited by Brian Speidal, Peter Fleming, John Anderson *et al.* 3rd edition 1998. Arnold Publishers, London.
5. Textbook on neonatal resuscitation, 4th edition, 2003. Editor John Kattwinkel based on original text by Ronald S. Bloom and Catherine Cropley, American Academy of Pediatrics and American Heart Association.

Table 30.1: Preparation of fluid with required glucose concentration

Glucose conc.	*10% Dextrose +*	*25% dextrose*	*Resultant solution 5% dextrose*
7.5%	435 ml	65 ml	500 ml
9.0%	400 ml	100 ml	500 ml
10%	375 ml	125 ml	500 ml
12.5%	310 ml	190 ml	500 ml
15%	250 ml	250 ml	500 ml
17%	200 ml	300 ml	500 ml
20%	125 ml	375 ml	500 ml

Table 30.2: Conversion table

Glucose (mg/kg/min)	Fluid ml/kg/min/day 5%	7.5%	10%	12.5%	15%	20%
4	115	77	58	46	38	29
6	172	115	86	69	58	43
8	230	154	115	92	77	58
10	288	192	124	115	96	72
12	345	230	173	138	115	86

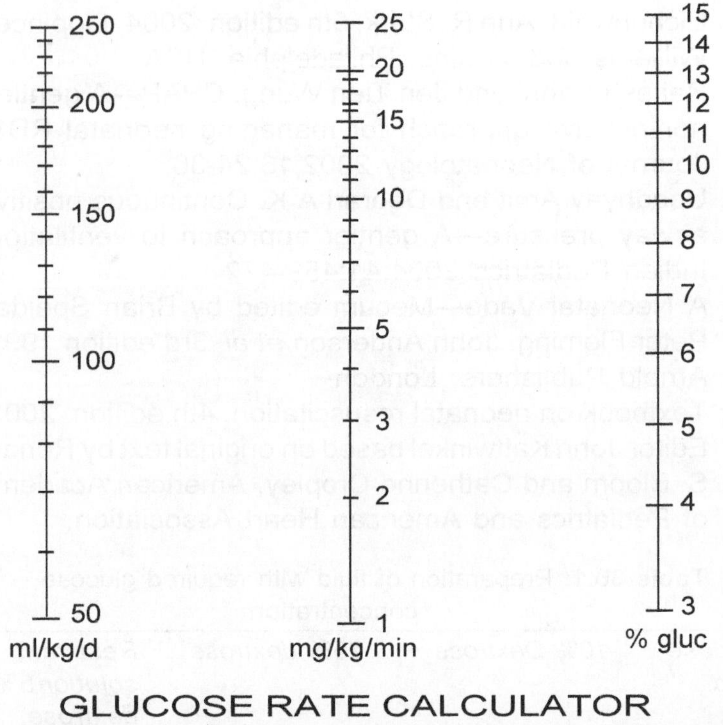

Use a straight edge to determine the volume required per 24 hours

Fig 30.1: Glucose rate calculator (*Source:* Klaus MH, Faranoff AA (Eds), Care of the High risk Neonate, 2 nd ed. Philadelphia: Saunders, 1979, Page 430)

Drugs and Dosage commonly used in newborn

Gautam Medhi

Drugs	*Dose*	*Route and frequency*	*Comments*
ANTIBIOTICS			
1. Ampicillin	Nondisseminated disease 50 mg/kg/dose	(IV q 12 hrly < 7 days IV q 8 hrly > 7 days) of post natal age	• Rash, hemolytic anemia • Interstitial nephritis • Pseudo-membranous
	Meningitis 100-150 mg/kg/dose	IV q 6 hourly	
2. Penicillin G Potassium Aqueous	Meningitis/Group B Streptococcus 75,000 to 100,000 U/kg		
	<2kg, 0-7 days	q 12 hours	
	<2kg > 7 days	q 8 hours	
	>2kg 0-7 days	q 8 hours	
	>2kg > 7 days	q 6 hours	
3. Penicillin G Procaine	50,000 unit/kg IM as single dose for preterm and term neonate	IM	
4. Cefotaxime	<1200gms> 7days 100mg/kg/day	IV q 12 hrly IV q 8 hrly	• Positive Coomb's test
	>1200gms> 7days 150mg/kg/day	IV q 6 hrly	• Good CNS Penetration
	Meningitis 200mg/		•
Nephrotoxicity •Neutropenia			kg/day
5. Ceftazidime	<1200 gms> 7 days 100mg/kg	IV 12 hrs IV q 8 hrs	• Adjust dose for renal impairment
	>1200 gms> 7days 150mg/kg		• Allegic rash • False positive Coomb's test
6. Ceftriaxone	50-100 mg/kg/day	IV q 24 hrs/ IV q 12 hrs	• Excellent penetration in CSF, Bile & lung • Monitor prothrombin time and serum bilirubin

Contd.

Contd.

7.	Cefipime	50 mg/kg/dose	IV q 8 hrs	
8.	Gentamycin	1200-2000 gm & < 7 days 2.5 mg/kg	IV q 12-18 hr.	Nephrotoxicity and auditory toxicity
		1200-2000 gm & > 7 days 2.5 mg/kg	IV q 8 hr.	
9.	Amikacin	1200-2000 gm & < 7 days 7.5 mg/kg	IV q 12 hrs	Renal and auditory toxicity
		> 2000 gm & < 7 days 10 mg/kg	IV q 12 hr.	
		1200-2000 gm & > 7 days, 7.5 mg/kg	IV q 8-12 hr.	
		> 2000 gm & > 7 days 10 mg	IV q 8 hr.	
10.	Aztreonam	< 2000 gm < 7 day 60mg/kg/24 hrs	IV q 12 hr.	Rash Thrombophleties
		>2000 gm < 7 days 90 mg/kg/24 hr	IV q 8 hr.	
		>2000 mg > 7 days 120 mg/kg/24 hrs	IV q 6-8 hr.	
11.	Imipenem cilastatin	< 1200 gm & < 7 days 20 mg/kg/24 hrs	IV q 18-24 hr.	Rash Eosinophilia, seizure
		> 1200 gm & < 7 days 40 mg/kg/24 hr.	IV q 12 hr.	
		1200-2000 gm & > 7 days 40 mg/kg/24hr.	IV q 12 hr.	
		> 2000 gm & > 7 days 60 mg/kg/24hr.	IV q 8 hr.	
12.	Piperacilin	> 7 days 150 mg/kg/24 hr.	IV q 8-12 hr.	Rash Eosinophilia
		> 7 days 200 mg/kg/day	IV q 6-8 hr.	
13.	Rifampicin	10 mg/kg/day	Q 24 hr.	Hepatotoxicity
14.	Isoniazid	5 mg/kg	P.O. q 24 hrs	Monitor liver functions & peri peripheral neuropathy Vit. B_6 depletion
15.	Pyrizinamide	20 mg/kg/day q OD	P.O.	Hepatotoxicity good CSF Penetration
16.	Ethambutol	25 mg/kg/24 hr q OD	P.O.	Ototoxicity, Nephrotoxicity
17.	Metronidazole	7.5 mg/kg >2kg <7 days	IV q hrly	
		15 mg/kg > 2kg >7 days	IV q 8 hrly	

Contd.

Contd.

18.	Vancomycin	<1200 gm & < 7 days 15 mg/kg/24 hr.	IV q 24 hr.	Ototoxicity Nephrotoxicity
		1200-2000 gm & < 7 days 15 mg/kg/24 hr.	IV q 12 hr.	Thrombo- phlebitis
		>2000 gm & < 7 days 30 mg/kg/24 hr.	IV q 12 hr.	Hepatic dysfunctions
		1200-2000 gm > 7 days 15 mg/kg/24 hr.	IV q 8-12 hr.	
		>2000 gm & > 7 days 45 mg/kg/24 hr.	IV q 8 hr.	
ANTIVIRAL				
1.	Acyclovir	8-10 mg/kg/day		Renal dysfunctions, Phlebitis
2.	Nystatin	Test dose 0.1 mg/kg Initial dose 0.25 g/kg Maximum daily dose 1 mg/kg Orally 100,000 to 200,000 units 6 hrs. for Thrush Topically applied as 2% ointment	IV q 8 hr. IV: q over 4-6 hours as infusion in 5% dextrose	Hypokalaemia, Hypomag- nesemia, RTA, Renal failure, Bone marrow suppression
3.	Zidovudine	8 mg/kg 12 hr.	IV q 6 hrs.	

Respiratory system

	Drugs	*Dose*	*Route and frequency*	*Comments*
1.	Aminophylline	Apnea of prematurity, Bronchodilator	Loading 4-6 mg/kg/dose IV over 30 mins Maintenance 1-3 mg/kg/dose IV q 8-12 hour. Start maintenance 8-12 hours after loading dose Maintenance, neonate 0.2 mg/kg/hour 6 wk-6 months 0.2-0.9 mg/kg/hour	GI upset, arrhythmia, seizures, tachycardia
2.	Doxapram (Dopram)	Idiopathic apnoea of prematurity refractory to therapeutic level of methylxanthine	Loading dose 2-3 mg/kg followed by 0.5-1.5 mg/kg/hr stepwise increase in dosage at 24-48 hr. interval until response or neonate has received 2.5 mg/kg/hr. for 48 hours	Hypertensions, Tachycardia, skeletal muscle hyperactivity, Abdominal distension
3.	Naloxone	Narcotic induced respiratory depression in neonatal resuscitation	0.1-0.2 mg/kg/dose IV push. (over 30 sec.) ETT, IM or IV repeat as necessary q 3-5 mins.	Vomiting, sweating, hypotension, ventricular tachycardia, seizure and cardiac arrest

Drugs for seizures

	Drugs	*Dose*	*Comments*
1.	Diazepam	0.25-0.5 mg/kg/dose, IV bolus, Per Rectal Slow push over 3 min, repeat q 15-30 min for 3 doses. Maximum 2 mg/kg/day	Hypotension and respiratory depression Displacement of bilirubin by benzoate
2.	Lorazepam	Loading dose 0.05-0.1 mg/k/dose IV bolus q 15 min. Maintenance 0.05 mg/kg IV q 6-24 hours	Respiratory depressions
3.	Midazolam	Loading dose 0.5 mg-0.75 mg/kg/dose IV bolus q 15 min. Maintenance 0.05 mg/kg IV q 6-24 hours	Respiratory depressions
4.	Phenobarbitone	State 15-20 mg/kg IV over 20 min. Maintenance 2-3 mg/kg IV / P.O. q 12-24 hours	Respiratory depression with overdose
5.	Phenytoin	Loading dose 15-20 mg/kg IV over 20 mins. Maintenance 3-5 mg/kg IV / P.O. q 8-12 hours	Cardiac arrhythmia

Miscellaneous group

Drugs	Indications	Dosage and route of Admn	Comments
1. Acetaminophen	Fever due to any cause	10-15 mg/kg 4-6 hrly	Hepatotoxicity Adjust dose for renal impairment
2. Acetazolamide	Hydrocephalous unassociated with Arnold-chiari malformations	50-75 mg/kg/day q 8 hours oral	Hypokalemic acidosis
3. Albumin 5% (1gm/20 ml)	Hypoproteinemia	0.5-0.1 gm/kg/day IV over 24 hours	Chill, fever, urticaria
4. Calcium Gluconate	Symptomatic hypocalcemia Acute therapy Maintenance therapy	100-200 mg/kg/dose IV over 10 min (1-2 ml/kg/dose) 200-800 mg/kg/day (2-8 ml/kg/day)	Cardiovascular instability ventricular fibrillation, lethargy
5. Cisapride	Gastro-esophageal reflux	0.2-0.3 mg/kg P.O. q 6-8 hours 30 min before feed	Transient abdominal Cramping and Diarrhoea
6. Dexamethasone	Refractory neonatal hypoglycaemia Cerebral oedema	0.25 mg/kg/dose IV, P.O. q 12 hours Load 0.5-1.5 mg/kg IV, IM Maintenance : 0.2-0.5 mg/kg/day Q 6h. IV, IM	Short term adverse effect, seizure hypokalemia, leukocytosis, hypocalcemic alkalosis, sodium and water retention
	Broncho-pulmonary dysplasia	5 mg/kg/day q 12 hours x 3 days then 0.3 mg/kg/dy divided 12 hours x 3 days. Decrease by 0.1 mg/kg/day q 72 hours until reaching 0.1 mg/kg/day then administer OD for 1 week	Long-term adverse effect Nephrolithiasis osteoporosis, Cushing syndrome, Growth suppressions.

Contd.

Contd.

7.	Dextrose infusions	Hypoglycemia	2-5 ml/kg 10% dextrose IV bolus followed by 6-8 mg/kg/min continuous infusion for maintenance	Phlebitis Rapid IV administration causes bradycardia, apnoea, cardiac arrest
8.	Glucagon	Hypoglycemia	0.03-0.1mg/kg/dose IM, IV, SC Maximum single dose 1 mg	• Rebound hypoglycemia • Tachycardia • Vomiting • GI upset
9.	Gammaglobulin	A. Preventive i. Measles exposure ii. Hepatitis A	 0.25 ml/kg/IM one dose 0.15 ml/kg IM one dose	 • Transient hypoglycemia • Tachycardia • Hypotension
		B. Replacement therapy i. Hypogammaglobulinemia	 100 mg/kg/month i.e. 0.6 ml/kg/ month IV,IM	
		C. Treatment of ITP or Alloimmune Thrombocytopenia	400 mg/kg/day IV infusions over 6 hours for 5 days	
10.	Hydrocortisone	i. Acute adrenal insufficiency	1-2 mg/kg/dose or 50 mg/m^2 bolus over 3-5 min followed by 50-100 mg/m^2/day (25-30 mg/kg/day) IV q 4-6 hours	• Hypotension • Oedema • Cataract • Peptic ulcer • Hypokalaemia
		ii. Congenital adrenal hyperplasia	Initial 30-36 mg/m^2/day q 8 hrs. IV Maintenance 15-20 mg/m^2/day q 8 hr. 0.8-4 mg/kg/day q 6 hr. IV	

Contd.

Contd.

		iii. Anti inflammatory Immunosuppressive iv. Hypoglycemia	10 mg/kg/day q 12 hr. IV	
11.	Iron	Prevention of iron deficiency anemia in preterm	2 mg/kg/day P.O. after 6-8 weeks of postnatal age	
12.	Mannitol 20%	Cerebral oedema	1gm/kg/dose IV 4-8 hrs interval	
13.	Metoclorpropamide	Gastro esophageal reflux	0.1-0.3 mg/kg/dose P.O., IM	Extra pyramidal signs
14.	Potassioum chloride	Hypocalcaemia–Acute	0.5-1 meq/kg/IV. Diluted in 6-8 hr vol. of IV soln, and administer over 1 hr	• Arrhythmia • Respiratory paralysis
		Maintenance	2-4 meq/kg/day, diluted in 24 hr maintenance IV soln. and divided into feeding	• Hypotension
15.	Ranitidine	Gastro esophageal reflux	P.O. 2-4mg/kg/dose q 8-12 hours IV 0.1-0.8 mg/kg/dose q 6 hours	GI disturbance sedation Hepatotoxicity, vomiting
16.	Vitamin A	Preventive dose in premature baby	600-1500 unit/day P.O.	
	D	Preventive dose in premature baby	400-1000 unit/day P.O.	
	K1 oxide	Preventive of early hemorrhagic disease	1 mg IM at birth 0.5 mg IM at birth < 1500 g	

Cardiovascular drugs in newborn

Drugs	*Indications*	*Dose*	*Route and frequency*	*Comments*
1. Digoxin	Heart failure, paroxysmal A. V. nodal tachycardia, Atrial fibrillation/ Flutter	Digitalizing dose for Premature infants 0.04 mg/kg/day Full term neonate 0.06 mg/kg/day Parenteral dose is 2/3rd of this amount	P.O ½ of digitalizing dose in given stat. ¼th after 8 hours and ¼th after another 8 hrs daily maintenance dose is about ¼th of initial digitalizing dose	Anorexia, nausea, Vomiting, conduction defect
2. Dobutamine	Short-term support of neonates with shock and hypotension	2.5 mcg-25 mcg/kg/min Maximum recommended dose 40 mcg/kg/min	IV	Arrhythmia, cutaneous vasodilatation, hyper-tension and dyspnea
3. Dopamine	Shock refractory to adequate volume replacement	Low dose 2-5 mcg/kg/min- 'Renal dose' causes renal blood flow and urinary outflow **Intermediate dose** 5-15 mcg/kg/min **Cardio tonic dose**		
		High dose > 20 mg/ kg/min	IV	Arrhythmia, Tachycardia, Vasoconstrictions, widened

Contd.

Contd.

		Presser dose, Prominent alpha agonist effect causes increased systemic and pulmonary vascular resistance		QRS complexes
4. Adrenaline	Cardiac arrest during neonatal resuscitation	0.1-0.3ml/kg of 1:10,000 solution	IV, IC, ET q 3-5 mins	Oliguria, Prolonged episode of hypotension
5. Enalapril maleate	After load reductions in newborn with CHF	Initial dose: 0.1 mg/kg/day increase according to response to 0.12-0.43 mg/kg/day	P.O.	Mild non oliguric renal failure
	Neonatal hypertension	Dose 5-10 mcg/kg/dose	IV q 8-24 hours	
6. Adenosine	Supraventricular tachycardia	0.05-0.2mg/kg/dose If no response in 1-2 min double the dose and continue to double the dose every 1-2 mins until response occurs. Maximum single dose 0.25 mg/kg	Rapid IV bolus by flush	Heart block, bronchospasm, dyspnoea and hypotension

Contd.

Contd.

Cardioversion	Supraventricular tachycardia Ventricular tachycardia	Initial dose 0.5 J/kg Double dose each time for a total of three attempts		Myocardial burns, Congestive cardiomyopathy secondary to reduced contractility and death
DIURETICS				
1. Chlorothiazide	Fluid overload, Pulmonary oedema, Bronochopulmonary dysplasia, congestive heart failure and hypertension	20-40 mg/kg/day	IV, P.O.	Hypochloremic alkalosis Blood dyscrasias, hypokalaemia, hyper-glycaemia and hyperuricemia
2. Furosemide	Do	1-6 mg/kg/dose q 12-24 hours 1-2 mg/kg/dose q 12-24 hours 1-3 mg/kg/day	P.O. IV/IM	Fluid and electrolyte imbalance, hypocalcemia, hypercalciuria, hypochloremic alkalosis, interstitial nephritis, anemia, potential ototoxicity
3. Spironolactone	• Congestive heart failure • Pulmonary odema • Boncho pulmonary dysplasia		P.O. q 12 hours	Hyperkalaemia, vomiting diarrhoea, hyponatremia

INDEX

O

P

R

V